Integumentary Physical Therapy

Ji-Whan Park • Dae-In Jung
Editors

Integumentary Physical Therapy

Springer

Editors
Ji-Whan Park
Daejeon Health Sciences College
Daejeon
South Korea

Dae-In Jung
Gwangju Health University
Gwangju
South Korea

ISBN 978-3-662-47379-5 ISBN 978-3-662-47380-1 (eBook)
DOI 10.1007/978-3-662-47380-1

Library of Congress Control Number: 2016943112

Printed on acid-free paper

This Springer imprint is published by Springer Nature
The registered company is Springer-Verlag GmbH Berlin Heidelberg

Preface

There was a stonemason whose job was cutting and shaping stones. He worked hard, streaming with sweat under the blazing sun. After the stone was shaped, he inscribed the stone with the phrase "integumentary PT."

"Such a beautiful stone! We would like to inscribe our names on people's hearts. How can we do that?" asked the people who had been watching the stonemason working.

"That's not difficult at all. You can do it as long as you get down on your knees and stay up all night working," he answered.

How many times have the physical therapy professors in South Korea got down on their knees and stayed up?

Since its origin in 1949, Korean physical therapy has been developing for the last 66 years with academic and technical supports from the world academics of physical therapy. However, there has been little contribution of Korean physical therapy to world physical therapy. Therefore, those professors, who believed that they must return the supports from the world physical therapy, considered the way to return what they have been benefited from the world physical therapy.

This book is a practical guide to safe and effective physical therapy methods that can be applied to patients with diverse skin ailments, including scars, decubitus ulcers, burns, frostbite, photosensitivity disorders, inflammatory skin diseases, skin cancers, obesity-related conditions, psoriasis, herpes zoster, tinea pedis, and vitiligo. For each condition, physical therapy interventions – therapeutic exercises, manual physical therapies, and therapeutic modalities employed in rehabilitation – are described in detail. In addition, information is provided on symptoms and complications, examination and evaluation, medical interventions, and prevention and management methods. In the case of obesity-related skin problems, management is discussed from the point of view of Eastern as well as Western medicine. The text is complemented by more than 300 color photographs and illustrations. Knowledge of integumentary physical therapy will help the therapist to obtain optimal therapeutic results when treating patients with skin ailments. It will be of value for both practicing physical therapists and students of physical therapy.

We thank the staff of Springer for sparing no efforts in publishing this book.

Especially, we express our sincere thanks to Prof. Keon Cheol, Prof. Lee, and the authors from many universities who worked relentlessly.

Hopefully, this book will contribute to the advancement of world physical therapy.

Daejeon, South Korea Ji Whan Park, PhD, RPT
Gwangju, South Korea Daein Jung, PhD, RPT
February 2015

Contents

1 An Outline of the Integumentary System

Keon Cheol Lee and Dae-In Jung

ICD-10 Code
A18.4 Tuberculosis of Skin and Subcutaneous Tissue
I73.9 Peripheral Vascular Disease, Unspecified
L29 Pruritus
L30.2 Cutaneous Autosensitization
L50.9 Urticaria, Unspecified
L53.9 Erythematous Condition, Unspecified
L68.0 Hirsutism
L68.3 Polytrichia
L83 Acanthosis Nigricans
L85.0 Acquired Ichthyosis
O01.9 Hydatidiform Mole, Unspecified
R23.2 Flushing
R23.8 Other Unspecified Skin Changes
A18.4

Learning Outcomes
After completing this chapter, you should be able to describe the following:

- The skin types
- The skin damages and the recovery processes
- Skin aging
- Histopathology of the skin
- Assessment of the skin

Key Terms
Dermis
Epidermis
Skin test
Subcutaneous
Skin type
Skin property
Skin interpretation
Skin assessment

K.C. Lee (✉)
Professor, Department of Physical Therapy, Kyungnam College of Information and Technology, Busan, South Korea
e-mail: rptgeon@lycos.co.kr

D.-I. Jung
Professor, Department of Physical Therapy, Gwangju Health University, Gwangju, South Korea

J.-W. Park, D.-I. Jung (eds.), *Integumentary Physical Therapy*, DOI 10.1007/978-3-662-47380-1_1

1.1 Structure of Integumentary System

1.1.1 Anatomy of the Integumentary System

As the largest organ of the human body, the skin surrounds the body and comprises 16% of a person's total body weight. The skin protects the body from the external environmental stimuli and also has a metabolic function. The skin forms the functional boundary between the external environment and the internal environment of the body, participating in the maintenance of homeostasis. Oral cavity, nasal cavity, orbital cavity, anal cavity, and vaginal cavity are body cavities that open to the exterior of the body, and the skin forms a mucosal surface barrier by contacting with the mucous membranes that line such cavities. The thickness of the skin varies from 0.5 to 6 mm. In the trunk, the skin of dorsal surface and limbs is thicker than that of the ventral surface, and in the neck, the dorsal surface is thicker than the ventral surface. The skin is composed of the epidermis and the dermis, which are structurally distinguishable. The epidermis consists of tough stratified squamous epithelium, and the dermis is composed of dense connective tissue (Chung 2011).

1.1.1.1 Epidermis

The epidermis protects internal organs from dangerous chemicals and harmful microorganisms, regulates body fluid volume and body temperature, and eliminates body wastes. The epidermis consists of tough stratified squamous epithelium and does not contain blood vessels (Fig. 1.1).

Stratum Corneum

The stratum corneum is flat and does not contain nuclei. It is composed of thick keratinized layers of dead squamous epithelial cells and accounts for up to 75% of the epidermal thickness. Cells of the stratum corneum are so tightly bonded to each other that water evaporation is prevented and the skin is kept hydrated.

Stratum Lucidum

The stratum lucidum (Latin for "clear layer") is a thin, translucent layer that presents only in thick skin such as the lips, the palm of the hand, and the sole of the feet. It lacks nuclei and organelles but contains distinct desmosomes and a semifluid substance

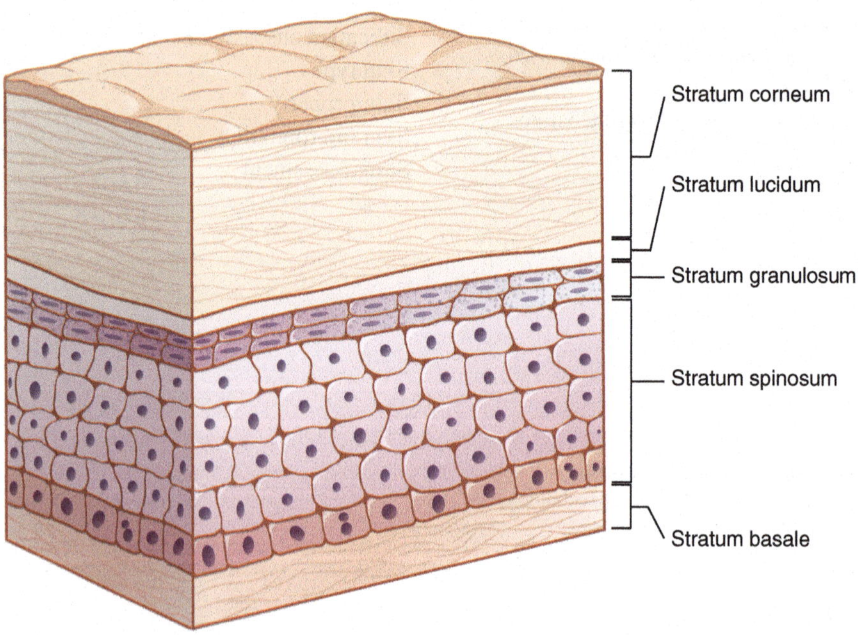

Fig. 1.1 Epidermis

called eleidin, which explains the histologically translucent character of the stratum lucidum.

Stratum Granulosum

The stratum granulosum is composed of three to four layers of flattened cells and contains irregular granules of keratohyalin.

Stratum Spinosum

The stratum spinosum consists of several layers of polygonal cells. It contains large oval nuclei and the cells undergo occasional mitosis. Spiny projections on the surface of the cells are connected to the projections of the adjacent cells and form intercellular bridges. Lymph fluid passes through the intercellular bridges and has a part in providing nourishment and immunity to the skin.

Stratum Basale

The stratum basale (basal layer) is composed of a single layer of columnar epithelial cells placed on the surface of the dermis, and its basal surface has a role to fix the epidermis to the dermis. Cells populating the stratum basale include keratinocytes, melanocytes, tactile cells (Merkel cells), and non-pigmented granular dendrocytes (Langerhans cells).

1.1.1.2 Dermis

The dermis is composed of two layers. The upper layer, stratum papillarosum, lies below the epidermis and consists of loose connective tissue. It accounts for 1/5 of the dermis. The deep thicker layer of the dermis is called stratum reticularosum (reticular layer). It is located beneath the stratum papillarosum and consists of dense irregular connective tissues containing cross-linked collagen and elastin fibers. Nerves are widely distributed in the dermis. Blood vessels provide nourishment to the stratum basale of the epidermis and have an important role in regulating body temperature and blood pressure (Fig. 1.2) (Faculty Committee of Korean Anatomy and Physiology 2011).

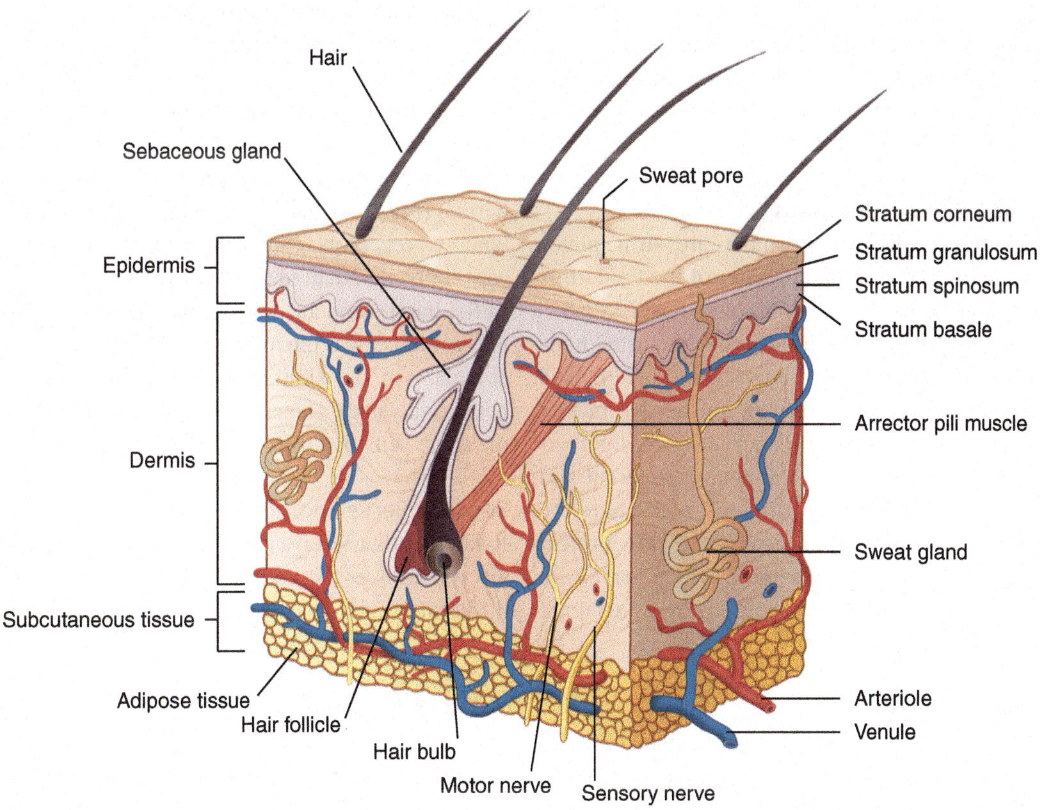

Fig. 1.2 Cross-section of the skin and subcutaneous tissue

1.1.1.3 Subcutaneous Tissue

The subcutaneous tissue consists of loose connective tissue, blood vessels, and adipose cells. It attaches the skin loosely to the underlying organs and muscles, so that the skin can slide over them. The adipose cells serve as a buffer between the bones and the tissues. Because blood vessels and nerves course through the subcutaneous tissue and are surrounded by the connective tissue fibers, they can withstand the pulling force applied to them.

1.1.1.4 Skin Appendages

The appendages of the skin include hairs, nails, sweat glands, sebaceous glands, mammary glands, and ceruminous glands. They are developed from the embryonic epidermis. While hairs and nails have very restricted functions, integumentary glands play a highly important role in body protection and homeostasis maintenance.

Hair

Hair is a thin and flexible filament produced by hair follicle. It consists of keratinized dead cells and contributes to maintaining body temperature and perceiving touch sensation.

Fingernails and Toenails

The fingernails and toenails are firm plates formed in the stratum corneum of the epidermis and consist of highly compressed and keratinized dead cells. While the growth rate of nails varies depending on individual's health and nutrition, fingernails grow at an average rate of 1 mm a week, and toenails grow slower than fingernails. Fingernails are almost transparent and colorless, but it appears slightly pink due to the capillaries running underneath. Nails protect sensitive fingertips and toes on which nerves are concentrated, and they help fingers' accurate movement.

Sebaceous Glands

Sebaceous glands developed from the follicular epithelium of the hair are a type of acinar holocrine glands, which secrete serum. They present in all skin except for the palms and soles.

Sweat Glands

Sweat glands are widely distributed over the skin except for the lips, nipples, and external genital organs. They secrete sweat to the surface of the skin. According to the structure and mechanism of excretion, they are classified into two types: eccrine sweat glands and apocrine sweat glands.

Mammary Glands

Mammary glands in female breasts are modified sweat glands lying in the subcutaneous tissue (Fig. 1.3).

Ceruminous Glands

Ceruminous glands are modified sweat glands that are found only in the external auditory canal. They secrete cerumen, whose role is to lubricate the ear canal and to protect the eardrum from bacteria, insects, and water.

1.1.2 Cutaneous Sensation and Innervation

1.1.2.1 Cutaneous Sensation

Sensory receptors that react to warmth, cold, touch, vibration, or pain are distributed in the dermis (Fig. 1.4), and they are also called subcutaneous receptors. Such sensory neurons are especially abundant in the skin on the face, palms of the hands, fingers, soles of the feet, and external genitals. On the other hand, they are less abundant in the skin of the back, back of the neck, and joints. Generally, the thinner the skin, the more sensitive it is.

Sensory Nerve Endings

Receptors that receive external or internal signals are spread over the body, but their structures are different to each other with no physiological relationship among them.

① Free Nerve Endings

Free nerve endings are unencapsulated and the most simple receptors. They are the primary nociceptors located beneath the epidermis. Free

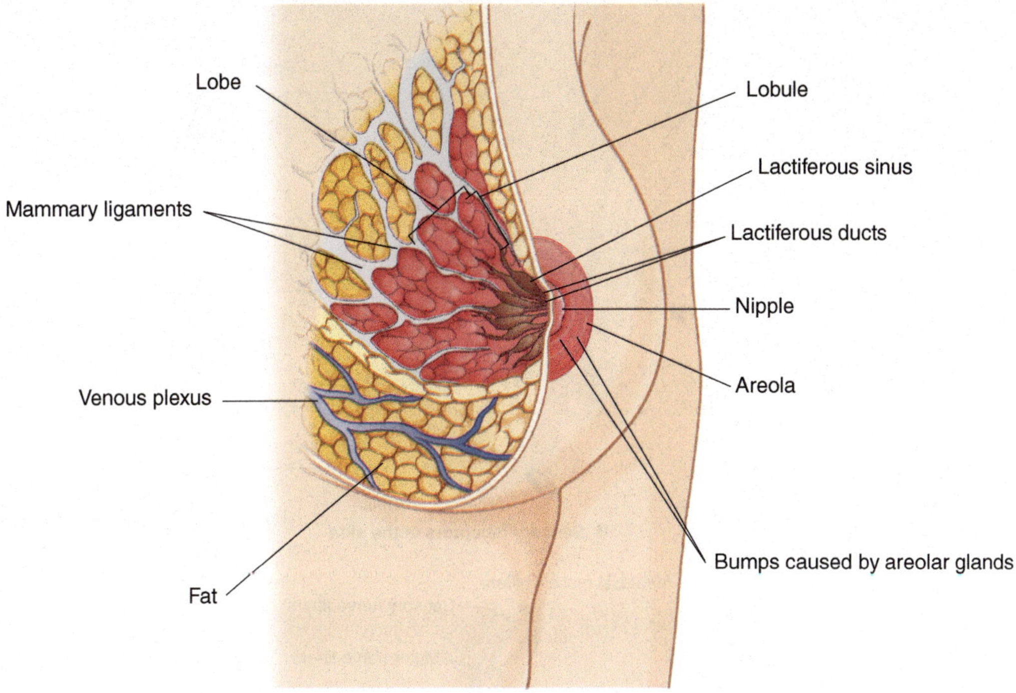

Fig. 1.3 The structure of mammary glands

nerve endings wrapped around hair follicle feel the sense of touch and pressure from the rough clothes (Faculty Committee of Korean Anatomy and Physiology 2012).

② Meissner's Corpuscles

Meissner's corpuscles exist in the stratum papillarosum of the dermis. They are encapsulated nerve endings and sense light touch. They are typical speed sensors and sense low-frequency vibrations. They are abundant in hairless skin such as the hands, feet, lips, mucous membrane of the tongue, front of the forearm, and external genitalia.

③ Pacinian Corpuscles

Pacinian corpuscles are encapsulated nerve endings and mechanoreceptors. They are found in the superficial fascia and abundant in the skin of the palms and fingers, soles of the feet, external genitalia, and chest. Generally, the tissues are stimulated by quick movements and play an important role in sensing deep touch and vibration.

④ Ruffini's Corpuscles

Ruffini's corpuscles, as mechanoreceptors, are similar to Merkel's disk. They are nerve endings surrounded by sheath and are found deep in the dermis and subcutaneous tissue. They respond to continuous pressure and stretching of the skin and detect the intensity and speed of the stimulus.

⑤ Krause's End Bulbs

The Krause's end bulbs are widely distributed throughout the body and can be considered as small Meissner's corpuscles. They are cold receptors and are located in the dermis.

⑥ Merkel's Disks

Merkel's disks are typical speed sensors. They are mostly found beneath the ridges of the fingertips and respond to light touch and constant pressure. Because of their low threshold of touch perception, they play an important role as

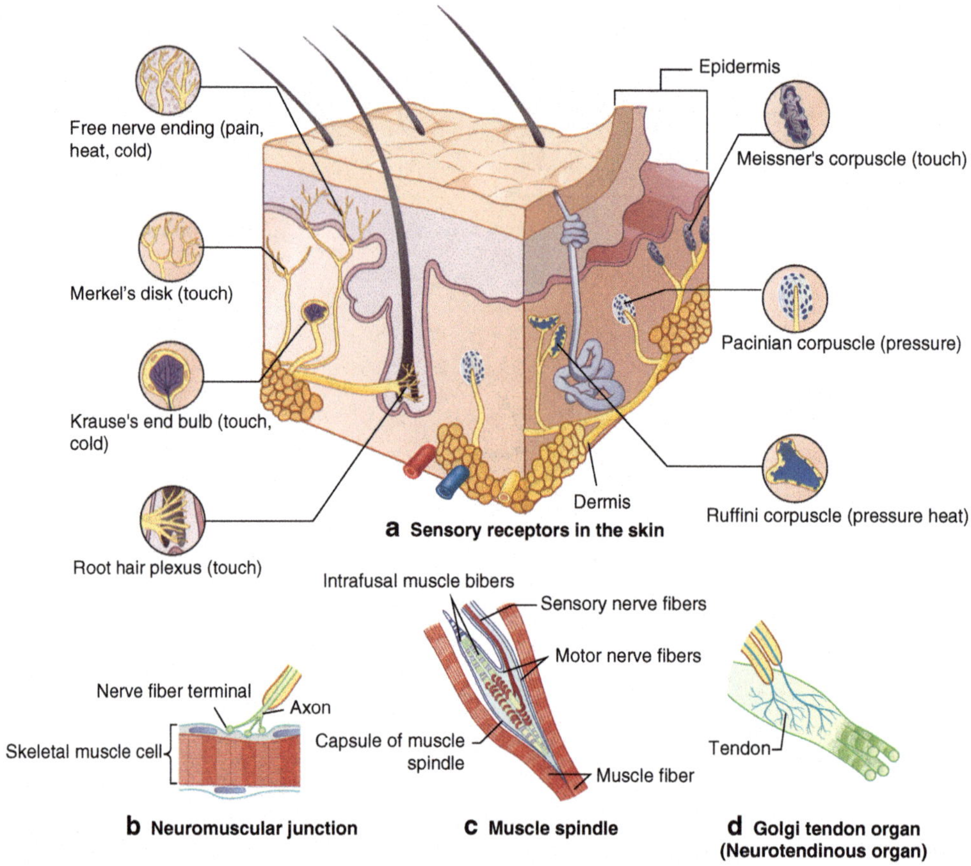

Fig. 1.4 Sensory nerve endings. (**a**) Sensory receptors in the skin. (**b**) Neuromuscular junction. (**c**) Muscle spindle. (**d**) Golgi tendon organ (neurotendinous organ)

a position sensor in pinpointing the location of a stimulus and two-point discrimination.

⑦ Muscle Spindles

Muscle spindles and Golgi tendon organs are called deep sensory receptors or proprioceptors, and they are found in muscles and tendons. Muscle spindles are pocket-shaped neural structures that detect the length of skeletal muscles and the speed of muscle contraction. Their sensory detection is related to the degree of muscle contraction, and the sensation is stimulated when muscle fibers are stretched.

⑧ Golgi tendon organs

The structure of Golgi tendon organ is not as complicated as that of muscle spindles, and there is no centrifugal innervation involved. Golgi tendon organs work as tension detectors by providing information about tension applied to tendons.

1.1.2.2 Cutaneous Nerves

Cutaneous Nerves of the Scalp

Concerning the sensory nerves of the scalp, the terminal branches of trigeminal nerves are distributed mainly on the front and sides of the head, while cutaneous cervical nerves are located in the neck (Fig. 1.5).

Cutaneous Nerves of the Face

Trigeminal nerves control facial sensation and are distributed on the scalp, teeth, and mucous membrane of the mouse and nose (Fig. 1.6).

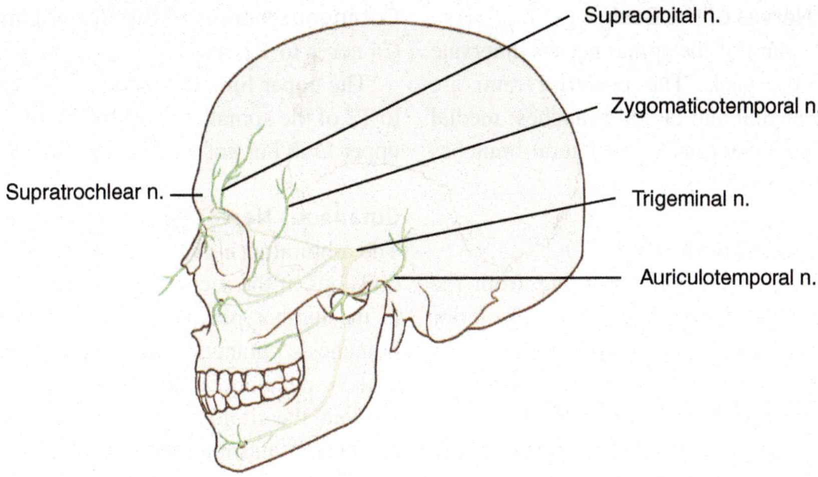

Fig. 1.5 The cutaneous branches of the trigeminal nerve

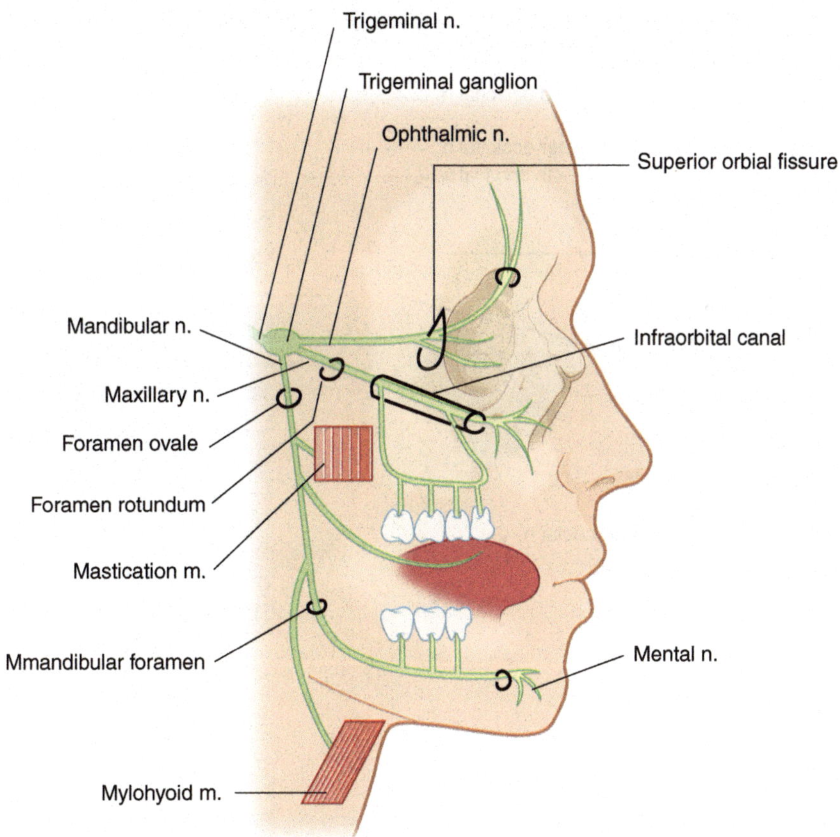

Fig. 1.6 Trigeminal nerve

Cutaneous Nerves of the Back

The posterior rami of the spinal nerves innervate the skin of the back. The posterior rami are divided into medial and lateral branches: medial branches in the upper back and lateral branches in the lower back (Fig. 1.7).

Cutaneous Nerves of the Chest

The supraclavicular nerves emerging from the cervical plexus (and from beneath the posterior border of the sternocleidomastoid muscle) are split into three branches in the posterior triangle of neck, cross in front of the clavicle, and innervate the upper part of the second intercostal space and the skin of the shoulder (Fig. 1.8).

Cutaneous Nerves of the Upper Limb

C4 nerve to T2 nerve.

The upper limb is innervated by segments C4 to T2 of the spinal cord with C5 to T1 only in the upper limb but not in the trunk (Fig. 1.9).

Cutaneous Nerves of the Lower Limb

The obturator nerves arising from the ventral divisions of the second and fourth lumbar nerves in the lumbar plexus are divided into muscular branches, cutaneous branches, and articular branches. Cutaneous branches are emerged from beneath the ilioinguinal nerves, pierce through fascia lata, and innervate the skin on the medial side of the thigh (Lee 2012).

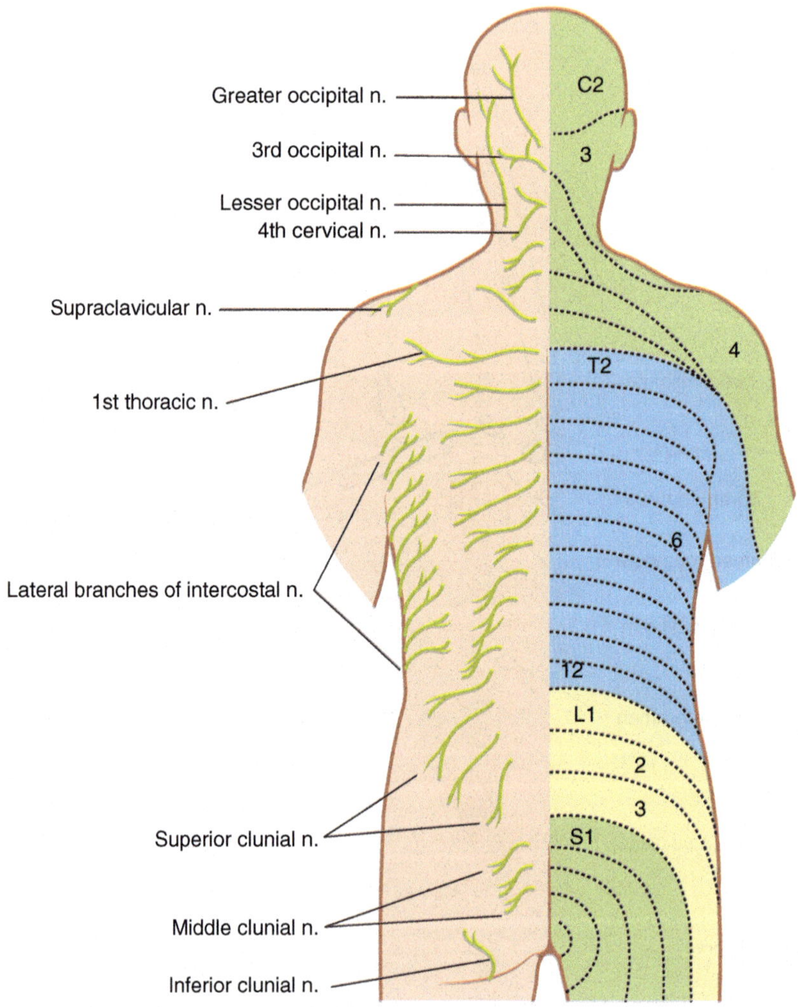

Fig. 1.7 Cutaneous nerves and dermatomes of the back

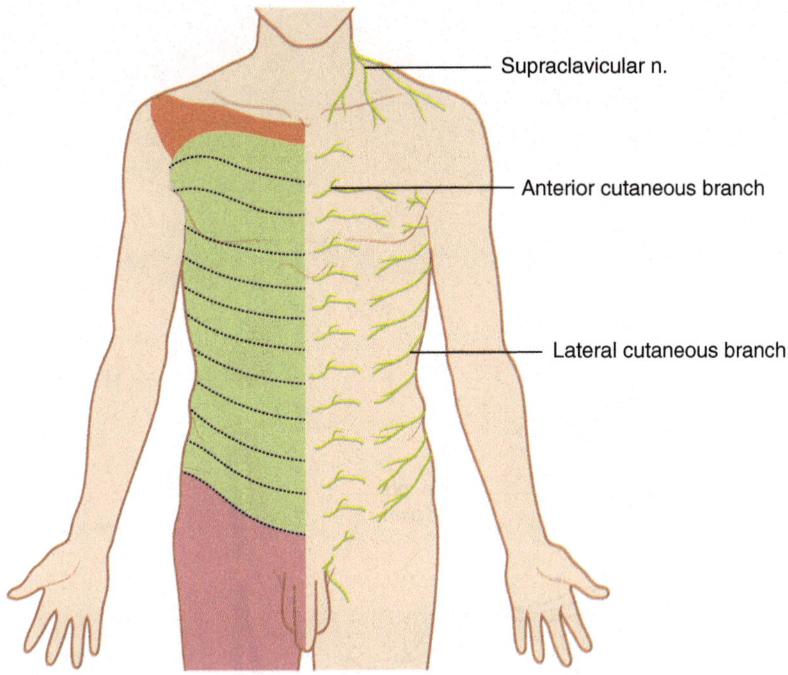

Fig. 1.8 Dermatomes of the chest

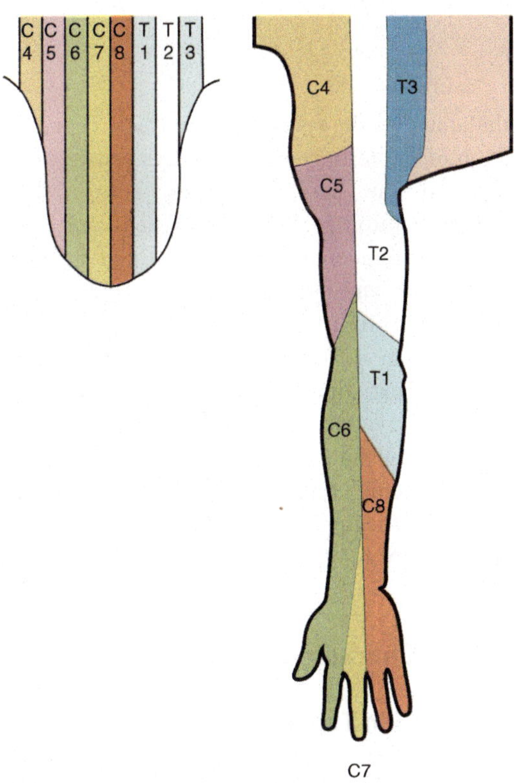

Fig. 1.9 Cutaneous nerve of the arm

1.1.2.3 Sensory Conduction Pathways

The four types of somatosensory stimuli received and perceived by the cerebral cortex are touch, proprioception, pain, and temperature. The conscious sensory pathways that relay signals from the spinal cord to the cerebral cortex include the posterior white column-medial lemniscal pathway and the spinothalamic tract. The posterior white column-medial lemniscal pathway relays discriminative touch information, and the spinothalamic tract conveys pain and temperature information (Fig. 1.10) (Chung 2000; Lee et al. 2012).

Posterior White Column-Medial Lemniscal Pathway

This pathway conveys discriminative touch information, with which the location and intensity of the stimulus can be discriminated; conscious proprioceptive information, with which the body's position and movement can be consciously determined; and stereognosis information, with which familiar objects can be recognized. The information carried through this pathway plays a crucial role in generating smooth movements and regulating fine movements (Fig. 1.11). Sensory receptors

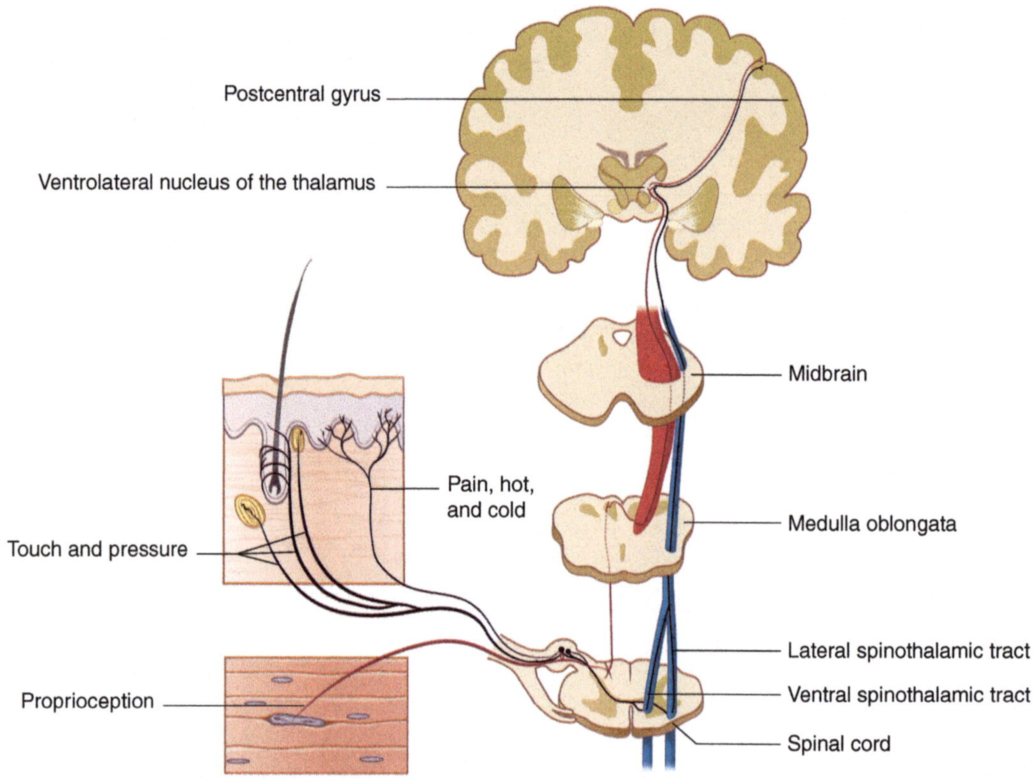

Fig. 1.10 Skin receptors and sensory pathways

include Merkel's disks, Meissner's corpuscles, Krause's end bulbs, Pacinian corpuscles, and Ruffini's corpuscles. Muscle spindles and Golgi tendon organs relay conscious proprioception through this pathway as well. When damage is done to above the medial lemniscus, the discriminative touch sense, vibratory sense, and position sense on the same side are lost or declined; on the other hand, when damage is done to below the medial lemniscus, those on the opposite side are lost or declined.

Spinothalamic Tract

Sensory information about heat, cold, and pain is conveyed to the spinal cord via unmyelinated sensory neurons. In the spinothalamic tract, the proximal axon of the primary neuron sprouts a new branch perpendicular to the adjacent spinal segment and forms a synapse with the secondary interneuron of the dorsal horn, and the secondary interneuron crosses over to the opposite side and gets connected to the thalamus via the spinothalamic tract. Then, the axon of the tertiary neuron relays sensory signals to the cerebral cortex (Fig. 1.12). Thermoception is the sense of heat and cold, and thermoreceptors are transmitted through myelinated and unmyelinated nerve fibers differentiated from free nerve endings. Aδ fibers transmit nerve impulses for cold, and C fibers conduct heat stimuli. Thermal and pain sensations conveyed through the spinothalamic tract are received by free nerve endings. When the spinothalamic tract is damaged, loss of pain occurs on the opposite side below the damaged segment (Ahn 1999; Ahn 2011).

1.2 Characteristics of the Skin

1.2.1 Skin Types

Skin types are classified into four types according to the sebum and moisture content of the

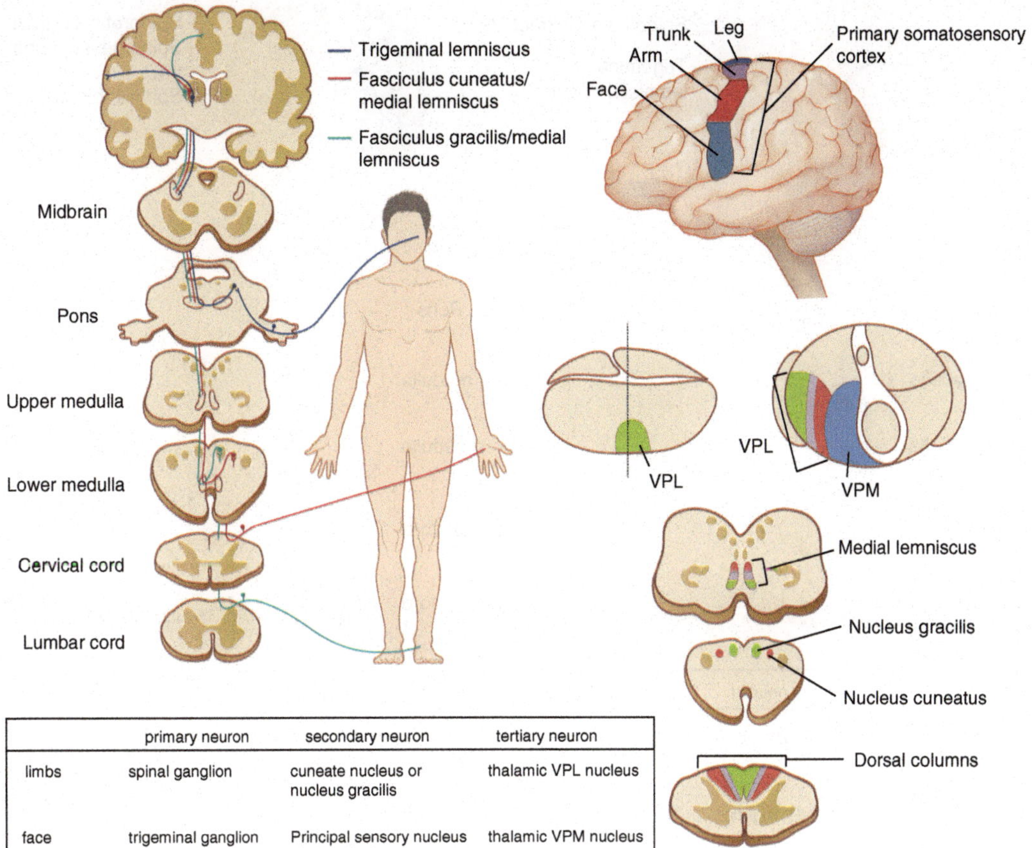

	primary neuron	secondary neuron	tertiary neuron
limbs	spinal ganglion	cuneate nucleus or nucleus gracilis	thalamic VPL nucleus
face (contact pathway only)	trigeminal ganglion	Principal sensory nucleus of trigeminal nerve	thalamic VPM nucleus

Fig. 1.11 Posterior white column-medial lemniscal pathway (relays discriminative touch information and conscious proprioception)

skin: normal, oily, dry, and combination. Further categories include sensitive skin, abnormal skin, and aging skin. However, the characteristics of the skin vary from person to person depending on the psychological, environmental, and pathological factors such as age, nutrition, air temperature, air humidity, air current, quantity and quality of sleep, eating habit, use of cosmetics, and stress.

1.2.1.1 General Classification of Skin Types

Normal Skin

Normal skin is the most ideal skin type with keratinization, desquamation, water loss, sebum excretion, and sweating in equilibrium. Normal skin is soft, elastic, and well moisturized (Fig. 1.13). It is not excessively oily or dry as well and appears mostly at young age. Consistent care is required because normal skin with high resistance and good tone can be changed to become oily or dry as a result of environmental changes.

Dry Skin

Dry skin is characterized by a lack of oil, which leads to lack of moisture. Dry skin has a rough surface and is often accompanied by the formation of the erythema, fissure, and scale (Fig. 1.14). The external factors that cause dry skin include dry air, wind, detergents, and chemicals such as organic solvents, excessive bathing or face washing, UV rays, treatment with drugs like retinoids, and physi-

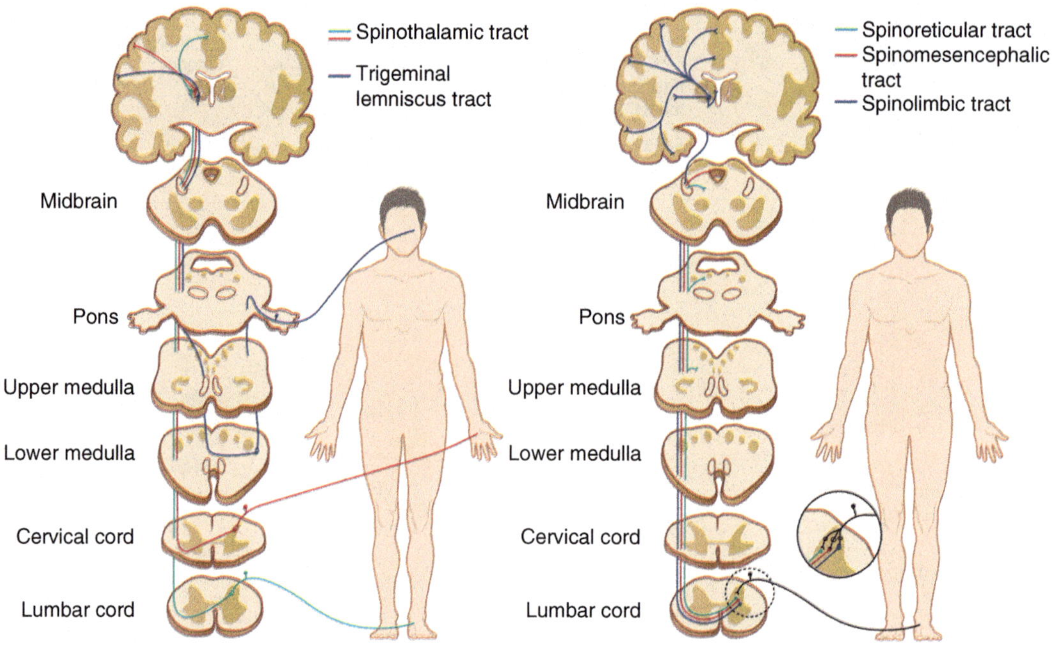

	primary neuron	secondary neuron	tertiary neuron
Limbs	spinal ganglion	Posterior horn of the spinal cord	thalamic VPL nucleus
Face (contact pathway only)	trigeminal ganglion	Spinal nucleus of trigeminal nerve	thalamic VPM nucleus

Fig. 1.12 Spinothalamic tract and its pain transmission

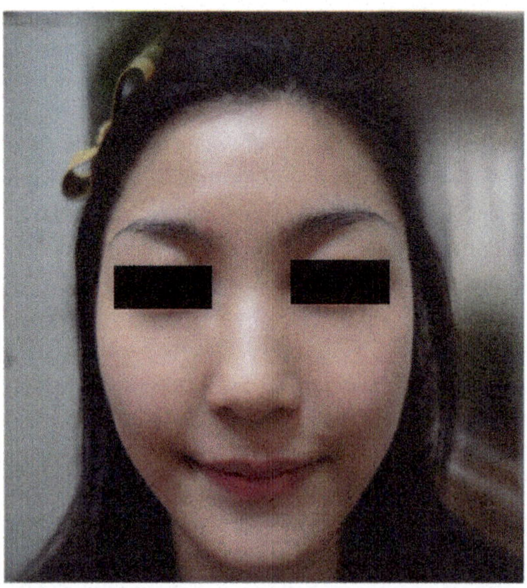

Fig. 1.13 Normal skin

cal stimulation. The internal factors include aging, atopic dermatitis, and chronic renal failure. Dry skin is caused by lack of natural moisturizing factor (NMF – function in maintaining moisture in the stratum corneum), reduced lipids in the stratum corneum (function in preventing moisture evaporation), and eliminated abnormal stratum corneum (scale formation by abnormal elimination).

Oily Skin

Oily skin refers to a greasy skin type with excessive sebum secretion due to overactive oil glands (Fig. 1.15). The excessive sebum secretion forms an oily film on the skin, which in turn blocks pores and induces pimples. Too much sebum also alkalizes the epidermis and increases the likelihood of bacterial infection; thus, sebum control is very important. The major causes of oily skin include

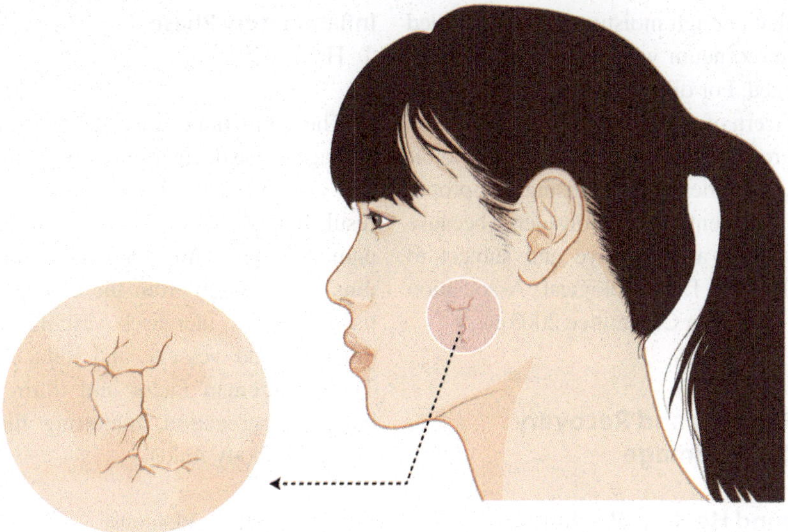

Fig. 1.14 Dry skin

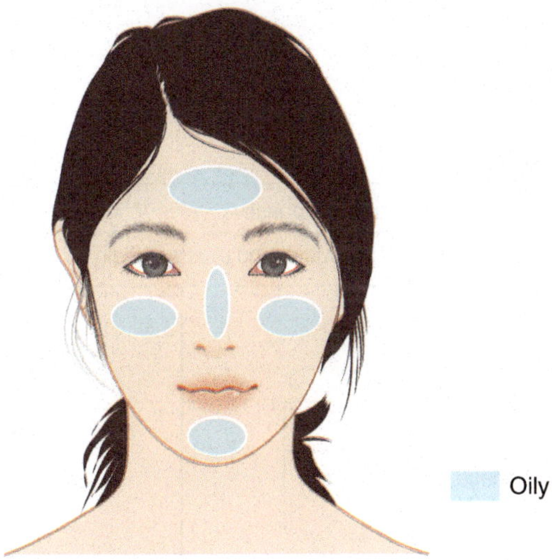

Fig. 1.15 Oily skin

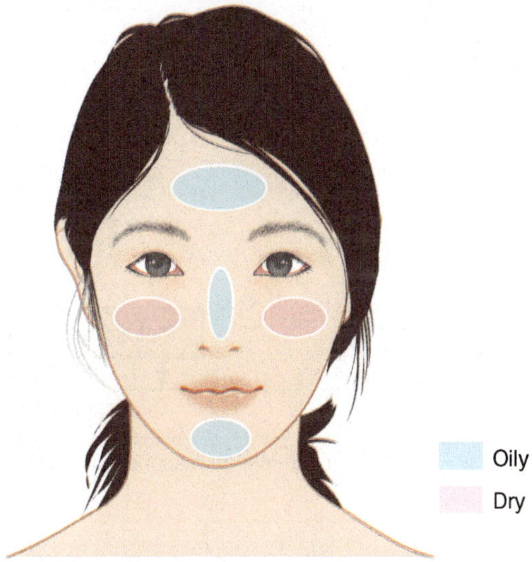

Fig. 1.16 Combination skin

excessive sebum secretion, genetic traits, puberty hormones such as androgen and progesterone, gastroenteric troubles, irregular eating habits (excessive intake of fats and carbohydrates), a lack of vitamin B_2 and B_6, and hot and humid air.

Combination Skin

Combination skin normally shows both characteristics of dry skin and oily skin due to the regional differences in sebum secretion, and it is sensitive to external stimuli and easily gets infected. Generally, the T-zone (nose, chin, and forehead) is oily while the cheeks are dry or normal (Fig. 1.16). This condition is common after the middle age due to the acquired factors such as the environment, lifestyle skin care habits, and hormone imbalances. It is important in integumentary physical therapy that each skin type characteristics are fully considered. For dry skins, appropriate moisturizing and cleansing are required so that enough moisture can be supplied to the stratum corneum while moisture evaporation is prevented. For oily skins, sebum removal is the major concern of the treatment to deal with the excessively greasy condition. In the case of combination skins, hypoallergenic cleansing and proper antibacterial treatment must be considered because combination skins are sensitive and subject to infections (Korean Dermatological Association Textbook Compilation Committee 2008).

1.2.2 Pathology and Recovery of Skin Damage

1.2.2.1 Wound Healing Mechanism

Wound healing after skin damage goes through the inflammatory phase, proliferative phase, and maturation phase (Fig. 1.17) (Park 2010).

Inflammatory Phase

① Hemostasis

The immediate vascular response to tissue damage is vasoconstriction, by which blood vessels are contracted in several minutes, and as a result hemorrhage is stopped. Once the tissue is damaged, serotonin, histamine, and prostaglandins are released from the damaged site of the tissue, which increases vascular permeability, dilates blood vessels, and induces congestion. Then, Hageman factor and fibrin take part in platelet aggregation, inhibiting further loss of blood and body fluids.

② Inflammatory Response

A. Vascular Response: Prostaglandins, bradykinin, leukotriene, and histamine dilate blood

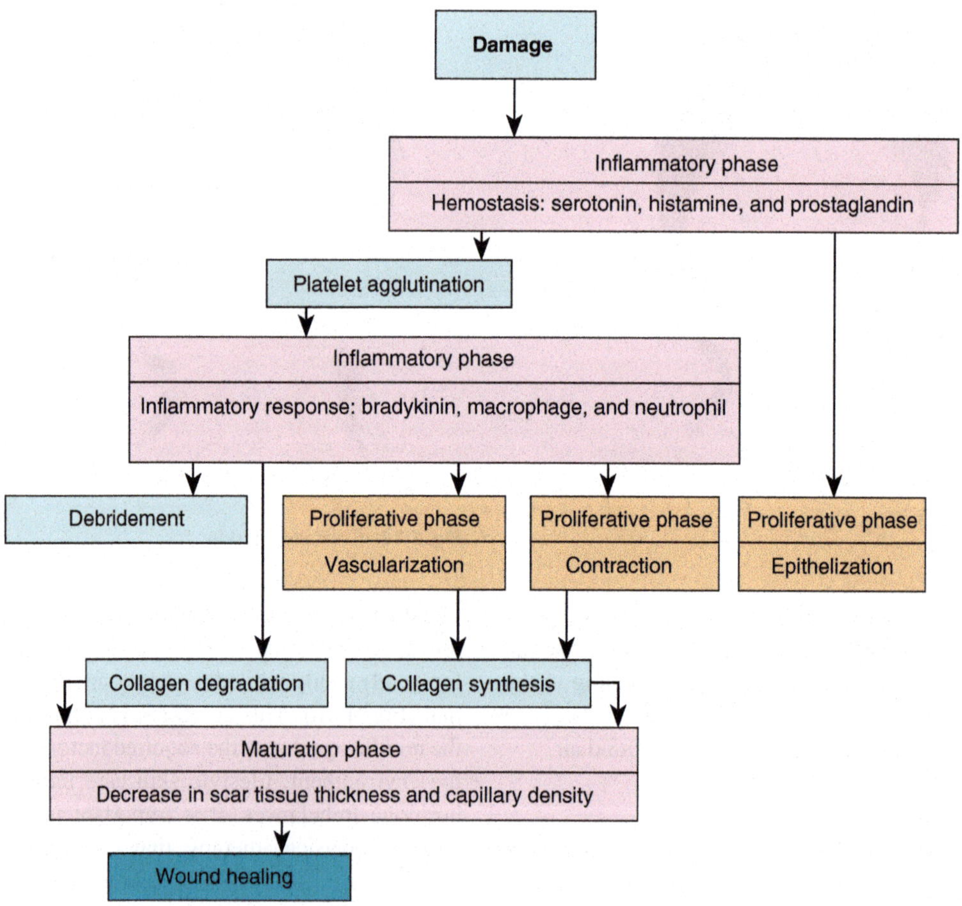

Fig. 1.17 Mechanism of wound healing (Lee 2010)

vessels, increase vascular permeability, and induce congestion. As serous exudate flows into the wound site, erythema, edema, pyrexia, pain, or dysfunction may occur.

B. Cellular Response: Neutrophils, macrophages, and monocytes on the wound site eliminate bacteria and foreign substances and boost phagocytosis and purification. The inflammatory phase usually lasts 3–5 days, but it may take longer depending on the severity of the infection. When the contamination of the wound continues, the activation of monocytes and neutrophils is maintained, which hinders the process from the inflammatory phase to the proliferative phase.

Proliferative Phase

① Granulation Tissue Formation

A. Vascularization: Vascularization or angiogenesis refers to the process in which endothelial cells near the necrotic tissue start proliferation within two days after the skin damage and grow into the damaged tissue so that oxygen and nutrients can be provided to the site.

B. Collagen Synthesis: When cellular regeneration within 24 h after the damage is difficult, vascular endothelial cells proliferate, and subsequent granulation tissue fills the wound site. Granulation tissue includes fibroblast, lymphocyte, mastocyte, and macrophage. Its branches are proliferated from capillaries, and they cause edema due to imperfect permeability and water leak.

② Contraction

Myofibroblasts pull the wound edges together decreasing the size of the defect.

③Epithelization

Epithelization is a process of closing the wound by the migration and replication of epithelial cells. Molecules of collagen, elastin, and glycoproteins are newly synthesized in the process of eliminating the damaged matrix, and after cross-linking of collagen, the initial scar tissue is formed. When the scar tissue is not eliminated by proteases, granulation tissue is formed on the wound surface, and after the continuous epithelization, keloid is developed.

Maturation Phase

In the maturation phase, as unnecessary fibroblasts and capillaries diminish, the scar tissue is replaced with soft and dense tissue which is not easily destroyed by external stimuli, and the color of the skin returns to normal. However, if the scar tissue remains, the skin becomes vulnerable to external stimuli since the scar tissue is 20–30 % less elastic than normal tissue.

1.2.3 Skin Aging

1.2.3.1 Classification of Skin Aging

Skin aging is classified into intrinsic aging caused by biological factors and photoaging caused by exposure to the sun. Intrinsic aging makes the skin thin and smooth; on the other hand, photoaging, which is generally accelerated by intrinsic aging, makes the skin dry, rough, and thick and is accompanied by deep wrinkle, pigmentation, telangiectasia, and purpura (Table 1.1) (Lee and Noh 2010).

Table 1.1 The comparison of clinical manifestations between intrinsic aging and photoaging

Clinical manifestations	Intrinsic aging	Photoaging
Skin texture	Soft	Rough and thick
Wrinkle	Shallow wrinkle	Deep wrinkle
Epidermis	Thinning	Thinning after thickening
Elasticity	Slight decrease	Significant decrease
Grenz zone in the papillary dermis	Not present	Present (solar elastosis)
Microvascular structure	Decrease in severity	Significant decrease, capillary dilation
Skin tumor	Benign	Malignant

1.2.3.2 Causes of Skin Aging

Causation Theory of Skin Aging

Two most acknowledged theories are "the programmatic theory" and "the stochastic theory," but there are also many other ongoing researches with different approaches.

① Programmatic Theory

This theory argues that aging process is genetically decided, that is, an individual's aging and lifespan are results of a process that is set and controlled by a genetic program. Suggested evidences are a limited number of cell division cycles, the existence of certain aging genes, and telomere shortening.

② Stochastic Theory

The theory claims that the continuous environmental stimuli destroy genes and proteins, and as cell damages accumulate, the cells become dysfunctional or deformed, which eventually leads to aging. In the process of using oxygen, the reactive oxygen radicals such as oxide ion, hydrogen peroxide ion, and hydroxide ion are produced, and they cause oxidative damages to normal proteins, lipids, and DNAs. The human antioxidant defense system has the function of minimizing the damage from oxygen radicals. However, cell damages accumulate as free radicals exceed the functional capacity of the antioxidant defense mechanism, and as a result of the functional decline of cells, aging proceeds.

Causes of Skin Aging

① Changes in the integumentary structure and function caused by intrinsic aging.
② Environmental factors such as the accumulation of ultraviolet radiation damage (photoaging).
③ Cutaneous changes or diseases related to the aging of other organs or age-related systemic diseases (diabetes, vascular insufficiency, and neurological syndromes).
④ Skin problems due to environmental changes: with more spare time, people make physical contact with more diverse range of materials.
⑤ Living conditions such as living alone, nutrition deficiency, poor hygiene, lack of energy, and financial difficulty make it difficult to receive medical cares.
⑥ Problems on physiological functions or cognitive functions: those with these problems tend to be stubborn and reluctant to listen to other people's advices (amnesia and dementia).
⑦ Declined motor ability: proper disease prevention and therapeutic activities (e.g., applying ointment to a wound) are difficult.

1.2.3.3 Skin Changes Due to Aging

Aging on the Epidermis

As aging progresses, regeneration of epidermal cells declines. As regeneration slows down, keratin synthesis of keratinocytes drops, and production of natural moisturizing factors such as filaggrin and keratohyalin granule decreases, resulting in severe dehydration and buildup of dead skin cells. Furthermore, moisture deficiency in the stratum corneum becomes severe, moisture transfer from the stratum basale to the stratum corneum slows down due to the decrease of extracellular matrix, and skin's acidic film becomes weaker as sebum production declines. Melanocytes in the stratum basale decrease by 10–20 % per decade. Because aged skin does not produce melanin pigment evenly, the color of the skin becomes uneven and irregular.

Aging on the Dermis

As the dermis undergoes aging, collagen and elastin, which are, respectively, responsible for keeping the skin firm and elastic, are hardened and become insoluble. The ground substance that fills the spaces between fibers and cells has high capacity to hold moisture. As aging proceeds, the number of this substance decreases, which leads to more and deeper wrinkles. Hyaluronic acids and mucopolysacharides are examples of ground substances, and they are called glycosaminoglycans (GAG) due to their chemical composition in which proteins and carbohydrates are combined. Hyaluronidase, an enzyme that breaks down hyaluronic acid, increases with aging, and subsequently the amount of hyaluronic acid in the dermis decreases.

Aging on the Subcutaneous Tissue

The subcutaneous tissue is composed of fat and water, and its roles include storing energy, thermal resistance, cushioning effect, and protecting the skin from sharp bones. With aging, the subcutaneous tissue becomes thin, and the veins become prominent, making the skin more vulnerable to damages.

Aging on the Skin Appendages

① Pilosebaceous Follicles

Aging reduces female hormone levels and strengthens the effects of male hormone (testosterone); as a result, sebaceous glands are stimulated, and overall sebum production declines. Reduced sebum levels and subsequent lack of acidic film lead to dehydrated, dry skin.

② Sweat Glands

The size and number of eccrine sweat glands and apocrine sweat glands decrease with aging.

The sweat glands secrete natural moisturizing factors such as lactic acids, urea, sodium PCA, minerals, and trace elements, and their production declines as well. Apocrine sweat glands, which secrete sweat through hair follicles, and eccrine sweat glands experience decline in the function of secretion (Park et al. 2006).

1.2.3.4 Functional Changes of Aging Skin

Reduction of Wound Healing Capacity

The epidermal cell division rate and the regeneration rate of the aged skin decline rapidly after the age of 50. Accordingly, the skin's wound healing capacity drops. Extra caution is required because reduced wound healing rate causes the secondary infection.

Increase in Benign and Malignant Tumor

Benign tumors such as seborrheic keratosis are observed in most elderly individuals, but there can be other problems such as the deterioration of the immune function caused by long-term exposure to ultraviolet light, reduced number and function of Langerhans cells, the deterioration of the skin's protective function caused by the decline in the number and function of melanocytes, and malignant tumors (basal cell carcinoma and squamous cell carcinoma) caused by the decline in the ultraviolet light sensitivity.

Decrease in the Skin's Immune Function

Deterioration in overall immune function in elderly individuals can cause malignant skin tumors by increasing the risk of the infectious diseases resulted from viruses or fungi. Aging causes the reduction in Langerhans cell numbers in the epidermis and the decline in the division and function of T lymphocytes. They lead to the damage to the skin immune cells and the deterioration in the contact hypersensitivity reaction, which in turn cause various skin diseases.

Decrease in Vitamin D Synthesis

As aging proceeds, the process converting 7-dehydrocholesterol to previtamin D by ultraviolet light is not effective resulting in problems of calcium and phosphorus metabolisms, which eventually lead to osteoporosis and rickets.

1.2.4 Histopathology of the Skin

Histopathology in the skin is divided into epidermis, dermoepidermal junction, dermis, and subcutaneous fat (Rotter et al. 2005; Spence and Mason 1984).

1.2.4.1 Changes in the Epidermis

Hyperkeratosis

Hyperkeratosis means an abnormal thickening of the stratum corneum and is classified into relative hyperkeratosis and absolute hyperkeratosis. Relative hyperkeratosis is the stratum corneum in the upper epidermis, and absolute hyperkeratosis is observed in chronic discoid lupus erythematosus and lichen planus.

Parakeratosis

Parakeratosis, characterized by incomplete keratinization, retains nuclei within the keratin layer, and this is often found in psoriasis and Bowen's disease. It is observed in warts, chronic simple lichen, atopic dermatitis, seborrheic dermatitis, pityriasis rosea, and pityriasis lichenoides.

Hypergranulosis

Hypergranulosis, observed in lichen planus, lupus erythematosus, wart, and lamellar ichthyosis, is characterized by a thickened stratum granulosum.

Hypogranulosis

When the thickness of stratum granulosum is decreased or lost, the state is called hypogranulosis, and it is found in psoriasis, Bowen's disease, and ichthyosis vulgaris.

Acanthosis

Acanthosis denotes increased thickness of the Malpighian layer (stratum basale and stratum spinosum). Acanthosis with a thickened epidermis is observed in wart, epidermal nevus, sebaceous nevus, seborrheic keratosis, acanthosis nigricans, actinic keratosis, and cutaneous tag. Acanthosis with regular elongation of rete ridges is found in psoriasis, and papillomatosis implies projection of adjacent dermal papillae with severe acanthosis. Pseudoepitheliomatous proliferation is an irregular downward proliferation of epidermal cells into the dermis. It is observed mostly in chronic eczema, tuberculosis, and deep-seated mycosis and responds to foreign substances.

Epidermal Atrophy

Epidermal atrophy is Malpighian layer with decreased thickness and is observed in poikiloderma, lichen planus atrophicus, lupus erythematosus, lichen sclerosus et atrophicus, and acrodermatitis chronica atrophicans.

Spongiosis

Spongiosis is caused by intercellular edema and refers to a condition of widening the intercellular spaces resulting in many small holes irregularly connected together, which impart the epidermis, a sponge like appearance. It can be found in acute contact dermatitis, nummular eczema, dyshidrotic eczema, vesicle autosensitization dermatitis, vesicle dermatophytosis, incontinentia pigmenti, allergic contact dermatitis, insect bite, bullous pemphigoid, herpes gestationis, and pemphigus.

Reticular and Ballooning Degeneration

Reticular degeneration is characterized by the mesh-like appearance of the epidermis due to many vacuoles and vesicles in the epidermis. It is generally accompanied by degenerative cellular changes and found in an acute blister response of contact dermatitis and herpes infection.

Ballooning degeneration implies cellular swelling caused by edema in the epidermis and is found in herpes and other viral blisters. Ballooning degeneration and multinucleated giant cells are the characteristics found in herpes.

Granular Degeneration of the Epidermis

In epidermolytic hyperkeratosis, clumping of immature tonofilament turns cytoplasm around the nucleus into edematous vacuoles, and cell dissociation occurs due to the failure of desmosomal adhesion. The excessive amounts of immature keratohyalin granules cause granular degeneration. This is observed in epidermolytic hyperkeratosis, epidermal nevus, palmoplantar hyperkeratosis, wart, and epidermolytic acanthoma.

1.2.4.2 Changes in the Dermoepidermal Junction

1. Hydropic degeneration is resulted by small vacuoles above and below the basilar membrane. It is found in lupus erythematosus, lichen planus, lichen sclerosus et atrophicus, incontinentia pigmenti, lichenoid eruption, polymorphous light eruption, erythema dyschromicum perstans, and erythema multiforme. Histological cleft observed by microscopy in the dermoepidermal junction is called Max-Joseph space and found in lichen planus and lichenoid eruption.
2. Tissue Changes in Blistering Diseases

   Blisters with serous or inflammatory exudates in or under the epidermis are moisture-containing spaces. The major pathologies include spongiosis; vacuolar, reticular, and ballooning degeneration; acantholysis;

epidermal cell necrosis; and sweat duct rupture. Subepidermal blisters can be subdivided into basilar membrane defect, severe denaturation, basilar membrane disruption by basilar necrosis, and inflammatory response which invades subepidermal connective tissue and basilar membrane; however, there is no perfect classification.

3. Lichenoid Infiltration

   Lichenoid infiltration is characterized by unclear dermoepidermal junction and band-like, diffuse infiltration composed of lymphocytes in the papillary dermis. It occurs as basal cells undergo erosion and is observed in lichen planus, lichenoid keratosis, acute lichenoid eruption, melanodermatitis toxica, secondary syphilis, pityriasis lichenoides, and chronic capillaritis.

1.2.4.3 Changes in the Dermis

Dermal Proliferation

Dermal proliferation denotes individual or collective proliferation of fibroblasts, blood vessels, lymphatic vessels, or nervous tissues and is found in traumatic neuroma, pyogenic granuloma, and keloid.

Dermal Atrophy

Dermal atrophy implies atrophy of the dermis resulted from general aging, and it can be caused by abuse of steroid ointments.

Dermal Degeneration

Dermal degeneration is observed in necrotizing angiitis, lupus erythematosus, and colloid degeneration, in which infiltration of homogenized gelatinous substances (in colloid milium or epithelioma) is found. It includes fibrinoid degeneration, in which granular substances (composed of fibrinogen, plasma protein, immunoglobulin, and dermal matrix) infiltrate the surrounding tissues, and myxoid degeneration, in which the dermal connective tissue is replaced by amorphous, basophilic mucus.

Vasculitis

Diseases that invade vessel walls are collectively called vasculitis. This can cause vascular necrosis and vaso-occlusion and shows thickening of vessel walls in the dermis and panniculus adiposus, proliferation of endothelial cells, and cell wall infiltration of inflammatory cells. Vasculitis, according to the types of infiltrated cells, can be classified into neutrophilic vasculitis, lymphocytic vasculitis, mixed vasculitis, and granulomatous vasculitis, but there is no standard classification system.

Granuloma

Granuloma refers to a collection of histiocytes (also lymphocytes, epithelioid cells, or giant cells) with excessive cytoplasm and is observed in Langerhans islets. It is accompanied by polymorphic leukocytes, plasmacytes, and eosinocytes, infiltration of fibroblasts, vascular degeneration, and proliferation and necrosis of connective tissues.

1.2.4.4 Melanocytic Neoplasms (Tumors)

Benign growth of melanocytes is called junctional nevus, compound nevus, or intradermal nevus depending on the location of nevocytes. Melanocytes in the subcutaneous layer are smaller and denser compared to those in the stratum basale. The malignant melanoma is suspected when the infiltration of inflammatory cells or atypical and abnormal growth of melanocytes is observed.

1.2.4.5 Panniculitis

An inflammatory condition of subcutaneous fatty tissue is called panniculitis and is classified into the panniculitis with granuloma, lymphocyte infiltration, neutrophil infiltration, and vasculitis; the panniculitis with septal, indurative, lobular characteristics but without vasculitis; and the panniculitis with vasculitis as well as septal, lobular characteristics.

1.3 Assessment of the Skin

1.3.1 General Symptoms and Signs Related to the Skin

Diagnosis of skin diseases can be difficult due to the similar symptoms and signs, but it can be also relatively easy because of the unique characteristics. Various examination methods that consider subjective symptoms, clinical sings, medical history, and skin biopsy are required (Ahn et al. 2009).

1.3.1.1 Cutaneous Symptoms

The major cutaneous symptoms include pruritus, pain, anesthesia, hypoesthesia, hyperesthesia, burning, tingling, and formication (Choi and Hong 2006).

Pruritus

Pruritus is an unpleasant sensation that causes an urge to scratch or rub. It is the most common type of cutaneous symptom and is caused by lightly stimulating the cutaneous nerves. It can be experienced as a light tingling sensation, but it can also become unbearably itching. Pruritus occurs suddenly or constantly with a great deal of variability among the individuals. The anus and genitals are especially prone to pruritus. It is usually accompanied by eczematous dermatitis, urticaria, bullous dermatitis, scabies, lichen planus, and mycosis fungoides. Senile pruritus and winter pruritus resulted mostly from skin dryness. Pruritus can be accompanied by systemic diseases such as diabetes, biliary obstructive diseases, uremia, hypothyroidism, and a state of endocrine imbalance such as menopause.

Pain

Herpes zoster causes stitching pains along the nerves and is a typical pain related to the skin diseases. Dermalgia and arthralgia are found in cellulitis, squamous cell carcinoma, malignant melanoma, lupus erythematosus, systemic sclerosis, and polymyositis.

1.3.1.2 Cutaneous Signs

Cutaneous lesions or skin manifestations are divided into the primary lesions and secondary lesions. The primary lesions are visible to the naked eye and refer to the lesions appearing for the first time. When the primary lesions progress or undergo modification by recovery, injury, or other external factors, those lesions are called the secondary lesions.

Primary Lesions

① Macule

Macules denote circumscribed changes in the color of skin and mostly occur in petechia, scarlet fever, measles, freckle, and nevus. Macules can appear as hypopigmentation like vitiligo, pigmentation like freckle, or erythema like hemangioma (Fig. 1.18).

Macules display circular or oval shapes without elevation or depression. Their borders can be well defined or fade out into the surrounding

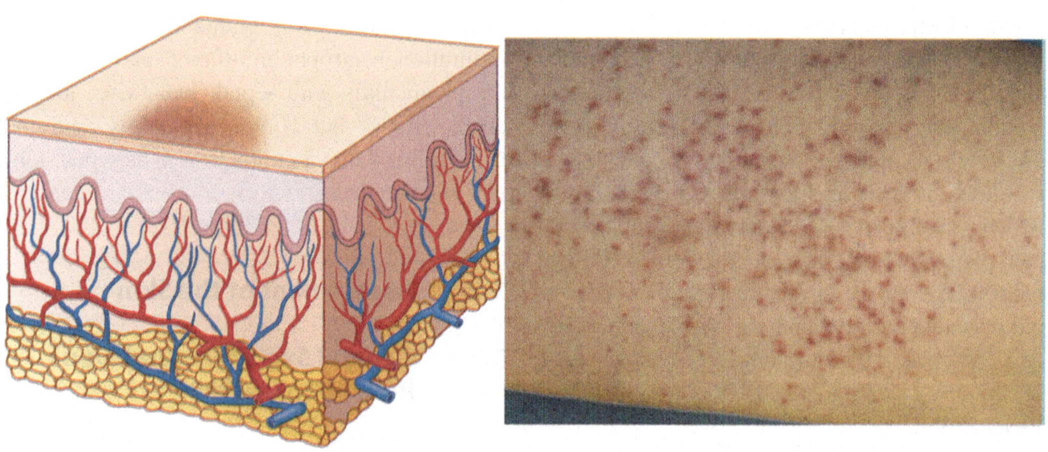

Fig. 1.18 Macule

skin. Macules can also appear as hyperpigmentation, hypopigmentation, erythema, or purpura.

② Papule

Papules are small, solid elevation of the skin with diameters less than 5 mm. Papules can be flat as lichen planus, dome-shaped like xanthoma, or pointed when they are related to hair follicles (Fig. 1.19).

They can also have depressed center in the case of molluscum contagiosum. Papules are usually present in the epidermis or upper dermis around the sebaceous glands or openings of hair follicles. In the course of diseases, papules may continue to exist without any changes, but when inflammation is involved, they can form vesicles, pustules, or ulcers.

③ Nodule

Nodules are similar to papules, but their diameters are normally larger than 5 mm, and they can invade any layer of the skin (Fig. 1.40). Nodules can appear in edematous or sclerogenic conditions and often present in the form of erythema nodosum or lipoma as in dermatofibroma or deposition. Nodule is an intermediate form between papules and small tumors, and unlike papules, the lesions appear on the dermis or subcutaneous fat layers (Fig. 1.20) (Terminology FCoA 1998).

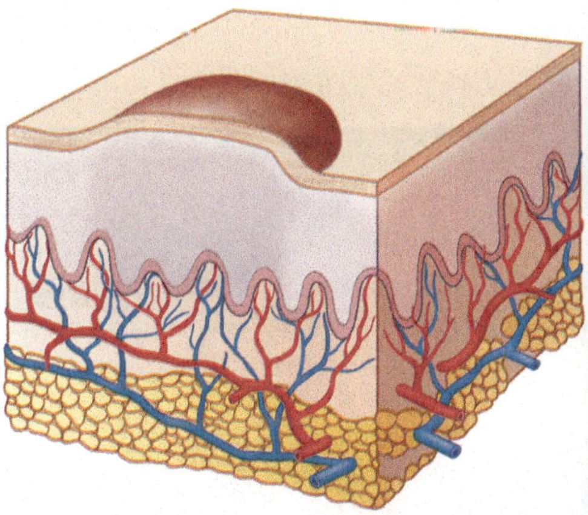

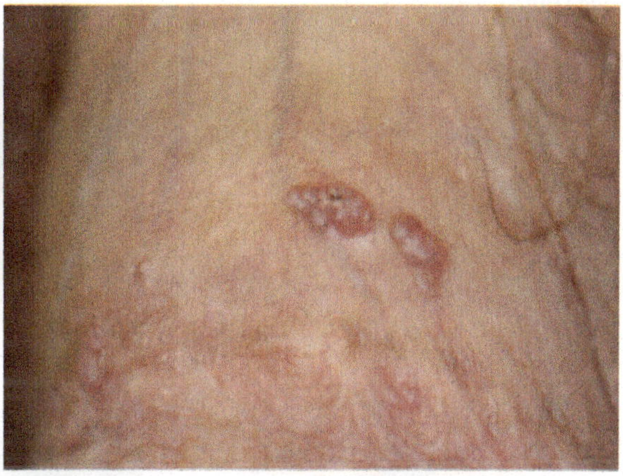

Fig. 1.19 Papule

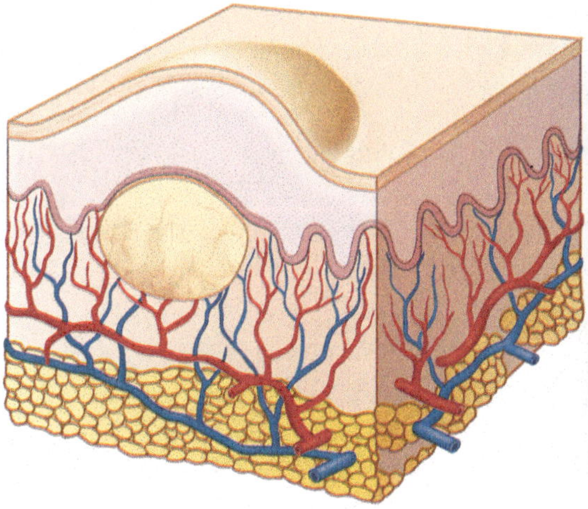

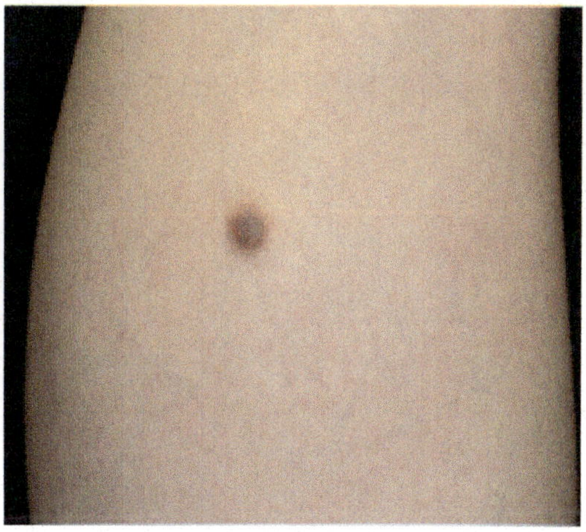

Fig. 1.20 Nodose

④ Bulla

Bullae have diameters more than 1 cm, and they are exemplified by bullous pemphigoid and pemphigus (Fig. 1.21).

⑤ Vesicle

Vesicles are small blisters less than 1 cm in diameter. They develop when fluid get trapped under or in the epidermis and are observed in varicella or herpes zoster (Fig. 1.22).

⑥ Pustule

In pustules, pus is observed with the naked eye (Fig. 1.23).

Pustules are pus-filled blisters, and pus implies inflammation. However, they can be observed without inflammation in the case of psoriasis.

⑦ Cyst

Cysts refer to epidermal nodules containing fluid or semisolid materials (Fig. 1.24).

⑧ Wheal

Wheals are temporarily developed papules or plaques caused by urticaria or allergic reaction. They are observed in red or white (Fig. 1.25).

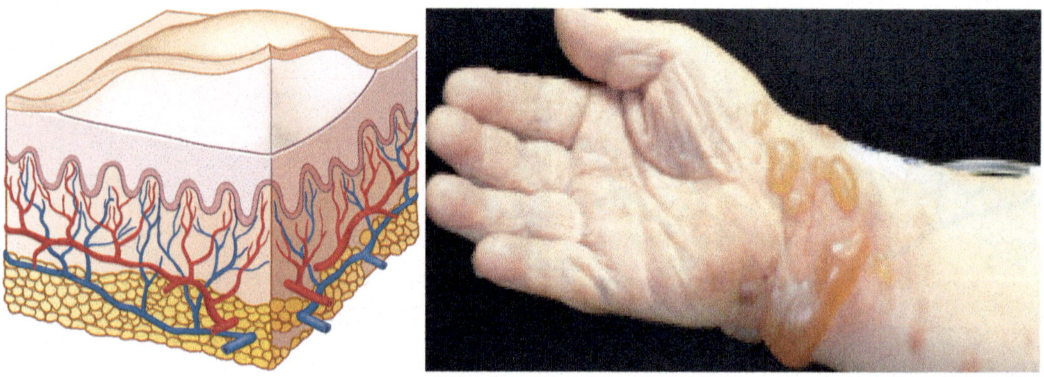

Fig. 1.21 Bulla

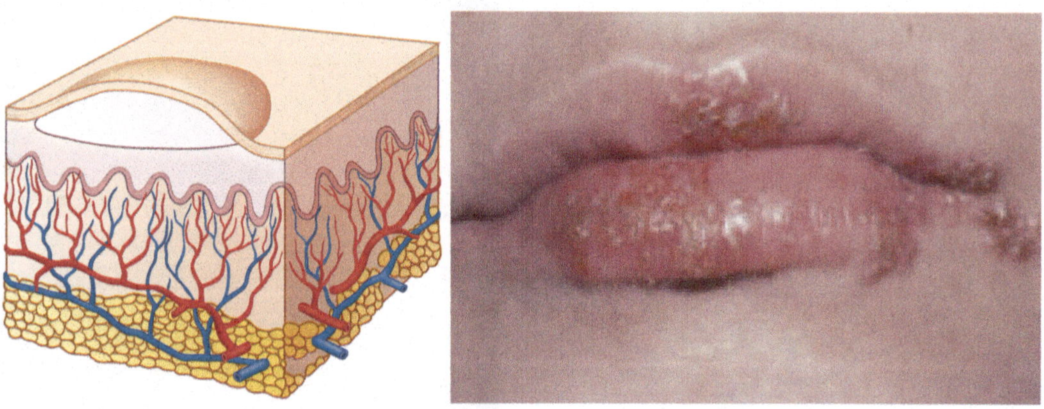

Fig. 1.22 Vesicle

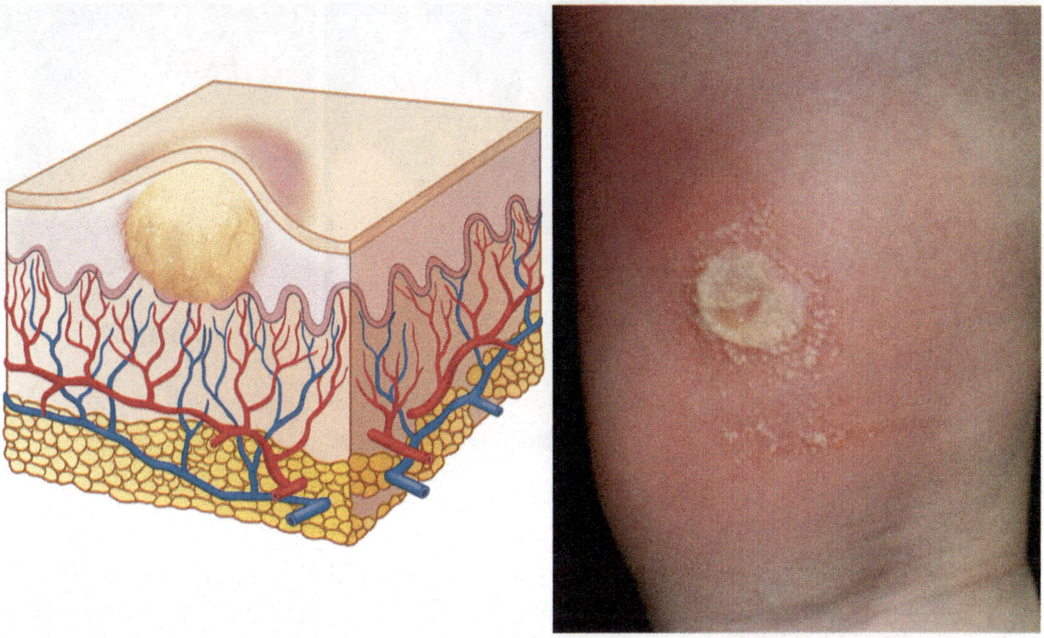

Fig. 1.23 Pustule

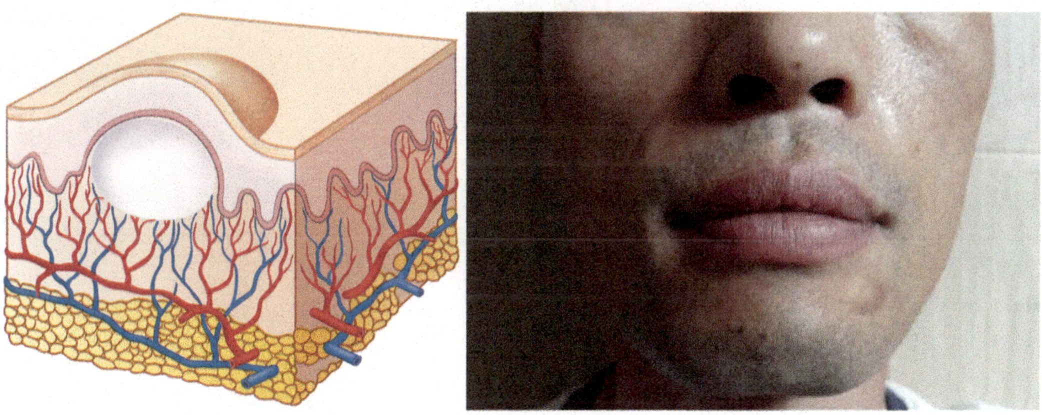

Fig. 1.24 Cystoma

⑨ Plaque

Plaques are elevated skin with 2 cm in diameter. They can be considered as grown papules, and they occur in psoriasis or mycosis fungoides (Fig. 1.26).

Secondary Lesions

① Scale

Scales are aggregates of keratin debris in the stratum corneum. Generally, they are observed to be very small in pityriasis. In psoriasis, scales look white or silver, and they may appear similar to fish scales (Fig. 1.27).

② Excoriation

Excoriations are caused by mechanical traumas or repetitive scratching to ease pruritus. Their sizes and shapes vary, but normally they are small lesions with punctate or linear shapes. Excoriations are often developed in scabies.

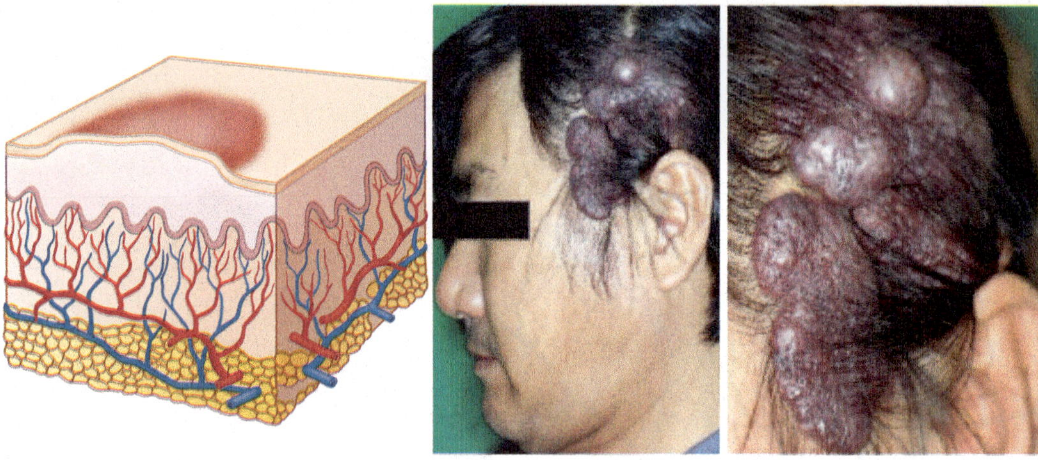

Fig. 1.25 Wheal

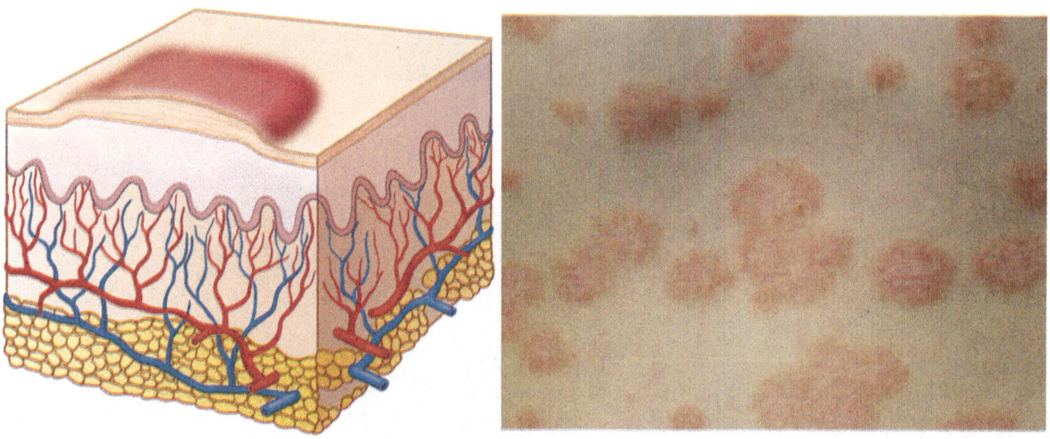

Fig. 1.26 Plaque

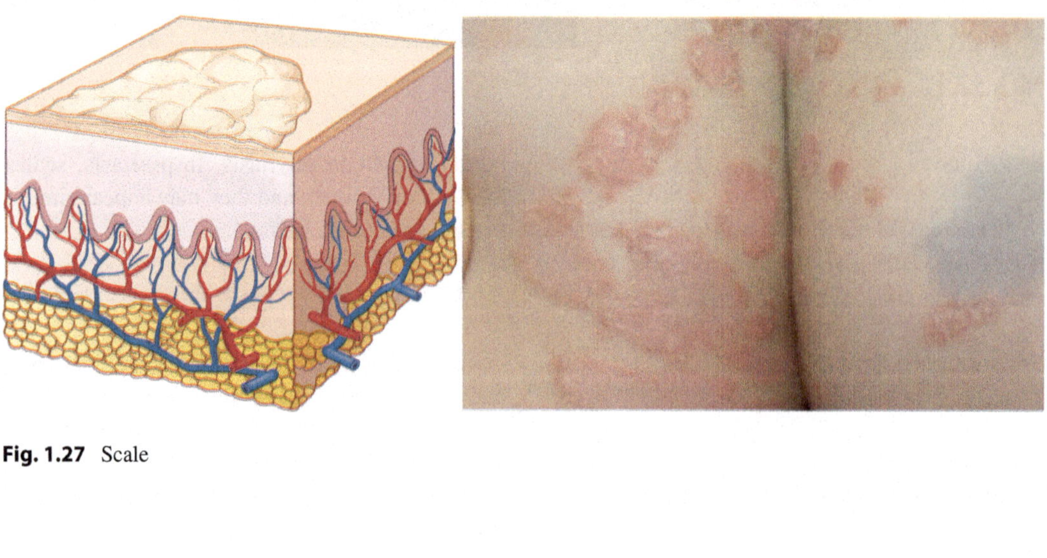

Fig. 1.27 Scale

Excoriations may reach the papillary dermis, but mostly they are abrasions occurring in the epithelial tissue. They are covered with red or yellow, dried blood components, and inflammatory annulus fibrosus is frequently formed around the excoriations. The infected excoriations form pustules and may cause hypertrophy of lymph nodes (Fig. 1.28).

③ Erosion

Erosions occur by bursting of vesicles in varicella, variola, impetigo, or herpes simplex resulted in epidermal loss and cutaneous depression making the skin humid and glossy. Regardless of the presence of crusts, no scar remains after the wound have healed (Fig. 1.29).

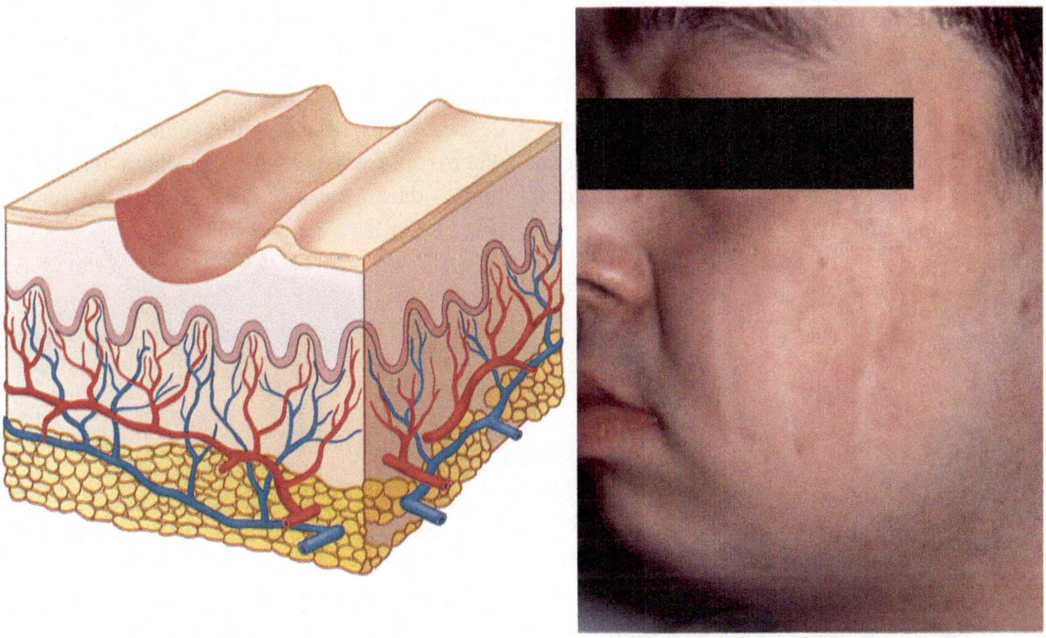

Fig. 1.28 Excoriation

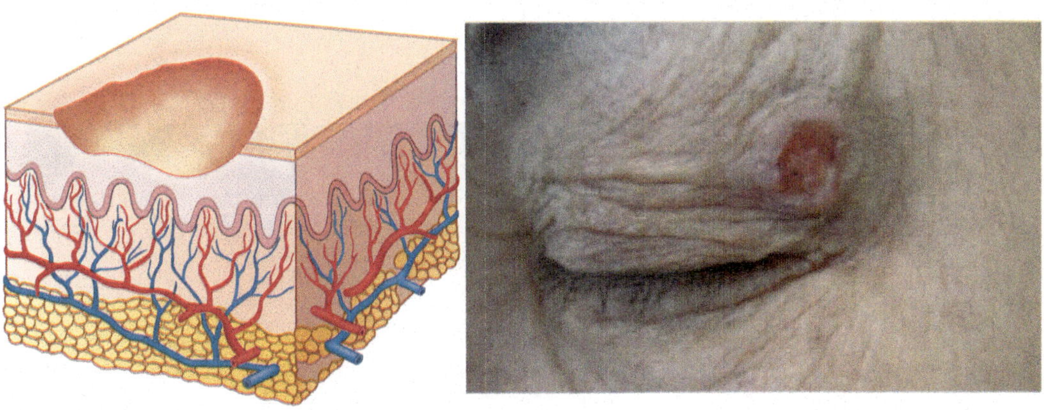

Fig. 1.29 Erosion

④ Ulcer

Ulcers imply skin loss extending through the epidermis and part of the dermis, which leads to a breach in epithelial continuity. They are generally caused by impaired or restricted supply of blood or nutrition due to the peripheral vascular diseases (Fig. 1.30).

⑤ Fissure

Fissures are linear cleavages of the skin which sometimes extend into the dermis. They are frequently developed around the flexural side of finger joints, finger tips, palms of the hands, lateral sides of the fingers and toes, oral angles, nostrils, auricles, and anus when the skin thickens and loses elasticity due to the inflammation or dryness (Fig. 1.31).

⑥ Crust

Crusts are dried layers of serum, blood, or purulent exudate and are composed of bacteria and epidermal debris. Their size, thickness, shape, and color depend on the composition and amounts of the secretion. Impetigos are identified by the formation of soft, breakable, dry, and golden crusts in the epidermis. Thick, hard, and tough crusts are related to the third-degree burns, and syphilis can be suspected when rupia exists, which is characterized by thick, dark, raised, and lamellated crusts (Fig. 1.32).

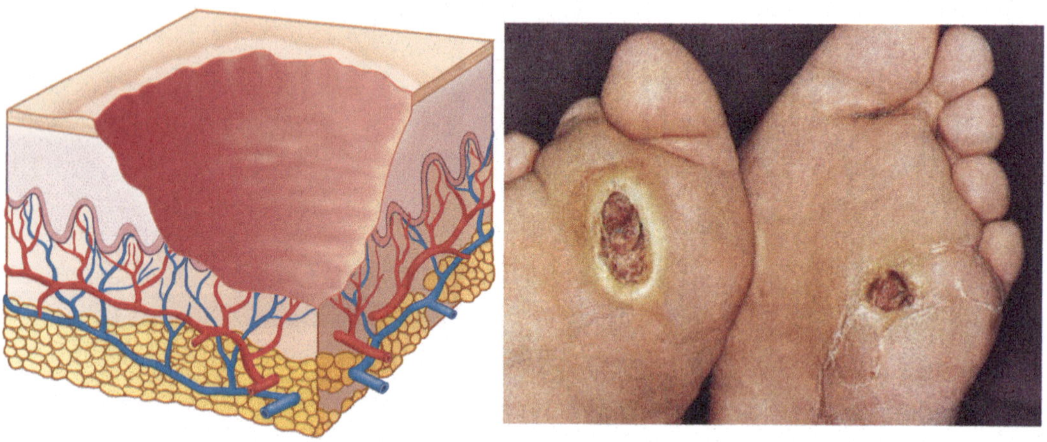

Fig. 1.30 Ulcer

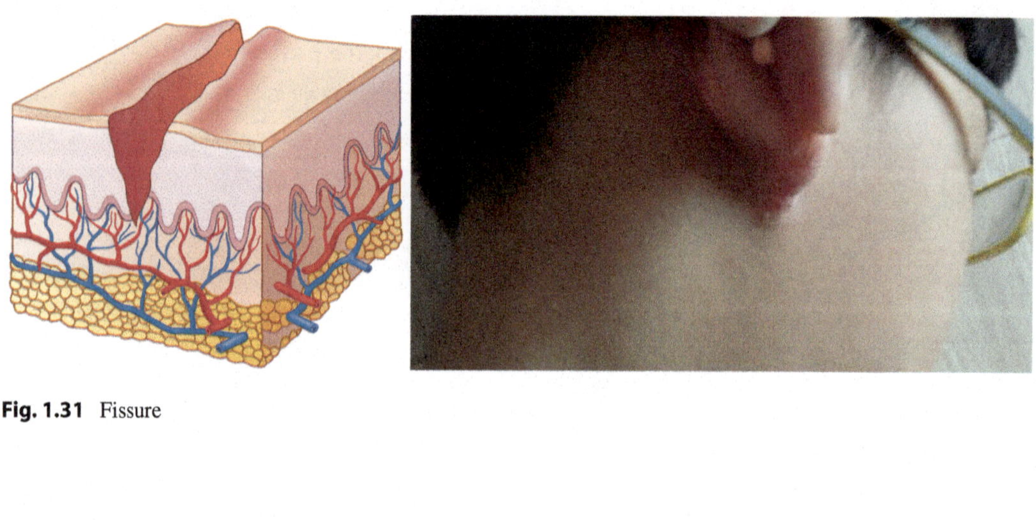

Fig. 1.31 Fissure

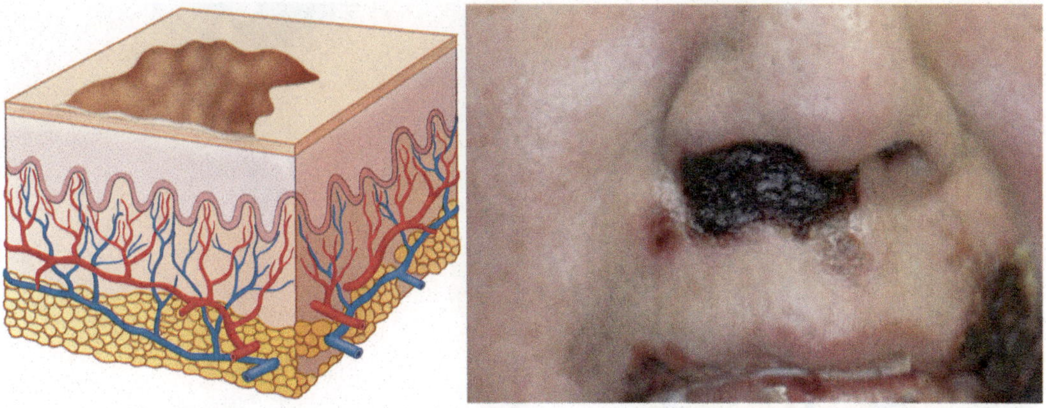

Fig. 1.32 Crust

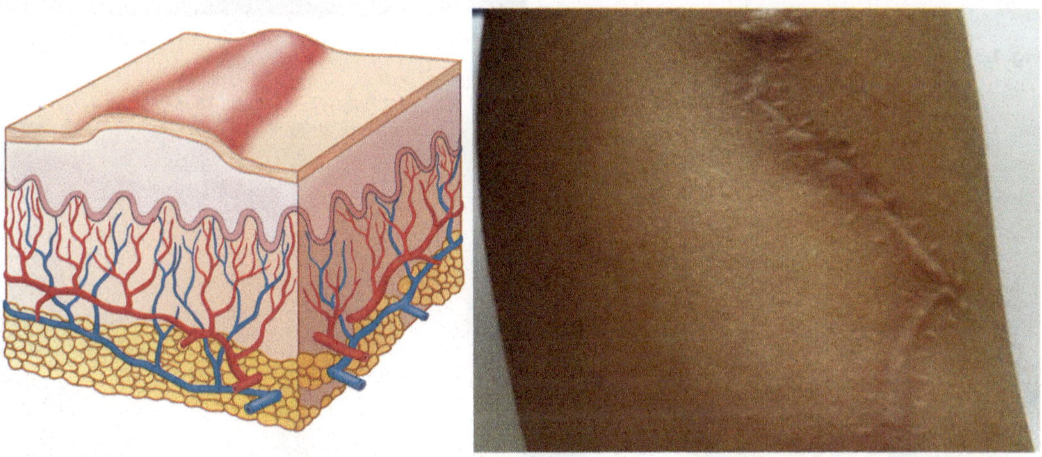

Fig. 1.33 Scar

⑦ Scar

Scars, as a part of the healing processes, replace the damaged skin tissues. Their shape and size are determined by that of the defect. Thin atrophic scars are observed in syphilis and lupus erythematosus. Keloids occur by overgrowth of the scar tissue (Fig. 1.33) (Park 2010).

⑧ Atrophy

Atrophy is a symptom with a decrease in cell size due to the loss of organelles and substances. This does not necessarily mean cell death, but functional decrease. The causes of atrophy include decreased blood supply, chronic inflammation, loss of stimulation by endocrine hormones, loss of innervation, malnutrition, and aging. Atrophy is not permanent, and the condition returns to normal once the causes are removed (Fig. 1.34).

⑨ Lichenification

Lichenification refers to a condition in which a part of the dermis thickens. As a result, the skin loses flexibility, and the wrinkles become prominent. It is frequently observed in chronic pruritus such as chronic simplex nuchae, atopic dermatitis, and prurigo nodularis (Fig. 1.35).

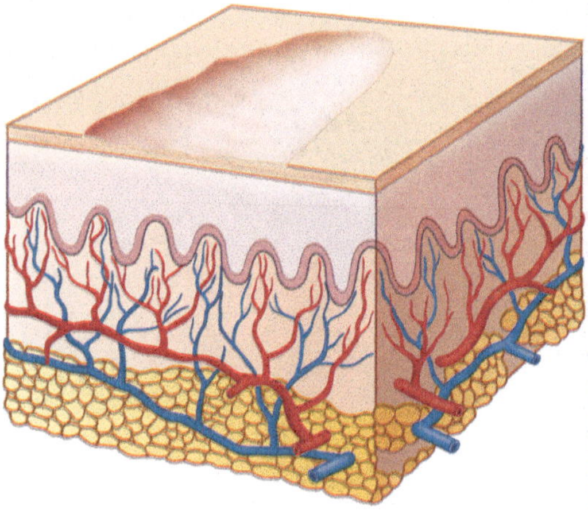
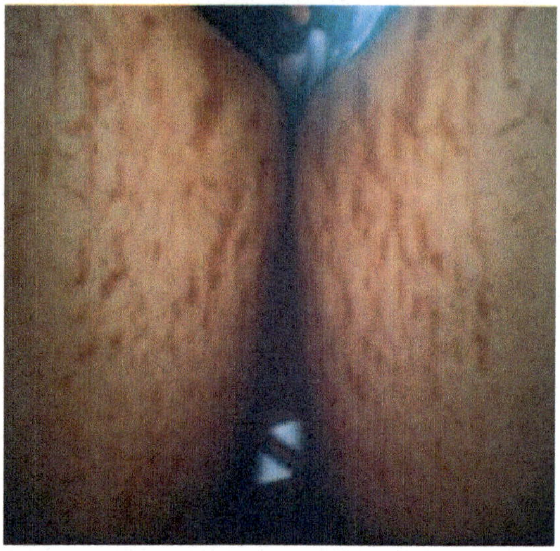

Fig. 1.34 Atrophy

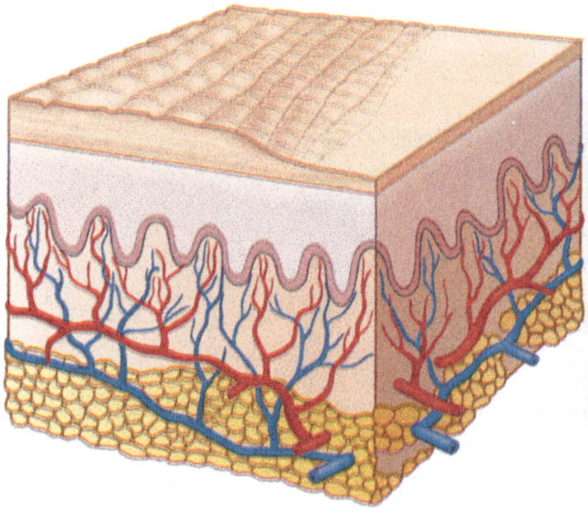
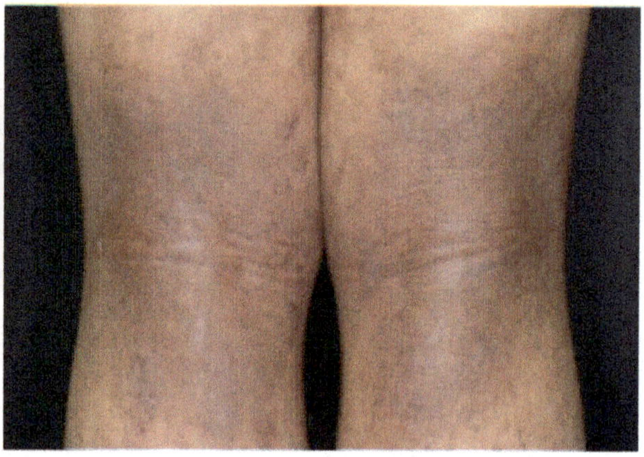

Fig. 1.35 Lichenification

1.3.2 Cutaneous Symptoms in Systemic Diseases

Cutaneous symptoms help confirming the presence of benign or malignant systemic diseases.

1.3.2.1 Pruritus

Pruritus is the most typical symptom among the dermatologic diseases. Severe pruritus and hyperpigmentation occur simultaneously in primary biliary cirrhosis, and systemic pruritus is involved with leukemia, metastatic cancer, myeloma, polycythemia vera, iron deficiency anemia, lymphoma, cholestatic jaundice, thyroid diseases, and drug hypersensitivity. Itchy sensation of diabetes is generated from the dry skin or the disease itself.

1.3.2.2 Eczema

Eczema is a term for several types of dermatitis. Its acute phase is involved in small blisters with pruritus, erosion, erythema, and edema; on the other hand, its chronic phase shows less edemas and vesicles and is marked by lichenification, squama, and hyperchromatism.

1.3.2.3 Erythroderma

Inflammatory diseases involved in both exfoliation and reddening of the entire skin surface are called pityriasis rubra pilaris, exfoliative dermatitis, or erythroderma. It appears as the secondary symptom when exposed to toxins or chemicals that interfere with the immune system. The diseases that cause erythroderma include psoriasis, atopic dermatitis, seborrheic dermatitis, eczema, scabies, and lichen planus, and it can also be developed from adverse drug reactions, lymphoma, leukemia, and internal malignancies.

1.3.2.4 Urticaria

Urticaria is a skin vascular reaction to an irritant and is marked by glossy, pale, red, raised, and itchy bumps. It shows an oval or irregular shape in many different sizes. Urticaria is accompanied by severe pruritus.

1.3.2.5 Nodule

When there is a tumor or malignant melanoma, metastatic nodules are often developed in the skin and the scalp. The numerous and firm nodules with 2–10 mm in diameter are sometimes found in the fingers, hands, joints, and tuberosity regions, and about 25 % of the nodules are related to cancers.

1.3.2.6 Vascular Lesion

Intravascular lesions that are related to malignant tumors include bleeding point, ecchymosis, and pressure purpura. In the elderly individuals, amyloidosis is frequently observed in the flexural side of the arm skin. Pressure purpura, which is often developed in an acute leukemia condition, is related to solar elastosis and systemic administration of steroids.

1.3.2.7 Flush

This results from carcinoid syndrome, adverse drug reactions, and hyperthyroidism. The symptoms appear on the face or neck and last for 10–30 min. Along with redness, there are edema around the face and eyes, excessive secretion of tears and saliva, tachycardia, and hypotension.

1.3.2.8 Vesicle and Bulla

Vesicles and bullae are present simultaneously in the case of lymphoma in the small intestine, herpes zoster, AIDS infection, leukemia, and systemic infections.

1.3.2.9 Hypertrichosis and Hirsutism

In these conditions, vellus hair grows excessively, which is related to malignant diseases in the adrenal gland, ovary, lung, large intestine, cystic duct, and uterus.

1.3.2.10 Acanthosis Nigricans

This condition is marked by melanotic macules in body folds and creases like armpits and groin. The discoloration is caused by thickening of the skin. Acanthosis nigricans develops due to the drug abuse (nicotinic acid) or endocrine diseases such as obesity, Cushing's syndrome, and diabetes. Once these diseases are cured, acanthosis nigricans disappears subsequently. Malignant acanthosis nigricans is accompanied by malignant tumors in the internal organs, so this can be a sign of tumor development.

1.3.2.11 Acquired Ichthyosis

This is a hereditary keratosis characterized by dry, and "fish-scale" skin. The cause of this condition is thickening of the stratum corneum due to hyperkeratosis or molecular defects in keratin. When ichthyosis develops in an adult, lymphatic tumors, solid tumors, pityriasis rotunda, hepatocellular carcinoma, and leprosy must be suspected.

1.3.3 Dermatologic Diagnosis

With the skin, it is easy to test and to collect the specimens with the minimum damage to the body. Moreover, it is of high value in terms of diagnosis. Results of many skin tests can be obtained in a clinic; those tests that have difficulties in obtaining their results should be taken in a microbiology laboratory or a pathology laboratory.

1.3.3.1 General Diagnosis

Chief Complaint

Before making a diagnosis of a skin lesion, it is essential to figure out the nature of the early lesion (when, where, and how the lesion started) and its progress. Dermatological symptoms including pruritus must be recorded. Effects on daily activity need to be assessed. In the case of chronic cutaneous diseases, evaluation of the influence on patient's quality of life and psychological conditions can be helpful. Each factor's degree of influence can be assessed by a scoring system.

Past Medical History

Patients must be asked about a history of cutaneous diseases, allergic rhinitis, asthma, or atopic symptoms such as juvenile eczema. Internal diseases can be involved with particular cutaneous diseases. Skin lesions can occur from prescription drugs or self-medication. Food diary may be important to some patients with atopic dermatitis, but food is often mistaken for the causes of cutaneous diseases (http://health.mw.go.kr).

Social History and Occupational History

Many social factors can influence on cutaneous diseases. The patients' occupational history must be identified because it can cause contact dermatitis or other skin changes. If a patient's condition improved after he/she quit his/her job, occupational factors must be taken under consideration. A hobby to collect specific objects or chemicals can lead to contact dermatitis as well. Understanding the patients' lifestyle or home environment can be helpful in determining therapeutic plans. Especially, when drugs with hepatotoxicity are used, patients' drinking habits must be considered along with other factors.

Family History

Family history must be fully understood. Diseases like epiloia are inherited and have clear cutaneous signs. Psoriasis and atopic dermatitis have distinct congenital causes. Family history is important not only in terms of its congenital correlation but also in regard to the possibility of infection among the members of the same household. Occasionally, the information on sexual contacts is also needed.

Drug History

Prescription drugs or self-medication can cause drug eruption. Most patients have experienced with over-the-counter topical agents, and many of them have been prescribed with improper, irritant, allergic drugs. Over-the-counter drugs in an oral or cream form are considered safe by patients; however, the safety of all drugs must be questioned. Cosmetics, cleansing agents, and moisturizing creams can cause dermatitis, so it is necessary to ask patients detailed questions.

1.3.3.2 Physical Examination

Direct examination or visual inspection of the lesion must be performed in a well-illuminated room. The ideal lighting is natural daylight. Overall lesion distribution can be visually inspected when the patients are undressed. Certain diseases need to be inspected under ultraviolet light, and a Wood's lamp (maximum output 365 nm) helps diagnosing tinea capitis, tinea versicolor, erythrasma, and vitiligo. A dermatoscopy can be useful in identifying a minute lesion. Palpation is important for checking a lesion's mobility and stability. Urticaria pigmentosa, commonly seen in infants, can be diagnosed by Darier's sign, which involves rubbing or scratching the lesion. The distribution of rash and characteristics of an arrangement are helpful in diagnosis.

Visual Inspection

Proper lighting is essential for visual inspection, and the possible considerations for visual inspection include a lesion's color (Table 1.2), shape, spatial arrangement, distribution (Fig. 1.36), symmetry, differences among the body parts, and differences between sun-exposed skin and sun-protected skin.

Palpation

Palpation is for assessing the skin's humidity, temperature, texture, level of tension, mobility, depression, and elevation. Keratinous lesions occur especially when the texture of the whole body becomes rough. Palmoplantar keratinization develops as a result of a systemic reaction to toxic chemicals.

When a section of skin is pinched and released, dehydrated skin springs back to the original position slower than the normal skin does. Skin with edema or scleroderma shows decreased mobility (Fig. 1.37).

Table 1.2 Diseases according to skin color

Skin color	Cause	Distribution	Typical disease
Brown	Increase in melanin concentration	Systemic	Diseases in hypophysis, adrenal gland, and liver
		Topical	Phacomatosis and neurofibroma
White	Absence of melanin	Systemic	Albinism
		Topical	Vitiligo
Red	Increase in erythrocyte concentration	Systemic	Fever, hives, rash, polycythemia
		Topical	Inflammation
Yellow	Increase in bile pigment	Systemic	Liver diseases
	Increase in carotenoid pigment	Systemic	Hypothyroidism and excessive intake of carotene
Blue	Decrease in oxidized hemoglobin	Systemic	Anemia and chronic renal diseases
	Increase in hemoglobin concentration caused by hypoxia	Lip, mouth, nail bed	Cardiovascular diseases and pulmonary diseases

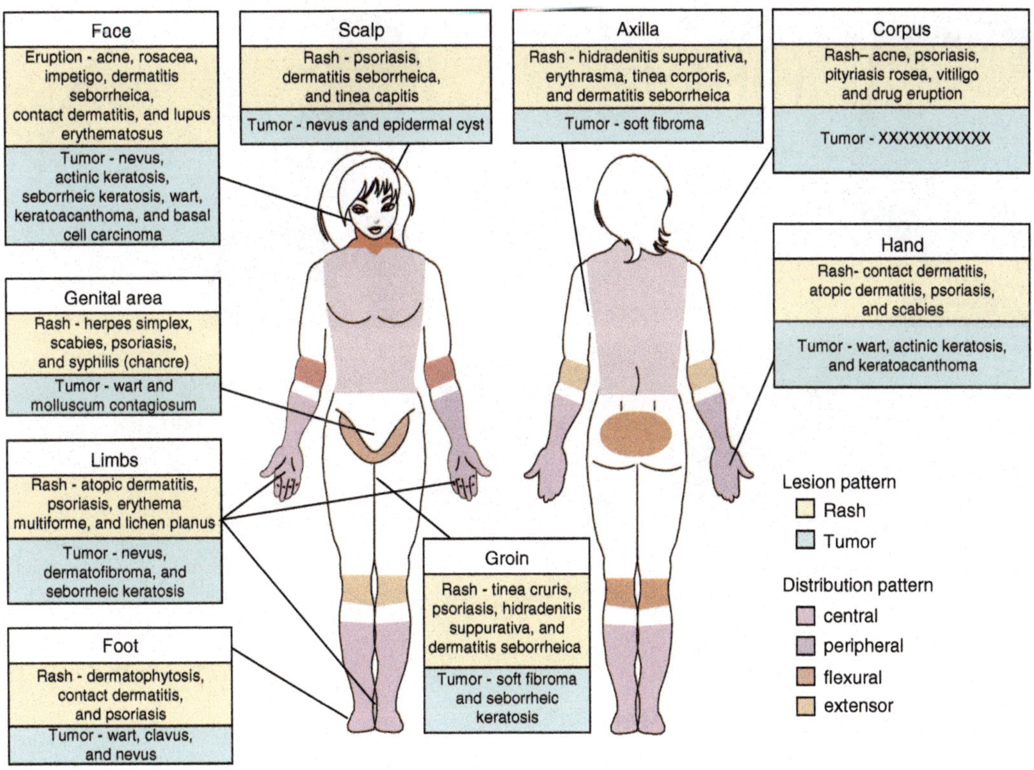

Fig. 1.36 Distribution of skin diseases

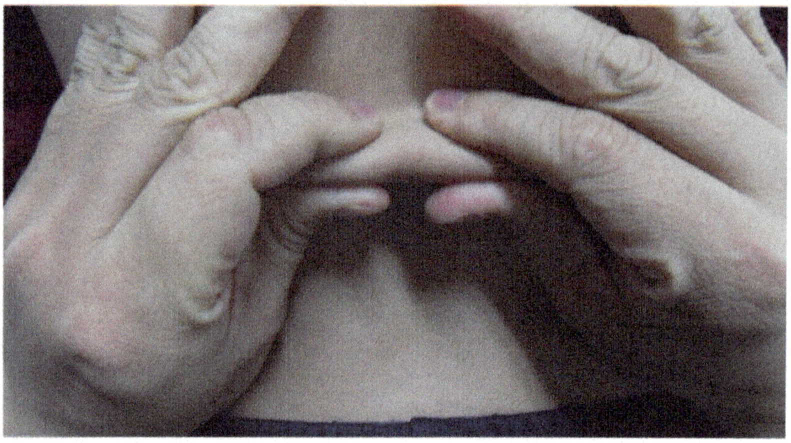

Fig. 1.37 Skin turgor test and skin mobility test

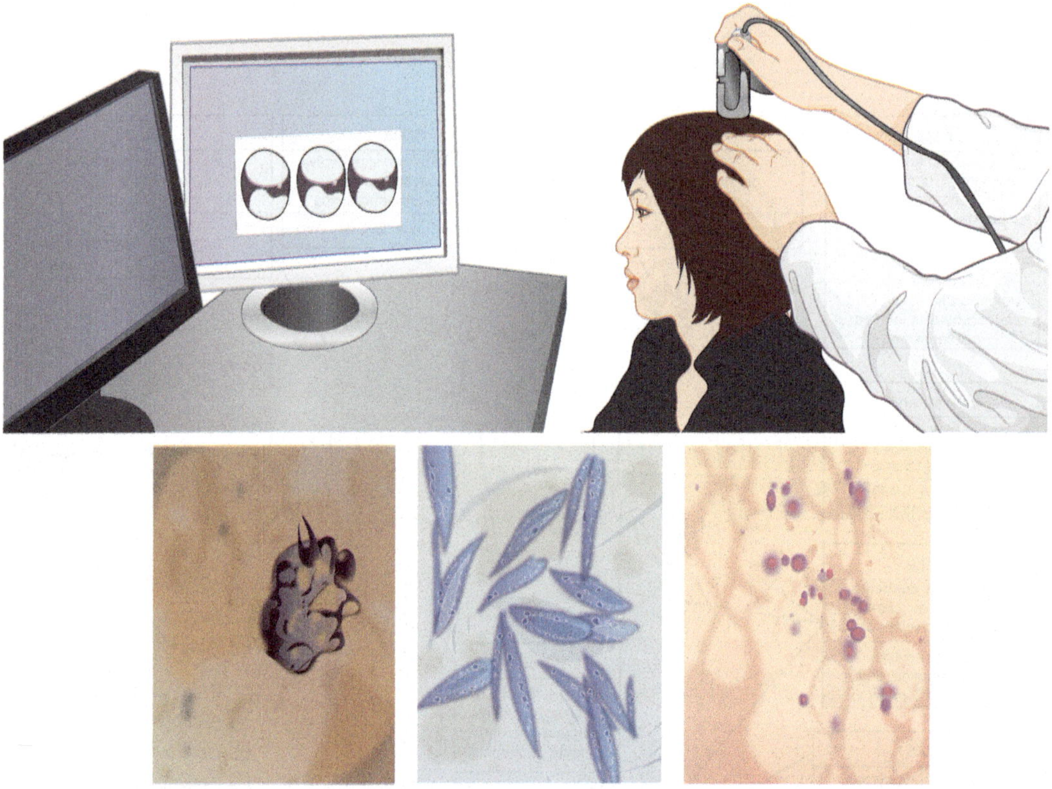

Fig. 1.38 Dermoscopy. (**a**) Scabies. (**b**, **c**) Mycete

1.3.3.3 Skin Tests with Diagnosis Supporting Devices

Dermoscopy

Dermoscopy, which uses a convex lens with 3.5–5× magnification, is an examination method that allows detailed evaluation of fine wrinkles, pigmentation, comedo, and acne. A dermatoscope with 7× magnification is used to observe minute morphological changes on the surface of the skin, and it helps diagnosing erythematosus lupus, lichen planus, basal cell carcinoma, and melanoma (Fig. 1.38).

Wood's Lamp Examination

Wood's lamp examination uses ultraviolet (UV) light in the wavelength range of 340–450 nm with a peak at 365 nm. It is helpful in the diagnosis of various skin conditions because infected skin shows a unique fluorescence reaction under the light of a Wood's lamp. This is also used for determining the size of vitiligo, observing varied skin types and a hypopigmented macule of tuberous sclerosis, diagnosing microbial infection and tinea capitis, and testing urine samples from patients with porphyria or pityriasis versicolor. Tinea capitis, pityriasis versicolor, and erythrasma are tinged with yellowish green, golden yellow, and coral red, respectively (Fig. 1.39) (http://www.derma.or.kr/guest/).

Diascopy

Diascopy is a method used for examining brown papule and nodule in sarcoidosis, scrofuloderma, lymphoma, and granuloma annulare and differentiating the causes of erythema and purpura. It is performed by pressuring a transparent, flat, firm object against the surface of the lesion (Fig. 1.40).

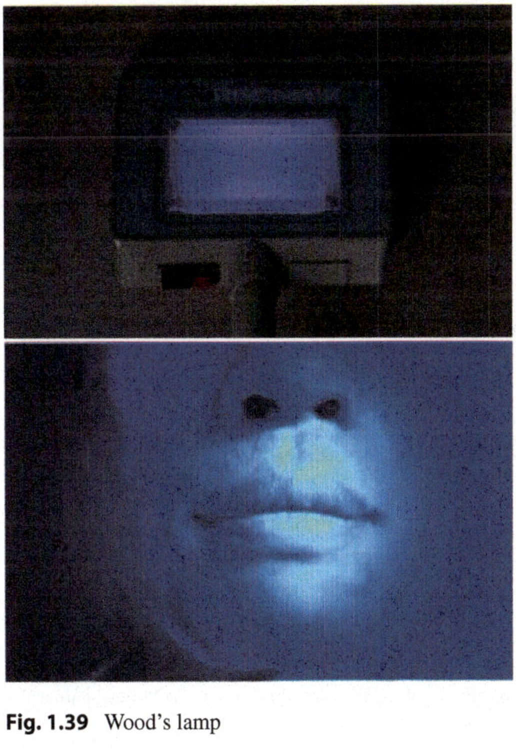

Fig. 1.39 Wood's lamp

1.3.3.4 Microbiological Examination

KOH Test

The purpose of the KOH (potassium hydroxide) test is to compensate the error of the Gram-staining procedure, switching between Gram-positive and Gram-negative microorganisms. Scale, hair, nail, and vesicle contents are collected and placed onto a glass slide and are covered with 10–20 % KOH solution. For 20–30 min, the slide is left or heated until the sample dissolves. Then, the solution on the slide is observed under the microscope (Fig. 1.41).

Gram Staining

Gram staining, the most typical method in bacteriological examination, is used to differentiate bacteria into two groups, Gram-positive and Gram-negative, and to test whether a pustular disease is bacterial or abacterial. Gram-positive bacteria, which are stained in purple, include *Staphylococcus*, *Streptococcus*, *Mycobacterium leprae*, *Corynebacterium diphtheriae*, *Clostridium tetani*, *Bacillus anthracis*, and *Actinomyces* and Gram-negative bacteria, which are stained in pink, include *Salmonella*, *Shigella*, *Salmonella typhi*, *Escherichia coli*, *Vibrio cholerae*, *Yersinia pestis*, and *Neisseria meningitidis*.

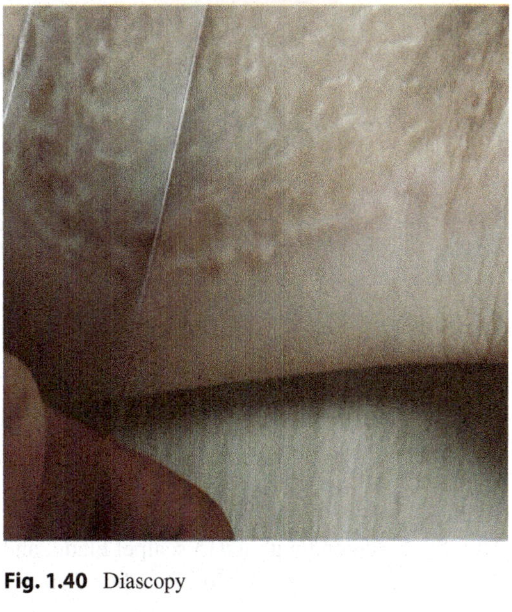

Fig. 1.40 Diascopy

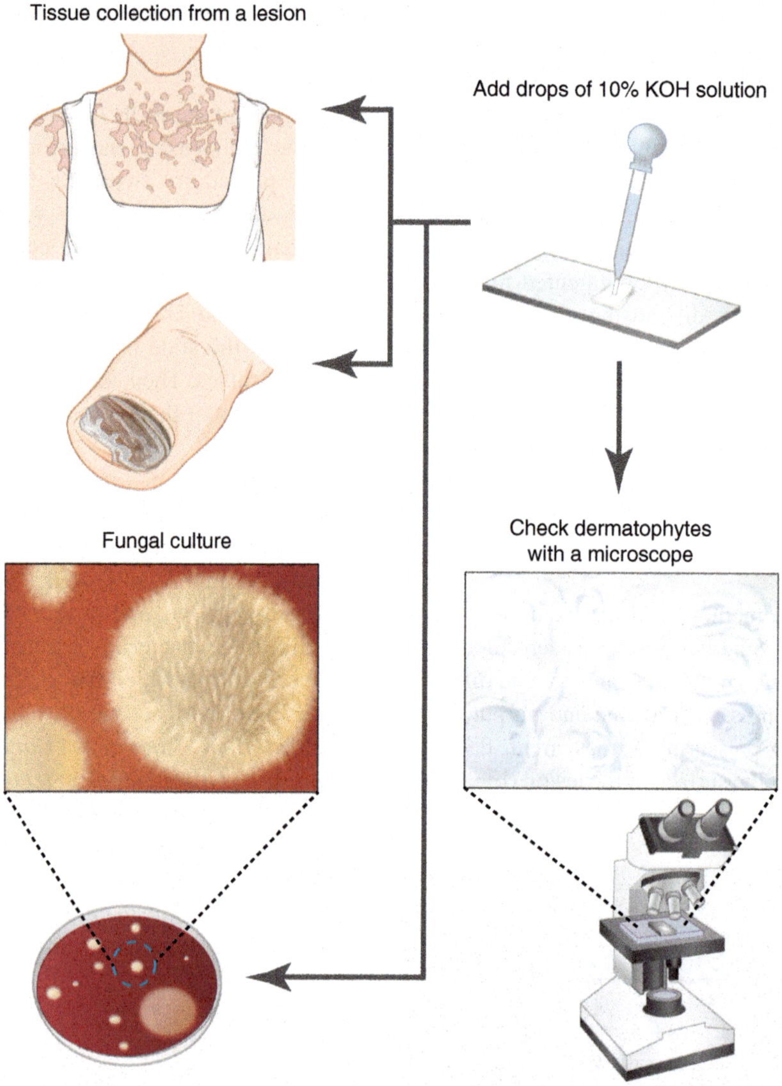

Fig. 1.41 KOH test procedure

Tzanck Smear

This test is used to confirm herpes zoster virus or chickenpox virus. An intact vesicle is bursted, and the specimen is placed onto a glass slide and dried at room temperature. It is fixed with methanol and stained with Giemsa, Wright, or toluidine blue, and then a viral infection is confirmed by the presence of multinucleated giant cell.

Scabies Test

The skin is scraped with a #15 scalpel blade, and the collected debris is placed on a slide. After a drop of oil is applied to the slide, the specimen is observed under a microscope.

Dark-Field Examination

This enables the direct observation of an ulcer and is a useful method of diagnosing syphilis. A clotted ulcer or the skin surrounding the secondary syphilis lesion is abraded with a curette[1].

[1] Curette: A spoonlike tool designed to scrape or debride tissues (endometrium or gingiva) by rubbing against the surface.

The serum from the lesion is taken on a slide. After a drop of saline solution is added, the serum is covered with a glass cover and examined.

Culture Test

Culture test is used to identify skin diseases related to fungus, bacteria, and virus, and it is done by culturing the exudates from pustule, bulla, or abscess.

1.3.3.5 Skin Biopsy

Skin biopsy is a means to gather information by examining skin tissue samples collected by a scalpel blade or a punch instrument. Skin biopsy methods include punch biopsy, incisional biopsy, and shave biopsy (Fig. 1.42).

1.3.3.6 Immunofluorescence Test

Autoantibodies can be detected and measured with this method. Deposited autoantibodies are tested with a direct immunofluorescence assay, and autoantibodies in serum are diagnosed with an indirect immunofluorescence assay. This is often used to diagnose pemphigus, pemphigoid, bullous diseases (e.g., herpes dermatitis), and lupus erythematosus.

1.3.3.7 Electron Microscopy

This is rarely used for skin test, but it is useful in diagnosing rare skin diseases such as histiocytosis X and several subtypes of epidermolysis.

1.3.3.8 Skin Reaction Test

In this method, the skin reaction is tested after various substances are applied or injected to the skin. The presence of positive reactions and their intensity are observed and analyzed.

Patch Test

Patch test is used to check whether the patient's skin is allergic to contact with certain biological or chemical substances. The test reagent diluted with water or Vaseline is applied to the skin of the upper back or upper outer arm and covered with an impermeable patch. Then the presence of allergic (hypersensitivity) reactions is detected after about 48 h. The result is scored ranging from 0 (no reaction) to 4(deep redness and blister formation) (Fig. 1.43) (http://www.wikipedia.org).

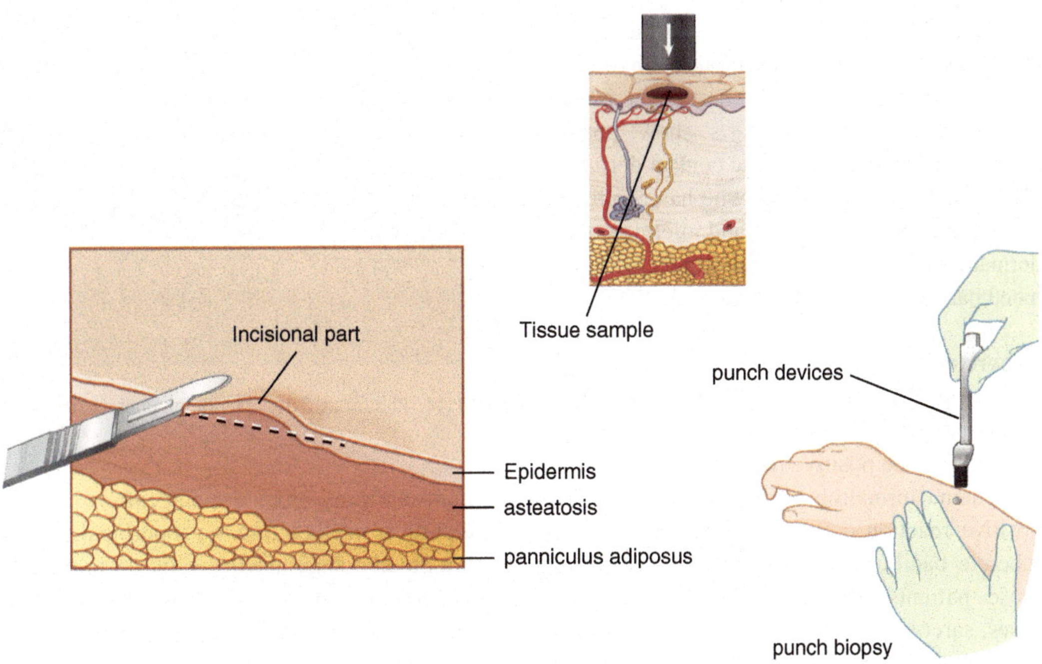

Fig. 1.42 Skin biopsy with a scalpel blade or a punch instrument

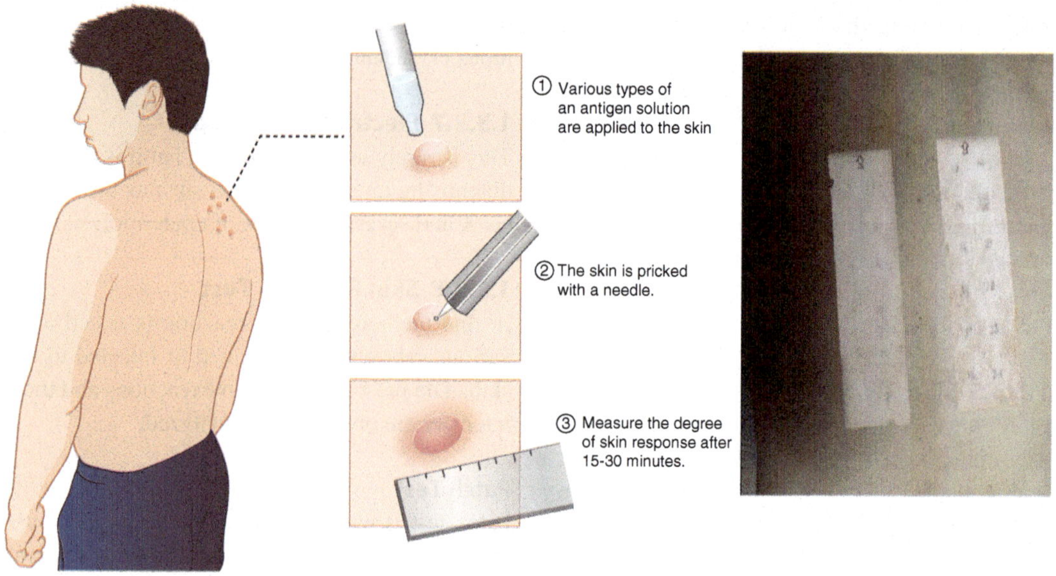

Fig. 1.43 Patch test

Photo Test and Photopatch Test

Photo test examines photosensitivity reactions of patients' skin by measuring the decrease of minimal erythema dose (MED) after the illumination with ultraviolet light or visible light. Photopatch test is used together with patch test for skin disease diagnosis. UVA (5–15 J/cm^2) is illuminated on a part of the patch. When only the illuminated part shows a positive reaction after 48 h, diagnosis of photoallergic contact dermatitis is confirmed, and when both parts show positive reactions, diagnosis of allergic contact dermatitis is confirmed. Those patients who have both photoallergic contact dermatitis and allergic contact dermatitis show a stronger reaction on the illuminated part (Fig. 1.44) (Bendova et al. 2007).

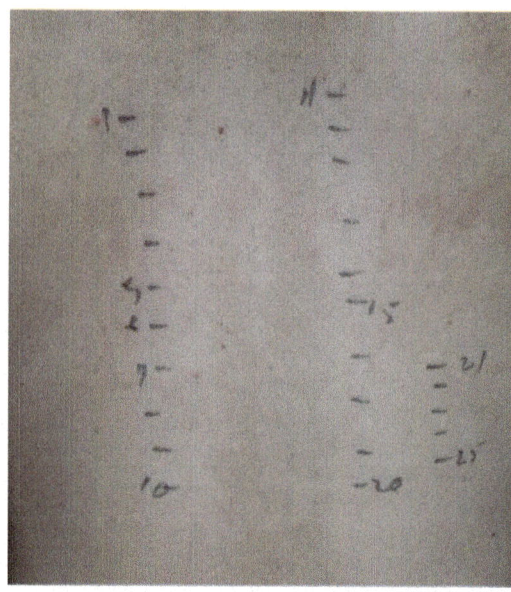

Fig. 1.44 Photosensitivity reaction on phototesting

Tuberculin Test

Tuberculin test is used to diagnose tuberculosis and is performed by injecting a small dose of tuberculin. The positive reaction shows redness and edema formation on the injected site. The positive reaction denotes cellular immunity to tubercle bacillus and may not be observed in those patients with lymphoproliferative diseases, sarcoidosis, measles, or AIDS as well as those patients who have been injected with immunosuppressant or steroid agents. 0.1 mL of tuberculin is injected into the superficial dermis with a 26–27 gauge needle. After 48 h, induration of 10 mm or more in diameter, 5–9 mm, and 4 mm or less are diagnosed as positive, false positive, and negative, respectively (Fig. 1.45).

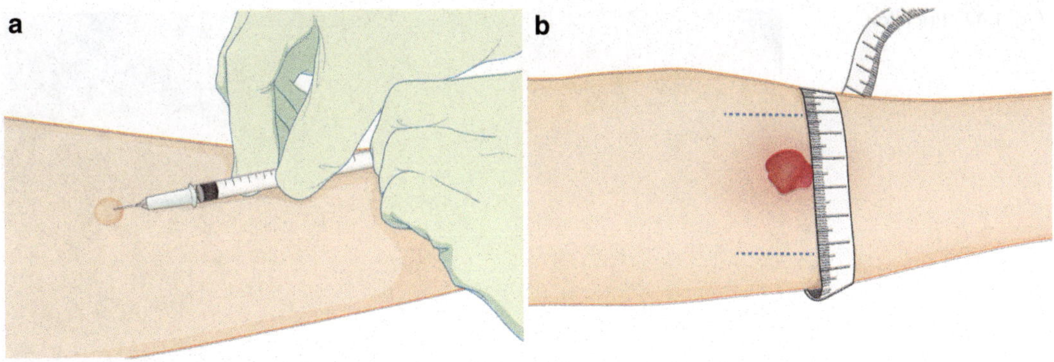

Fig. 1.45 Tuberculin test. (**a**) Tuberculin injection and (**b**) tuberculin response measurement

Immediate Type Skin Test

This method examines the presence of immunoglobulin E responding to allergens. Prick test and scratch test are performed preferentially, and the symptoms arose from wheal reactions can be suppressed with antihistamine drugs (Fig. 1.46).

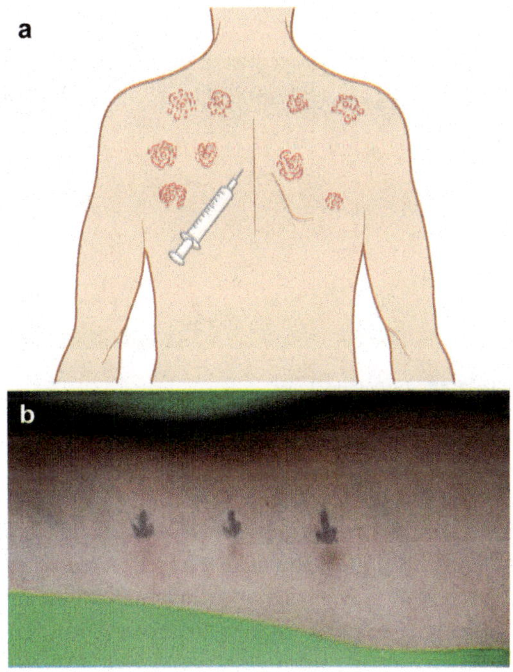

Fig. 1.46 Immediate response test. (**a**) Allergen injection and (**b**) wheal reaction measurement

① Prick Test

The skin is pricked with a needle after a solution with suspected allergens is applied. If type 1 allergic response is induced, the patient is allergic to the substance (Fig. 1.47).

② Scratch Test

Scratch test is performed by inspecting the specimen obtained by scratching superficial lesions.

③ Intradermal Test

The amount of allergen absorbed in the intradermal test is 100–1000 times greater than that in the prick test, which triggers much stronger local or systemic reactions. This test is carried out by injecting 0.1 mL of suspected allergen solution with a 26–27 gauge needle, and the result comes out after 14–20 min (Fig. 1.48).

Other Allergy Tests

Other tests that are designed to examine IgE responses in asthma, atopic dermatitis, urticaria, and hay fever include RAST (radioallergosorbent test), ELISA (enzyme-linked immunosorbent assay), MAST (chemiluminescence test), and ImmunoCAP system (fluorescent enzyme immunoassay).

1.3.3.9 Oral Provocation Test

Oral provocation test is used to diagnose the exact cause of skin rash and is performed by checking

Fig. 1.47 Prick test

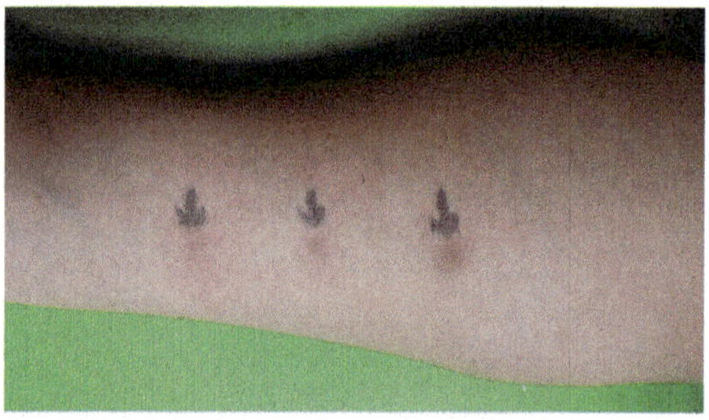

Fig. 1.48 Intradermal test

for the reactions after oral intake of drugs or foods. This tool is of value in finding the cause of drug eruption especially when the patients are allergic to multiple allergens. The suspected drugs or foods are given one at a time and following urticaria or atopic response is observed.

1.3.4 Physical Therapy Diagnosis and Evaluation Methods

1.3.4.1 Examination

Examination provides data gathered from medical histories, systematic reviews, tests, and measurements. It includes the process of collecting data from physical therapy evaluation forms, while physical therapy and intervention are ongoing (Fig. 1.49) (Kim 2012).

Medical History

This is the initial information that physical therapists obtain from the patient interview and the first step of the diagnosis, through which a treatment planning is facilitated. Medical history includes general details gained from history taking, family history, birth records, past health status, occupational history, marital history, pregnancy, menstruation, previous(and current) illnesses, injuries, surgeries, and medications.

Example/s) General details: Mr. A is a 16-year-old Korean man. He is a left-handed high school student. (He is suspected to be socially inexperienced due to young age, to have difficulties in using right-handed tools, and to be subject to skin damages like burns due to decreased concentration levels from engaging in study and social experience together.)

Social history: He is an only child living with both parents. (He is suspected to have communication problems due to lack of the experience of growing up with siblings, which may lead to traumatic skin diseases like burns.)

Occupational history: He is a part-time worker at a restaurant as an assistant to a chef. (He is suspected to be exposed to traumatic skin diseases like burns due to occupational characteristics.)

Family medical history: When he was 8 years old, he lost both his grandparents to a house fire. His father has diabetes and hypertension. (He is suspected to be vulnerable to traumatic skin diseases like burns because his psychological trauma may cause muscular rigidity when he manages fire.)

Previous illnesses: He had chickenpox in his childhood. (A connection between current skin diseases and chickenpox is suspected.)

Integumentary Physical Therapy Evaluation Form

Previous patient : ______

Name : ______

Age : ______

Address : ______

______

Insurance : ______

daytime phone # : ______

occupation : ______

______

previous skin treatment
topical :

light therapy :
photosensitizing meds :
radiation therapy :

skin assessment at first treatment

subjective
skin type :

duration :
factors causing :
flare
remission
itching :
discomfort :
history of 'cold sores'

objective :
lesion type :
hair/scaip :
nails :

Date : ______ time : ______

physician : ______

diagnosis : ______

Additional medical problems : ______

______

medications : ______

previous RX : ______

______

Therapeutic goal :
clearance of skin disease

family history of skin disease: ______

______

______

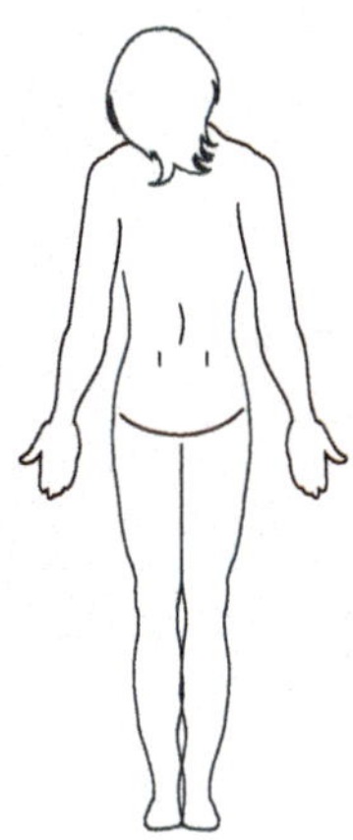

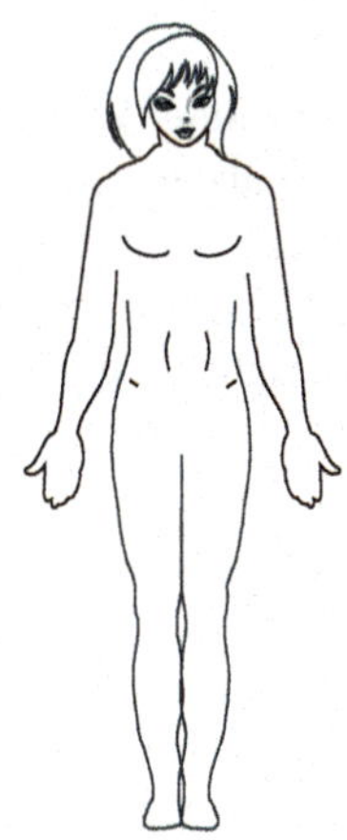

therapist :

Fig. 1.49 Integumentary physical therapy evaluation form (Moffat and Harris 2006)

Systematic Review

Systematic review, as the second step of diagnosis, is carried out after history taking. This includes the process of evaluating emotional status, learning type, communication, communicative competence, and cognitive status by making an observation on the cardiovascular system, integumentary system, musculoskeletal system, and nervous system. Blood pressure, heart rate, respiratory rate, and edema are evaluated in the cardiovascular system;

scar structure, skin color, and the skin integrity are accessed in the integumentary system; joint working range, gross muscular force, symmetry, height, and weight are estimated in the musculoskeletal system; and balance control, ambulatory ability, and locomotion are evaluated in the nervous system. Moreover, systematic review also includes patients' capacity with regard to emotional/behavioral responses, learning preference types, consciousness, and propensity.

Example/s) The integumentary system: There are defects on the right chest and the lower right arm. Red wounds are observed with no scar tissue formation.

Test and Measurement

Tests and measurements are performed based on the information gained from the history taking and systematic review. For the most proper test and measurement, pathophysiology, damages, functional restrictions, disorders, risk factors, prevention, physical health, and mental health need to be investigated.

Example/s) Skin color: Redness on the wound
Body hair: Normal
Nail: Normal
Body temperature: Warm on the wound
Skin texture and tension: Normal
Edema: None
Wound: Irregular-shaped scars on the right arm and the right chest
Burn: 5.5 % of the entire epidermis

Assessment

Physical therapists conduct overall evaluation of the problems obtained as a result of analyzing skin disease history, systematic review, and tests and measurements. The physical therapists' disease assessment includes the disease's progress, phases of symptoms and signs, stability of the disease, and correlation between the involved system and the damaged site. Clinicopathologic tests, radiologic tests, and neurologic tests are assessed and get associated with functional restriction, impairment evaluation, and examination status.

Example/s) According to patient A's medical history and risk factors, he is estimated to be a young man with 5.5 % burns on the right chest and the lower right arm.

Diagnosis

Diagnosis is information about the final result of examination and evaluation. This is a process of classifying the category of skin-related diseases and syndromes.

Example/s) Patient A have a burn injury on the skin of the right chest and the lower right arm. Accordingly, his daily life, social activity, and school life are restricted. This result agrees with the damage of the epidermis by burns.

Prognosis and Plan of Care

Prognosis refers to the process of figuring out the possible results of a patient's current status based on the collected data regarding the treatment of the patient or other patients with similar symptoms. A plan of care is a list of suggested intervention methods and their frequency and duration. Prognosis is determined by consideration of the patients' health status, disease risk factors, response to intervention, safety of the patients, needs, therapeutic goals, diagnosis, assessment results, suspected diseases, and progress of disease.

Example/s) The prognosis of patient A, as a result of analyzing the diagnosis, is that full recovery of the skin is expected. Thus, he will be able to return to his daily life and school life. Accordingly, the care plan for patient A is focused on achieving full recovery and improving proficiency in his daily life and school life. So as to attain the goals, the patient and his guardian will be educated with self-care instructions and will be provided with a treatment through functional trainings. There will be 5–6 times of home visiting treatment for 2 weeks.

Intervention

Intervention means various approaches and techniques of physical therapy designed to improve the patients' medical condition, which is determined by the therapist-patient interaction, assessment, diagnosis, and prognosis. Intervention requires the consideration of possible functional improvements, side effects, and expected costs.

Example/s) Patient A and his guardian are instructed to avoid skin irritation by wearing big clothes, keeping the wound site clean, trying not to scratch the burn, and being careful with the sun exposure. Recommended activities are weight-bearing exercises, cycling, running on a treadmill, and swimming. For the recovery and protection of the skin, use of moisturizer (especially after swimming), whirlpool bath, and wound dressing are required.

Reexamination

A reexamination is carried out to detect the changes after the treatment.

Example/s) Patient A was reexamined 2 months after he left the hospital. As a result of the diagnosis, his skin condition was considered to be fully recovered. Accordingly, he was told to return to the daily life and school life. The care plan is arranged to prevent recurrence, to achieve a full recovery, and to improve proficiency in his daily and school life. So as to attain the goals, the patient and his guardian will be educated with self-care instructions and will be provided with a treatment through functional training (Korean Physical Therapy Association 2006).

1.4 Problem Solving

1.4.1 An Overview of the Integumentary System

Choose the most suitable answer to each question.

Question 1

This is the layer of the epidermis that accounts for up to 75 % of the epidermal thickness. Its cells are so tightly bonded to each other that water evaporation is prevented and the skin is kept hydrated. What is this?

1. Stratum basale
2. Stratum lucidum
3. Stratum corneum
4. Stratum spinosum
5. Stratum granulosum

Question 2

Which cutaneous sensory receptor corresponds to the following characteristics?

- Receptors detecting compression sensation.
- Onion-shaped when cut in cross section.
- Abundant in the skin of the palms and fingers, soles of the feet, and chest
  1. Muscle spindles
  2. Free nerve endings
  3. Ruffini's corpuscles
  4. Pacinian corpuscles
  5. Meissner's corpuscles

Question 3

Patient A is known to a left-handed high school student. He is an only child and part-time worker at a restaurant as an assistant to a chef. Since he lost his grandparents to a house fire, it is suspected that he might have a burn injury. Thus, we intended to investigate his skin color, skin integrity, and scar structure. Which step of examination is this?

1. Diagnosis
2. Prognosis
3. Reexamination
4. Systematic review
5. Test and measurement

Question 4

What is the correct examination inspecting the condition of the scalp or the skin with ultraviolet (UV) light using 340–450 nm of the wavelength range?

1. Dark-field examination
2. Wood's lamp examination
3. Immunofluorescence test
4. Tzanck smear examination
5. KOH test

Question 5

What is the examination method that examines the causes of erythema or purpura by pressuring a transparent, flat, and firm object against the surface of the lesion?

1. Photo test
2. Diascopy
3. Dermoscopy
4. Dark-field examination
5. Wood's lamp examination

Answers

Question 1-③, Question 2-④, Question 3-④, Question 4-②, Question 5-②

References

Ahn DC, Hwang KS, Paik DJ, Han SH, Chung HS. The distribution pattern of the cutaneous nerves on dorsum of the hands in the Korean. Korean J Phys Anthrop. 1999;12:187–95.

Ahn S, Jang GH, Song JW, SH. C. Common skin disease of Koreans. Daijeon: Doctor's Books. 2009.

Ahn CS, Kho SS, Kim YN, Kim JH, Kim JS, Kim JH, et al. Human anatomy. Seoul: Jungmunkag; 2011.

Bendova H, Akrman J, Krejci A, Kubac L, Jirova D, Kejlova K, et al. In vitro approaches to evaluation of Sun protection factor. Toxicology in vitro : an international journal published in association with BIBRA. 2007;21(7):1268–75. Epub 2007/10/20.

Choi MA, Hong HS. Pathophysiology. Seoul: Gyechuk Munwhasa; 2006.

Chung IH. Human anatomy. Seoul: Hyunmoon Publishing Co; 2011.

Chung IH, Yim JH. Branching pattern and morphometry of the axillary nerve. Korean J Anatomy. 2000;33:373–9.

Faculty Committee of Korean Anatomy and Physiology. Human anatomy. Seoul: Hyunmoon Publishing Co; 2011.

Faculty Committee of Korean Anatomy and Physiology. Physiology FCoKAa. Human anatomy. Seoul: Hyunmoon Publishing Co; 2012.

Kim SH. Integumentary physical therapy. Seoul: Sky Yard Publishing Inc; 2012.

Korean Dermatological Association Textbook Compilation Committee. Dermatology. Seoul: Rho Moon Gak; 2008.

Korean Physical Therapy Association. Clinical cases in physical therapy. Paju: Koonja Publishing Inc; 2006.

Lee M, Noh H. Dermatology: an illustrated color text. Paju: Koonja Publishing Inc; 2010.

Lee HG, Kim MH, Kim BW, Kim JS, Kim HJ, Moon SG, et al. Human anatomy. Seoul: Hyunmoon Publishing Co; 2012.

Lee SH. Human anatomy. Seoul: Hyunmoon Publishing Co; 2012.

Moffat M, Harris KB. Integumentary essentials: applying the preferred physical therapist patterns. Thorofare: Slack; London: Eurospan [distributor], 2006. p. 2–3.

Park KH. Wound management. Paju: Koonja Publishing Inc; 2010.

Park BC, Choe YS, Kim DW, Lee WJ, Lee SJ, Na GY. Clinical study on dermatologic disease of the elderly. Korean Dermatological Association. 2006;44(7):818–23.

Rotter B, Bournier O, Nicolas G, Dhermy D, Lecomte MC. AlphaII-spectrin interacts with Tes and EVL, two actin-binding proteins located at cell contacts. Biochem J. 2005;388(Pt 2):631–8. Epub 2005/01/20.

Terminology FCoA, editor. Terminologia anatomica. Stuttgart: Thieme Verlag; 1998.

Reference Sites

National Health Information Portal. http://health.mw.go.kr/.

Korean Dermatological Association. http://www.derma.or.kr/guest/.

Wikipedia. http://www.wikipedia.org/.

2 Wounds

Eun Young Kim

ICD-10 Code
O86.0 Infection of obstetric surgical wound
O90.0 Disruption of caesarean section wound
S01 Open wound of the head
S01.0 Open wound of the scalp
S01.1 Open wound of the eyelid and periocular area
S01.2 Open wound of the nose
S01.3 Open wound of the ear
S01.4 Open wound of the cheek and temporomandibular area
S01.7 Multiple open wounds of the head
S01.9 Open wound of the head part, unspecified
S05.4 Penetrating wound of the orbit with or without foreign body
S05.5 Penetrating wound of the eyeball with foreign body
S11 Open wound of the neck

Learning Outcomes
After completing this chapter, you should be able to do the following:

- Classify wound types according to wound depth.
- Examine different types of wounds.
- Explain different types of wound healing.
- Describe physical therapy intervention during wound treatment.
- Solve problems concerning the wound treatment

Key Terms
Partial-thickness wound
Hypertrophic scar
Wound
Full-thickness wound
Keloid

2.1 Wounds

2.1.1 Overview

In our daily life, we experience various types of wounds. We may get pricked by a thorn, scratched by a sharp object, or burned by hot water. We may also suffer from sunburn while swimming at the beach. There are surgical wounds as well, and as we age, we may encounter ulcerating wounds on the toes from a circulatory disturbance. When the normal structure of the skin is destructed with varying degrees, we refer the condition as a wound. We get wounded as a result of uncontrollable accidents, and once damaged, the skin cannot be recovered completely due to the biological limitations. All wounds are healed with scars. The goals of wound treatment are to prevent

E.Y. Kim
Department of Physical Therapy, Gumi University, Gumi, South Korea
e-mail: cebuj@naver.com

J.-W. Park, D.-I. Jung (eds.), *Integumentary Physical Therapy*, DOI 10.1007/978-3-662-47380-1_2

complications, to restore the function, and to minimize the resulting scars, and they require time. Wounds can be classified into acute wounds, which can be healed in a timely manner, and chronic wounds, which do not follow the normal healing process. However, the exact time required for healing of acute or chronic wounds remains unknown. Affecting factors include the patient's age and physical conditions along with the wound's depth, location, and causes. Chronic wounds are defined as wounds that failed to have orderly and timely healing processes needed to achieve anatomic and functional integrity. Understanding of wounds' characteristic roles has been used in the researches of embryogenesis, carcinogenesis, and metastasis and helps understanding the reparative processes of other organs (Ahn 2009).

2.1.2 Causes

The causes are important determining factors for assessing inflammatory risks and for deciding treatment methods. The causes of wounds can be classified according to the types of forces applied to the skin: shearing, tension, and compression.

2.1.2.1 Shearing

A shearing wound occurs when tissue is cut or torn with a sharp object such as a knife or a piece of glass, and clinically observed laceration is an example of a shearing wound. Because the low energy is applied to the tissues, it causes a little or no cell destruction. It carries a low risk of inflammation and can be treated with the primary suture.

2.1.2.2 Tension

When a blunt object hits the skin at a diagonal angle, a triangular flap or a partial avulsion develops. Ischemia or necrosis can occur due to hindered blood supply to both sides of the flap. Blood runs through the bottom surface of the flap, so a careful procedure is required to maintain blood supply. If the bottom part of the flap is facing the end, hypostasis becomes more severe. The energy applied to the tissue is higher than that in a shearing wound, so greater damage is done to the skin cells. If the damage and potential ischemia act together, the risk of inflammation can become higher.

2.1.2.3 Compression

Compression or crushing injury occurs when a blunt object hits the skin perpendicularly. Resulting wounds have bumpy and fragmented texture and include a considerable amount of dead tissue. Inflammation occurs easily in this condition. Cleansing over a wide area and excision of the edge are required. In spite of the meticulous treatment, cosmetic prognosis is not expected.

2.1.3 Classification

Wounds are classified by depth. Skin is divided into the epidermis, the dermis, and the subcutaneous tissue. When only the epidermis is damaged, the wound is called an erosion, and when a deeper breach of the epithelium is involved, it is called an ulcer.

2.1.3.1 Partial-Thickness Wounds

Partial-thickness wounds are characterized by involving only the superficial part of the dermis. Acute partial-thickness wounds show the epidermal organization. The epidermal organization of acute partial-thickness wounds is different from that of full-thickness wounds in their mechanisms. The dermis in partial-thickness wounds and its appendages remain mostly intact. These structures can participate in restoring the lost epidermis.

2.1.3.2 Full-Thickness Wounds

In full-thickness wounds, the entire epidermis, dermis, and often the underlying structures (including muscles and bones) are involved. Since the appendages are lost, the epidermis, which can cover the wound, moves to the edge. Contraction takes place during the wound healing process. Contraction can be mediated by mechanical or biological factors, and the wound size diminishes during the contraction. This resulted from existing tissue's contraction movement and not from newly formed connective tissues. Except for the very tiny wounds, contraction is almost always imperfect. Moreover, contraction occurs in a predictable direction of the tension line. The tension line agrees with the direction of the gravity (Alloju 2008).

2.1.3.3 Other Classifications

Other classifications apart from the partial-thickness wounds and full-thickness wounds include stab wounds, incised wounds, lacerations, and abrasions (Fig. 2.1).

2.1.4 Symptoms and Complications

General symptoms and signs of wounds include erubescence, swelling, burning sensation, pain, and pus formation. Infected sites may become hard and tense showing lines come out of the wound. Especially, wound infection may cause fever when infection spreads through the bloodstream. Skin infection often results in skin discoloration, pain, pruritus, and pus formation.

2.1.4.1 Wound Infection

Wound infection means a topical damage by bacterial invasion and growth. Microorganisms that cause diseases are called pathogens, and the physiological responses to infection are referred to as inflammation. Bacteria exist in all types of wounds, but increased bacterial loading does not necessarily leads to the colony formation. The occurrence of infection depends on the number of bacteria, pathogenicity of bacteria, and the host resistance. When wounds are infected, bacteria consume oxygen and nutrients which are needed by normal cells for wound healing. This competition over oxygen and nutrients makes the normal cells lose function and die of starvation. Moreover, toxins and metabolites of bacteria destroy normal cells and tissue substrates, which leads to unsuccessful wound healing.

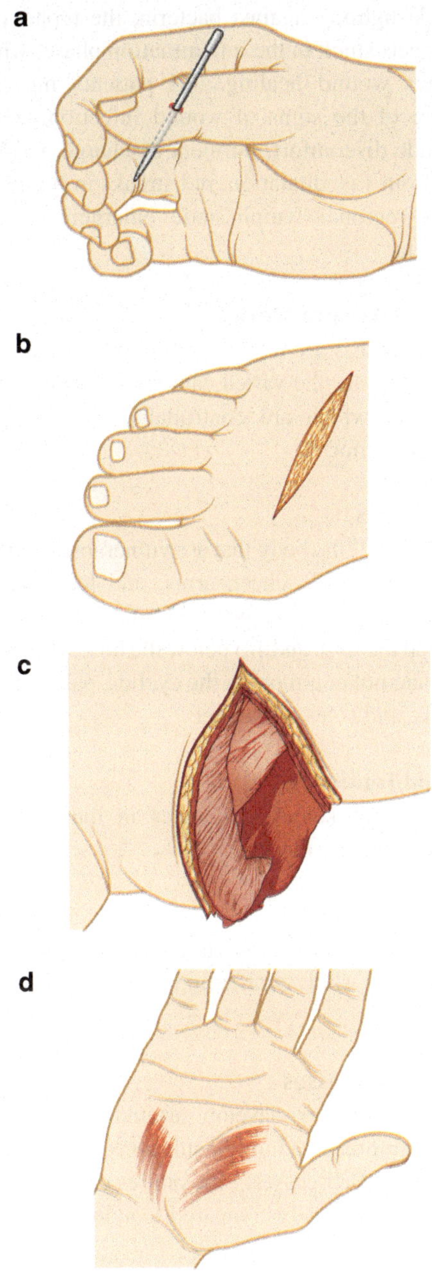

Fig. 2.1 Wound classification. (**a**) Pierced wounds. Wounds that occur when a sharp object such as a knife or an awl penetrates the skin. (**b**) Incised wounds. Wounds that are produced when sharp-edged objects cut the skin. (**c**) Lacerations. Wounds that are characterized by torn up skin with ragged skin edges. (**d**) Abrasions. Wounds are caused by superficial damage to the skin, which often occur when the skin is scraped in a fall

While fighting against bacteria, the repair process gets stuck in the inflammation phase, which delays wound healing. All patients must be aware of the signs of wound infection, which include discomfort, purulent discharge, reddening from vasodilatation, red streaks in lymphangitis, regional lymph node enlargement, and pyrexia.

2.1.4.2 Suture Marks

Suture marks are unpleasant complications. The following are the varied causes of suture marks, some of which are controllable and some of which are not.

Skin Types

The parts of the body that are vulnerable to suture marks are back, chest, arms, and legs. Suture marks are also frequently found on the skin around the nose and 1/3 below the nose. However, they are not common on the eyelids, palms of the hands, and soles of the feet.

Keloid Tendencies

Those with keloid tendencies in the skin are prone to suture marks.

Suture Tension

Excessive suture tension caused by knotting results in skin contraction and clear suture marks.

Suture Abscesses

Small abscesses develop around the sutures. Since sutures are foreign substances, they carry the risks of abscesses. Silk sutures cause inflammation more easily compared to nylon sutures or staplers.

Duration of Sutures

If sutures are no removed within 14 days, they leave marks. Epithelialization makes a progress along the suture lines, which leaves permanent marks. On the contrary, no marks remain if sutures are removed within 14 days. Between 7 and 14 days, it is difficult to predict the possibility of leaving marks. The shape of the needle or the size of the sutures is irrelevant.

2.1.4.3 Keloids and Hypertrophic Scar Formation

Keloids refer to inappropriate accumulations of scar tissues caused by lesions that extend beyond the injury margins. They are common in dark-skinned people, but they can occur on dark pigmented skin of other races. Keloids are prone to occur on the ears, arms, lower abdomen, and breastbone region (Fig. 2.2). Hypertrophic scars swell, but unlike keloids, they do not extend beyond the injury margins. These tend to occur on stressed sites such as intertriginous areas. Precise causes of excessive scars are yet to be discovered (Fig. 2.3).

2.1.5 Testing and Assessment

Evaluation on wounds is assessed according to the proper interventional methods of healing. Evaluation includes patient history, inspection

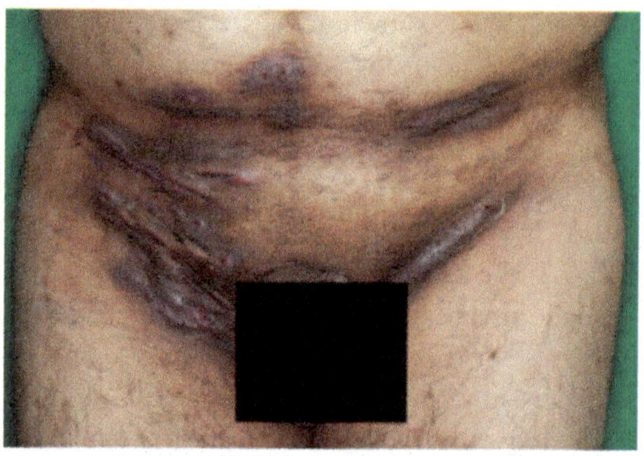

Fig. 2.2 Keloid

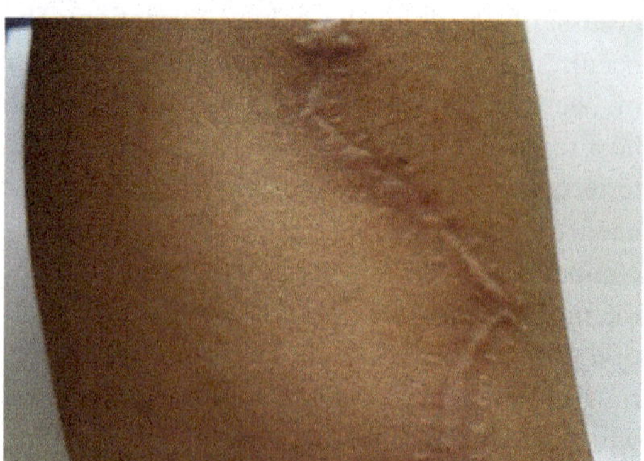

Fig. 2.3 Hypertrophic scar

coupled with the measurement, inspection used for wound evaluation, skin around the wound, and measurement methods for anatomic evaluation. Based on this evaluation, decisions concerning the data gained are made, and treatment plans are established. The following is based on clinical decision making for physical therapist (APTA 1997).

2.1.5.1 Early Assessment of Wounds

Medical History

Patient history, a part of subjective inspection, plays an important role in patient evaluation and further treatments. Physical therapists must build a strategy for essential evaluation factors along with gaining patient medical records from the patients or carers. Such simultaneous decision making process includes rearranging treatments, predicting the possible outcomes, and collecting data for determining relevant symptoms and prognoses (Table 2.1).

Occupational History

Occupation includes job requirements, group activities, job responsibilities, and educational requirements. The cooperation of the patients, families, and carers is essential for gaining this information. The causes of the wounds can be revealed based on the patients' job.

Table 2.1 Information concerning a patient's medical history

① Population statistics
② Social experience
③ Job/area
④ Growth/development
⑤ Living environment
⑥ Current status/past status
⑦ Functional status/degree of activity
⑧ Medication
⑨ Past tests/measurements
⑩ Past treatment experience/surgical records
⑪ Family history
⑫ Health status
⑬ Social tendency

*American Physical Therapy Association: Guide to physical therapist practice, 1997. http://www.apta.org.

Social Information

Social information helps setting up the practical plans concerning patients' lifestyle and value system. Therapeutic problems regarding patients, patient's family, and carer can be discovered with the knowledge of social information. Social roles of patients, patient's family, and carers come along with the patients' personal goals, demands, and needs.

Past Medical History

The past medical history of wounded patients is the information affecting the predicted outcomes. Various diseases can have negative effects on healing processes. For example, circulatory diseases affect oxygen supply to the tissue, nutrition, health, function, and mobility. Such effects of circulatory diseases delay healing processes and exert an influence upon patients' overall health and quality of life. Ultimately, patients' past medical records must be considered when the wound management is planned.

Current Health Status

Current health status includes general health, functional capacity, psychological happiness, current medication, nutrition and water supply, recent inspections or measurements, current wound status, and pain from wounds. These data are needed for proper wound care (Alloju 2008).

2.1.5.2 Wound Examination

During the wound examination, the size and location of the wound, characteristics of the wound basal layer, pus or exudate, and wound pain must be considered. Such factors are used to determine chronic signs or symptoms after the tests and assessments are done.

Wound Location

Wound location is one of the factors that should be considered first for the evaluation. A location can be marked on a body chart or be explained with proper terms and anatomical marks. Wounds by neuropathy are generally situated on the soles of the feet; on the other hand, pressure sores are often found on bony projections such as the sacrum, coccyx, greater trochanter, and ischemic regions.

Wound Size

① The surface area must be recorded regularly

Baseline measurement is required when healing process is going on or when the measurement accuracy is needed to be improved. Many measuring methods include measurement range for easy and quick use. Measuring the longest length and the largest area with the tape measurement is the simplest method with linear and two-dimensional characteristics. Consistent use of one measuring method is required while measuring wound surface areas. For example, length is measured in a head-to-tail direction, and the area is measured perpendicularly to the length. In the clinic, the clock face method, which overlaps the wound, is used. Pictures can be used in measuring the wound sites. Pictures with wound colors can be obtained from either a Polaroid or a digital camera, and video footage clips can be downloaded to a computer for the surface area analysis. Polaroid grid film helps measuring the wound surface area from the pictures taken (Fig. 2.4).

② Vertical, Horizontal, and Oblique Measurements

While the video footage clips of wound's length, area, and circumference are important in wound evaluation, they don't always provide perfect information. Information concerning ductus, tunnel, degree of fistula, and depth of wounds provides valuable information. These data require different measuring methods, so they need to be measured with the wound depth measurement (Fig. 2.5, Table 2.2) (http://www.ewma.org).

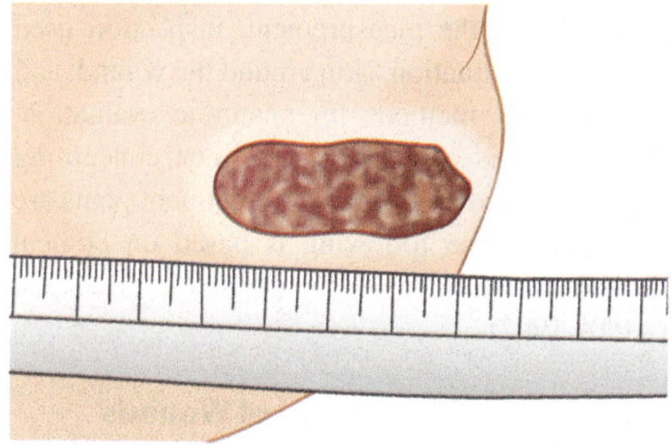

Fig. 2.5 Horizontal measurement of the wound

Table 2.2 Considerations for wound evaluation

Considerations for venous ulcer	Considerations for pressure ulcer
Location	Location
Pain	Size
Edema	Undermining
Size of the wound	Exudate
Odor	Epithelialization
Pulse palpation	Distribution of color
Surrounding skin tissues	Pain
Blood distribution of the ankle joint	Side effects
Circulation time of the capillary	Sinus pathways
Infection	Tunneling
Basic factors of the wound	Necrosis
Exudate	Granulation tissue
Venous circulation	Nutritional status

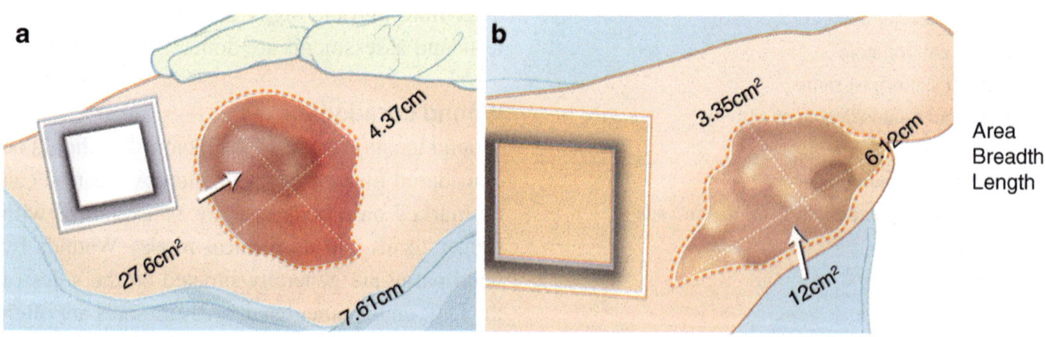

Fig. 2.4 Surface area measurement of the wounds. (**a**) Large size wound (**b**) small size wound

③ Depth Measurement

Sterilized cotton swab is inserted into the wound with gloved hand. The depth of the wound is marked on the stick of the cotton swab. The length from the tip to the marked point is measured in millimeters. This method is also used when the depth of sinus tract, tunneling, or undermining is measured (Fig. 2.6) (Pawar et al. 2010).

④ Volume Measurements

Patients are positioned in a way that the wound site becomes perpendicular to the gravity. The volume is measured by the amount of saline solution filled in the wound. However, it is not practical because it is difficult to make a position in which saline solution stays without overflowing. As an alternative method, an adhesive and transparent film is attached on the wound site, and then saline solution or amorphous hydrogel is injected through the film with a sterile syringe (Fig. 2.7a, b). For an accurate measurement, foam is eliminated, and the amount of solution injected needs to be appropriate. There is also a method of casting a mold on the wound side, but it is less frequently used (http://www.woundcare.or.kr).

2.1.5.3 Inspection of the Wound Surrounding the Skin

Wound surrounding the skin also requires regular evaluation and recording. Lack or overgrowth of hair, callus, hyperkeratosis, blister, and scar must be checked. Fissure may occur when the patients' skin becomes severely dry, so intervention regarding the skin moisturization is required. Ecchymosis or hemosiderosis, which develops when hemoglobin precipitates permanently, may be found while checking for the color of the wound surrounding the skin. Especially, color change to brown or purple is a sign of venous insufficiency. NPUAP (National Pressure Ulcer Advisory Panel) grade, which classified wounds according to the tissue destruction degree, and Wagner grade are most frequently used and will be discussed in Chap. 3.

2.2 Intervention

2.2.1 Intervention

2.2.1.1 Intervention Approach

Because wounds cannot be separated from the patients, the factors that delay healing processes such as lack of knowledge or decrease in

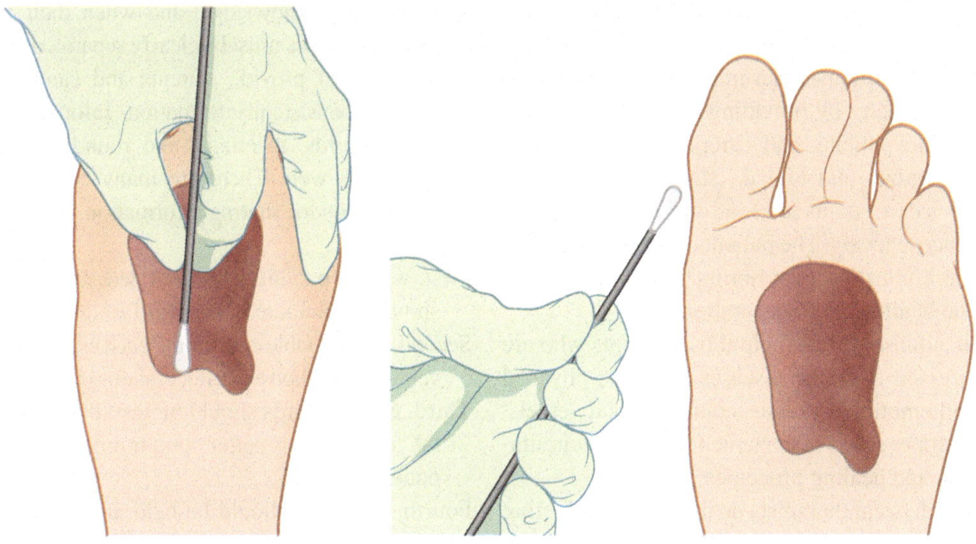

Fig. 2.6 Depth measurement of the wound

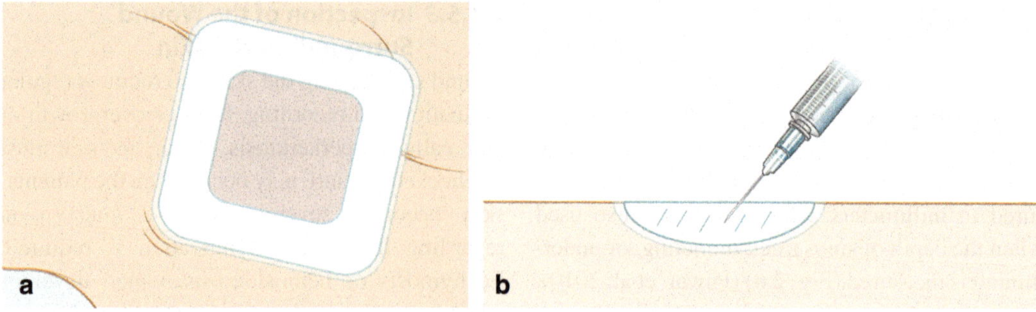

Fig. 2.7 Volume measurement of the wound. (**a**) Transparent film. (**b**) Sterile syringe

mobility must be considered. Interventional approach requires a team approach and cooperation among the patients, carers, doctors, pharmacists, nutritionists, counselors, physical therapists, occupational therapists, nurses, and medical social workers. Those who work together in medical intervention have the following roles.

First, patients must actively participate in treatment programs, and carers must encourage patients and have questions regarding the treatments.

Second, doctors must provide carers with information about patients' disease, infection, overall medical condition, and medical team's guidance.

Third, during pharmaceutical intervention, pharmacists must check the patients' therapeutic dose, possible interaction among drugs, and toxicity.

Fourth, nutritionists can improve patients' healing capacity by providing necessary information to patients and carers such as ways to maximize nutritional status and dietary advices to manage blood pressure and blood glucose levels. The patients with wounds need more nutrition than normal people to aid tissue healing and regeneration.

Fifth, counselors can help those patients who are stressed from the diseases. Because physical and emotional stresses contract blood vessels, a proper stress management can boost circulation and healing processes.

Sixth, physical therapists deal with strengthening muscular strength after the surgery, rehabilitating ambulatory function, and designing position change programs that team members must follow. Physical therapists need to communicate with occupational therapists because they share several areas such as exercise, mobility, and wheelchair prescription.

Seventh, nurses act as a communication bridge between patients and other medical teams. Nurses follow prescription orders, and they proceed with the position change, dressing, dead tissue elimination, and progress observation.

Eight, medical social workers provide information about medical devices and medical supplies and help patients to return to local communities by providing counsel about discharge planning and social situations.

Team members must respect other members' specialties and knowledge, and when their tasks overlap, their roles must be clearly separated. Team members must provide patients and carers with timely and consistent information. Information in medical records, meetings, and rounds must be consistent as well. There are many communicational methods for sharing information.

First, when a patient is hospitalized, all members should participate in the ward round.

Second, a result table concerning each expert's interventional method and effects should be made.

Third, notice boards should be installed in hospital rooms for better communication with patients.

Fourth, meetings should be held among the carers, doctors in charge, nurses, physical therapists, occupational therapists, and medical social workers, so that those who participate in wound management have enough chances to communicate. Cooperative approaches are required to achieve efficient teamwork, clear communication, and successful treatment.

2.2.1.2 Medical Management

Types of Wound Healing

Clinical wound healing is classified into primary closure, secondary closure, tertiary closure, and intention. A suturing method is chosen according to the degrees of contamination and tissue devitalization by time elapsed (Fig. 2.8) (Kloth and McCulloch 2001; Wound Therapy Research Group 2002; http://www.npuap.org).

① Primary Closure

Primary closure can be used only when the wound is minimally contaminated with little tissue damages. This type of wound is normally

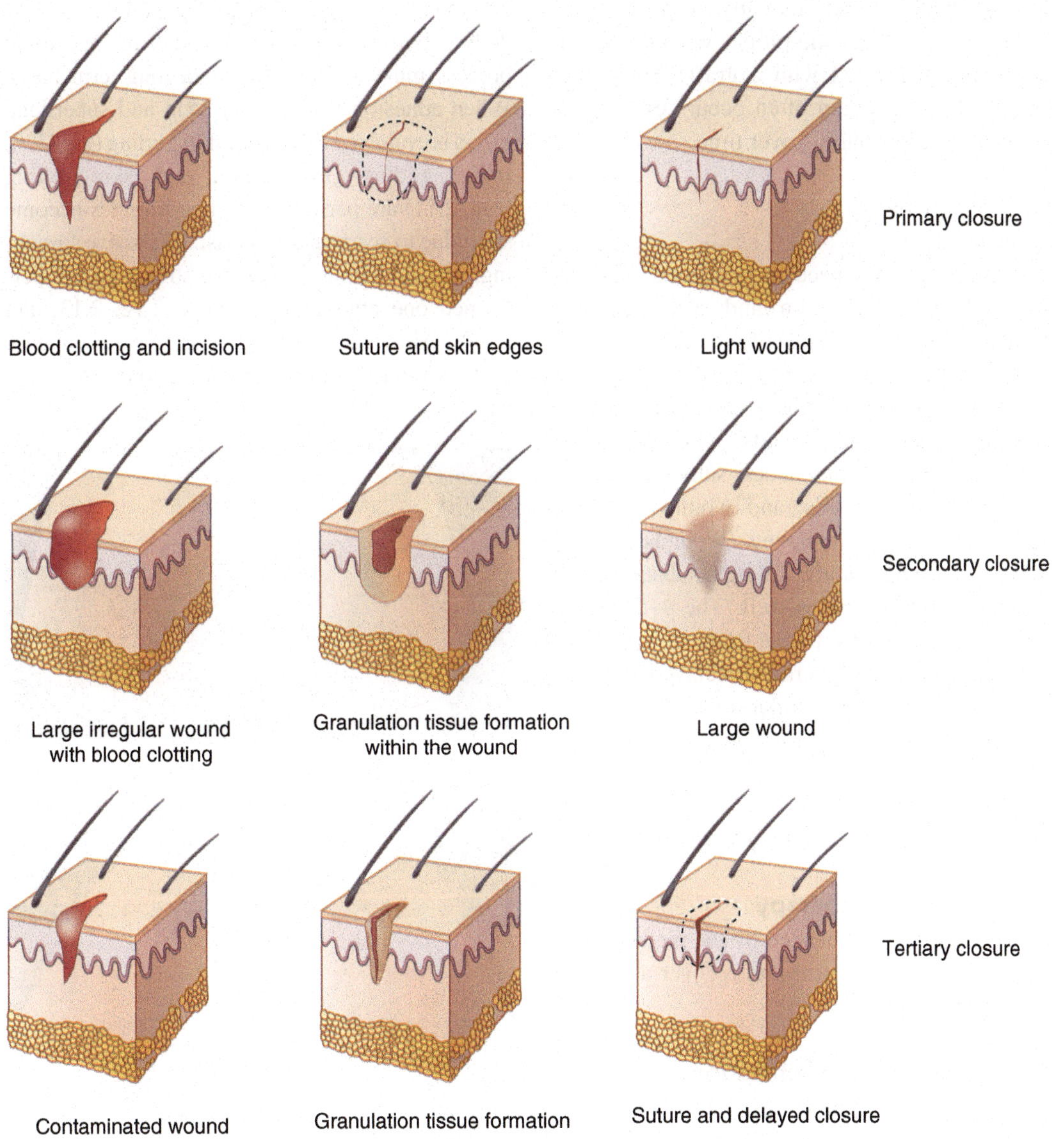

Fig. 2.8 Process of wound healing

caused by cutting with a sharp instrument and can be closed with a needle, a wound tape, or a stapler. The ideal timing for primary closure is within 6–8 h.

② Secondary Closure

Cosmetically less important wounds and partial-thickness abrasion with maintained basal dermis such as skin infarction, ulcer, abscess, pierced wounds, and bite wounds are better to be left for the secondary closure. Such wounds are not easily closed and gradually go through epidermalization. After the proper wound care, the skin can be covered with a graft if necessary. Inflammatory reaction often occurs excessively, so wounds may contract over time.

③ Tertiary Closure

Certain wounds need to be closed after 4–5 days of the observation and cleansing. The tertiary closure is considered when the wound is too contaminated to be sutured or when there is no severe damage to the tissue. This type of wound includes old wounds; wounds that are contaminated with dirt, feces, saliva, or vaginal secretion; bite wounds; and wounds by high-speed objects such as bullets. Wounds occurred while searching for the foreign substances are included in this type as well. The 4–5 days of waiting is determined by the frequency of wound infection. The infection rate of delayed closure is about 4 %, which is similar to the rate of the primary closure with clean wounds.

2.2.2 Physical Therapy Intervention

2.2.2.1 Exercise Therapy

Cells are greatly influenced by the methods used during healing processes and recover as the following stages.

Early Stage Before Inflammation

Skin tissues at this stage have very weak mechanical strength. If a force is applied, the end part of the wound will likely be broken, so the goal of treatment is promoting metabolism needed for the inflammatory cells by stimulating the flow of lymphatic fluid and blood. Rhythmic non-painful technique can be used at this stage.

Treatment Stage After Inflammation

At this stage, patients are required to do exercise on a regular basis, which affects the recovery and remodeling process. Tissues regain their stretching force, so the force application and the range of motion can be gradually increased. Because the treatment is performed until the patients can do daily activities, stimulation needed for reshaping process must be provided on a long-term basis. When adhesion between the skin and superficial fascia is evaluated or treated, skin gliding (Fig. 2.9), finger gliding (Fig. 2.10), and skin rolling (Fig. 2.11) are performed. When muscles become short due to scars or adhesions, the passive stretching, self-stretching, and active stretching are performed one after another (Figs. 2.12, 2.13, and 2.14) (American Physical Therapy Association 1997; Wound Therapy Research Group 2002).

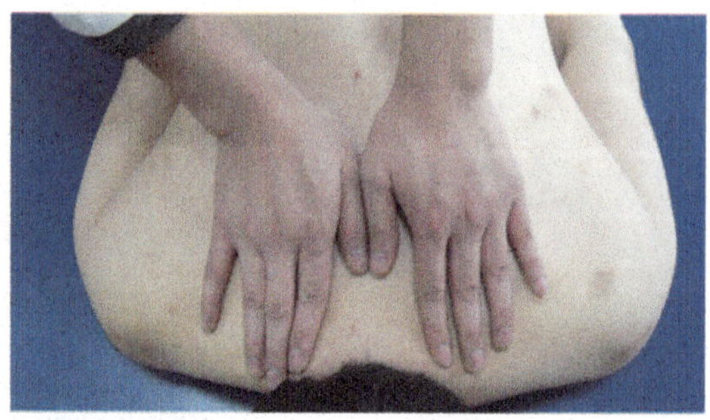

Fig. 2.9 Skin gliding

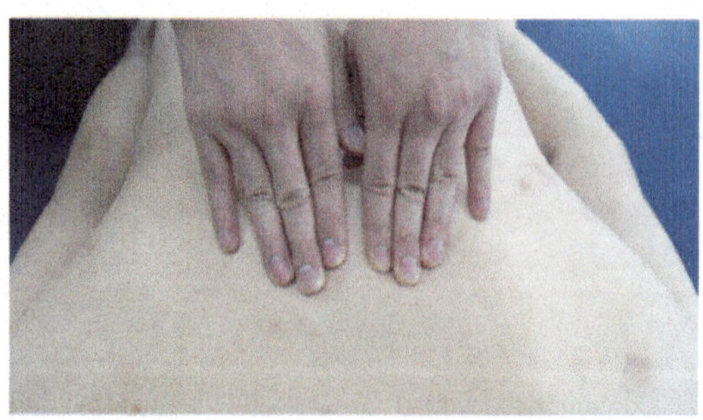

Fig. 2.10 Finger gliding

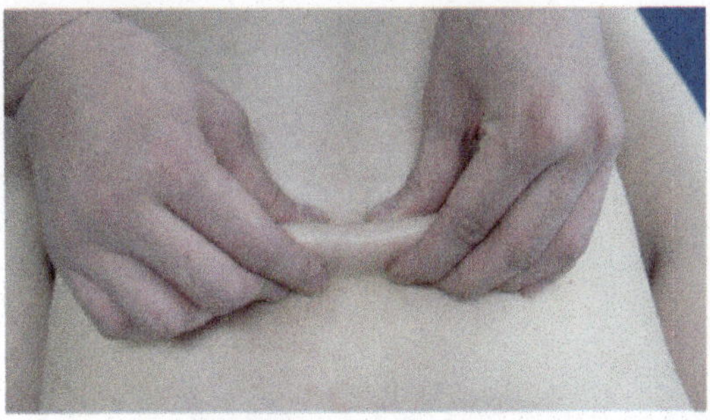

Fig. 2.11 Skin rolling

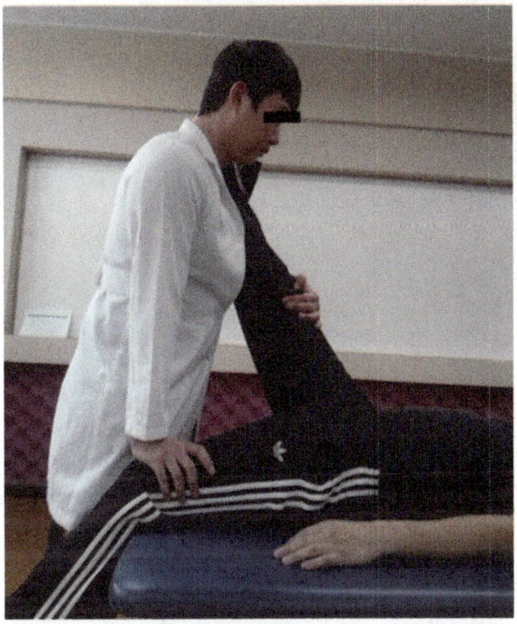

Fig. 2.12 Slow passive stretching

2.2.2.2 Manual Therapy

Functions of Manual Therapy

In manual therapy, therapists use their hands to detect tissue changes. Muscles, ligaments, tendons, articular capsules, articular surfaces, skin, and fascia are affected by manual therapy, and such manual therapy of tissue organs has many functions.

① When the normal tissues are damaged, different types of mechanical manipulation during the remodeling process can improve physical capacity of the entire tissues such as tensile strength and flexibility.

② When soft tissues become short due to adhesion and contracture, manipulation can be used to lengthen the shortened tissues and to decrease the abnormally enhanced strength and range of motion.

③ Viability, health, and regeneration of the tissues are greatly affected by the supply of blood and lymph. Metabolic demands increase especially during the regeneration process after soft tissue damage.

④ Boosting the flow of tissue fluid reduces tissue edema, which in turn relieves pain. Inflammation and exudates can be reduced by accelerating the flow of joint fluid and joint regeneration.

⑤ The skin's wound healing is influenced by mechanical stimulation. Scars with mechanical stimulation are stronger and more similar to the normal skins than those without any stimulation (Table 2.3).

Manual Therapy Classification

① Positional Release Technique

In positional release technique, tender points and scars are inspected for dysfunctions. After patients take a comfortable position, contact on the scar tissue is maintained until the tissue relaxation toward the distal end is sensed. It is more effective when the comfortable position is maintained for a long time (5–10 min). After slowly returning to the original position, the status of the scar tissue is rechecked. Patients are required to avoid intense exercises (Fig. 2.15) (Chang et al. 2008; Kim and Hwang 2002).

② Strain and Counterstrain Method

Strain and counterstrain methods are applied to relieve stiffness in perioperative patients or when direct therapeutic methods for muscle twitching are not performed. Whether acute or chronic, the ability of checking for dystonia and soft tissue change is required. After palpation of the most important therapeutic point, the minimal pressure is applied to the point. The most relaxed and comfortable position should be found, and there must not be any pain from other parts of the body (Hunt et al. 1984; Park et al. 2006).

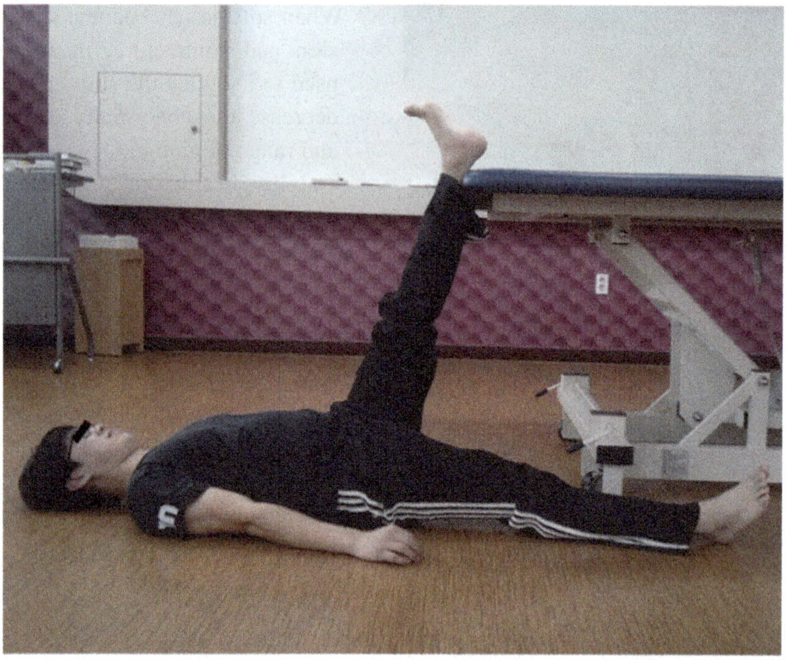

Fig. 2.13 Self-stretching of the lower extremity

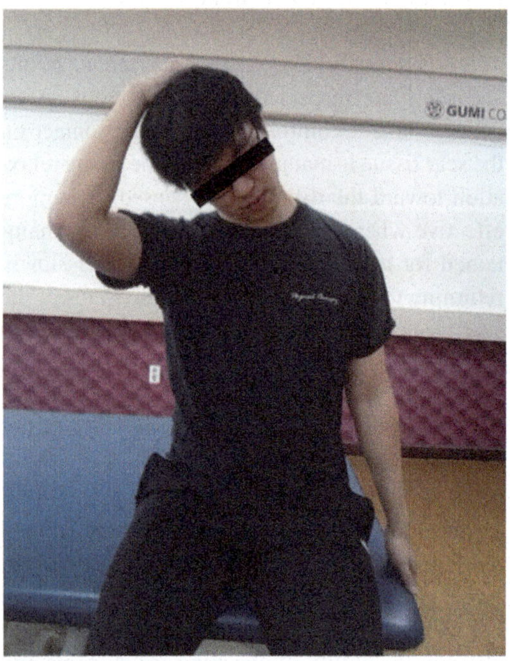

Fig. 2.14 Self-stretching of the neck

③ Scar Tissue Release Method

Scar tissue release methods are usually applied to thick wounds and adhered regions associated with the abdomen and chest. Patients are asked to take a deep breath because it causes sharp pain and increases the level of tissue tension. Blood pressure decreases and heat loss may occur after the performance, so patients need to take a moment of regaining homeostasis in a comfortable position. Because scars can be accompanied with adhesion and contracture or become a cause of trigger point formation, the possible methods for treatments are used including soft tissue techniques, soft tissue mobilization, cross-friction massage, muscle energy techniques, post-isometric relaxation, and myofascial release (MFR, Fig. 2.16) (Gong and Yun 2009).

2.2.2.3 Physical Agent Modalities

Whirlpool Bath Therapy

Whirlpool bath therapy is a water immersion with massage effects on the damaged regions. It is used to stimulate wound healing and to relax pain and muscle cramps, and it is also effective in massaging soft tissues and preparing stretching. A patient's body is soaked in a bathtub filled with warm water (105–110 °F or 93 °F). If the patient has infected wounds, 10 g of sodium sulfathia-

Table 2.3 Difference of manual therapy between acute phase treatment and chronic phase treatment (Moffat 2006)

Physiological process	Goal of treatment	Type of manual therapy
Acute phase Edema Inflammation Swelling Disturbance in circulation resistance	Tissue healing and nutritional improvement Improvement of humeral motion	Soft manual method Intermittent compression Joint exercise within painless range Application of minimal mechanical stretching
Collagen precipitation and remodeling process	Improvement of mechanical characteristics in tissues Adhesion and decrease in excessive cross-link formation	Stretching with low load on tissues Gradual increase in length and proper load
Chronic phase Tissue extensibility/ Flexibility loss	Increase of tissue flexibility and mechanical movement during load application	Increase of tissue flexibility and mechanical movement during load application Mid-high load Vertical or cross-fiber method Low repetition or continuous stretching Load application with varied methods
In case of adhesion and abnormal cross-link	Decrease in adhesion and cross-link formation	High load Vertical or cross-fiber method High-speed load Slow repetitive or continuous stretching

zole is dissolved in 8 gallons of water (Moffat 2006).

High-Voltage Pulsed Current Stimulation

High-voltage pulsed current stimulation (HVPCS) is used to speed up the inflammatory phase by stimulating phagocytosis in wound healing and to utilize both poles of the epithelialization phase as

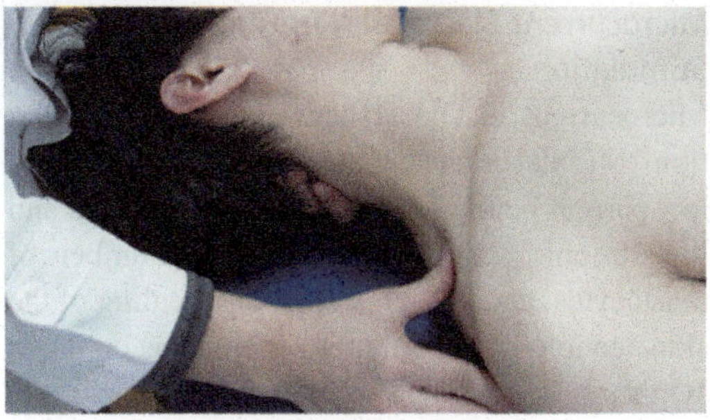

Fig. 2.15 Positional release therapy

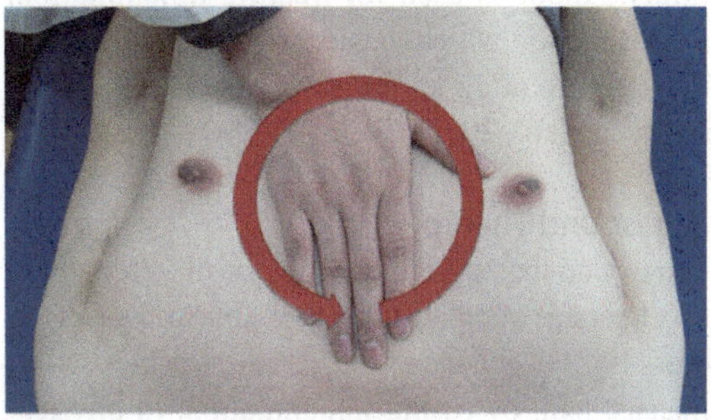

Fig. 2.16 Myofascial release

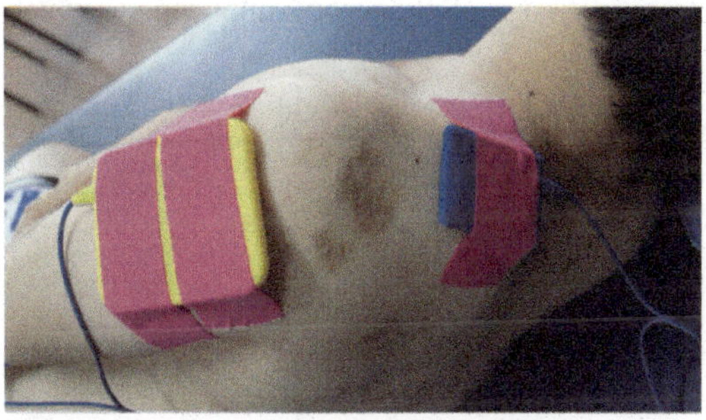

Fig. 2.17 High-voltage pulsed current stimulation

active electrodes. Making the cathode as an active electrode has effects of suppressing bacterial growth and increasing collagen synthesis by stimulating fibroblast cells. Because collagen synthesis and epithelialization occur almost simultaneously, the polarity can be changed at an interval of 3 days or every other day during the proliferative phase. During the remodeling phase, stimulation is applied once a day for 60 min with a frequency of 60–64 pulses per second. Water immersion technique can be used in the case of poor electrode contact due to crushing injuries or irregular shapes of bony prominences (Fig. 2.17) (Pliquett et al. 2002).

Microcurrent Electrical Neuromuscular Stimulation

Microcurrent electrical neuromuscular stimulation (MENS) is an electrostimulation that uses low current below 1mA. It decreases fibrosis and hypertrophic scar by reducing the number of mastocytes, and it can boost wound healing of the skin, tendon, and ligament by increasing collagen synthesis. The low pulse rate (0.3–0.9 pps) and current are used for acute tissue injury, and high pulse rate and current are used for chronic tissue injury. Anode is used for treating inflammation, and cathode, which has sterilization effect, is used for treating chronic diseases (Fig. 2.18) (Pliquett et al. 2002).

Ultrasound Therapy

Ultrasound therapy can increase tensile strength by accelerating wound contraction and strengthening cross-link of collagen, and it can also be used to manage pain by easing inflammation. In physical therapy, low-intensity ultrasound (20–120 kHz, 0.05–1.0 W/cm^2) is used to sterilize and eliminate necrotic tissues. Subaqueous application, which utilizes ultrasound in the water, is used to treat wounds with irregular surfaces such as bony prominences. In subaqueous application, therapists use an ultrasonic transducer in the warm sterilized water (37 °C) while wearing surgical gloves (Fig. 2.19) (Park et al. 2009).

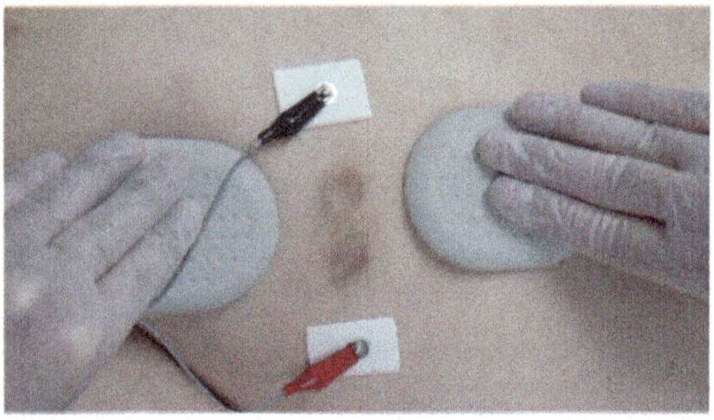

Fig. 2.18 Microcurrent electrical neuromuscular stimulation

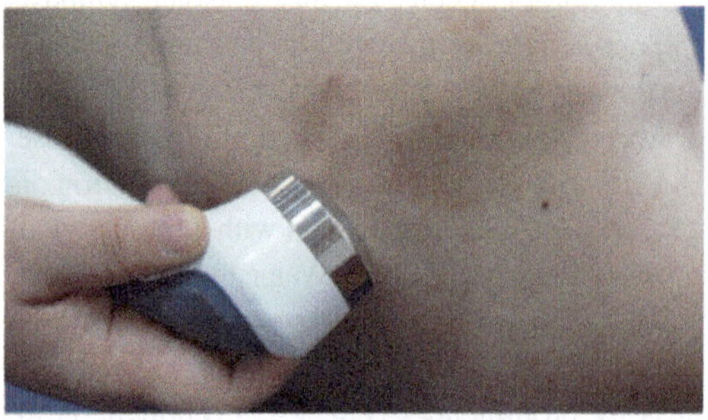

Fig. 2.19 Ultrasound therapy

Iontophoresis

Iontophoresis transmits ionic drugs through hair follicles and sweat pores by using the repulsive force between the same electric charges. Zinc ion is used when there are open wounds, ulcers, or dermatitis. A terminal with the same charge as the ionic drugs being used is connected and maintained for 15–20 min with low intensity (Fang et al. 2002).

Ultraviolet Therapy

Ultraviolet therapy utilizes photochemical effects on the skin, which helps treatment by activating substances on the skin. Sterilizing effects are effectively used to treat skin wounds or infections, and third-/fourth-degree erythema doses are mainly used as a therapeutic dose. Cold quartz mercury lamps emit 95 % of 2,537Å wavelength, so it is mainly used for sterilization. In the case of pressure ulcer patients, 10–15 min of infrared radiation along with ultraviolet therapy can help drying the waste from ulcer (Kang et al. 2007).

Negative-Pressure Wound Therapy

Negative-pressure wound therapy (NPWT) is a wound healing method which boosts wound contraction and wound intention by increasing the capillary blood stream and lymph flow. It can be applied to acute/chronic wounds, diabetic ulcers, traumatic wounds, cut wounds, and wounds from vasogenic edema. Before treating negative-pressure wounds, dead tissues like eschars are eliminated, and sterilized foam is cut to the wound size and placed on the wound. If the wound site is dented or undermined, the thicker size of the foam is used to fill the wound. A hydrogel plate is attached to protect the skin around the wound by fixing the foam and exudates. Then, a tube is inserted, and as negative pressure is applied by a pump, exudate is removed into a canister. The range of the negative pressure is 50–175 mmHg, and the pressure is to be increased gradually according to patients' conditions.

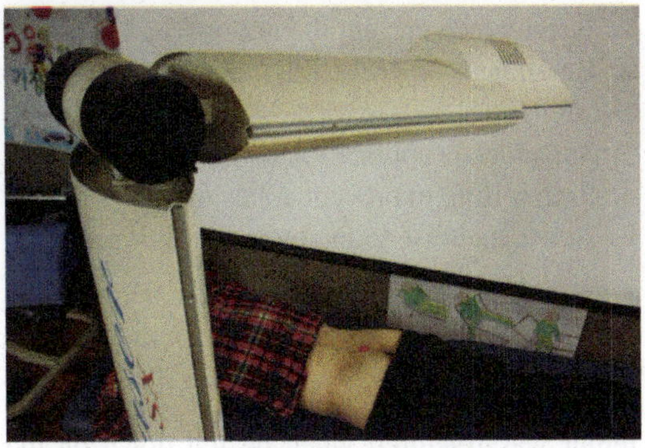

Fig. 2.20 Laser treatment

Laser Treatment

Laser is effective in treating skin diseases and endermosis consistent. Laser treatment helps collagen formation, blood circulation, and cellular regeneration on the wound site. It is also used to treat ulcers, to minimize keloid formation, and to improve nutritional status. Low-strength laser (He-Ne, 632.8 nm/GaAs, 904 nm) is applied to 6–8 spots for 3 min per spot, which is performed 10–12 times. Noncontact methods are used to prevent contact infections and to avoid external damages such as keloid wounds (Fig. 2.20) (Han 2008; Park et al. 2005).

2.2.3 Prevention and Management

2.2.3.1 Prevention

1. Patient education is required to prevent skin trauma.
   ① Patients should avoid pressure on the skin and provide compressive force at regular intervals.
   ② Patients should keep the skin clean and healthy and minimize the skin friction and the shearing force.
   ③ Patients should wear gloves or proper clothes to protect the skin from harmful substances.
2. Physical therapists are required to provide proper education to relieve skin problems.
   ① Therapists should make patients comfortable by loosening their clothes.
   ② Therapists should teach patients how to move weight in a way that vulnerable regions are not pressured.
   ③ Therapists should make an assessment of patients' occupational condition and skin condition before treatment.
3. After injury, immediate compression, elevation, and ice pack are used to relieve pain and edema.
4. Therapists should develop regular exercise programs so as to keep patients' fitness and health.

2.2.3.2 Management

Important principles for wound management are protection, elevation, and cleanliness.

1. Patients instinctively protect the wound from other injuries, but therapists need to remind patients that unexpected pressure or mechanical force on the wound may open the sutured wound or cause infection.
2. Elevating the wounded part is very important especially for wounds on the limbs. Legs and hands are subject to edema from pooling of lymph fluid. Elevation prevents such complications, relieves pain, and improves wound healing process. Probability of complications from infection, edema, and pooling is comparatively high on leg wounds.
3. Recently sutured wounds are easily damaged from sun exposure. Excessive exposure can cause permanent discoloration and pigmentation to the epidermal tissue. Sun exposure to the wound should be avoided for a year, and the use of sunblock is recommended (American Physical Therapy Association 1997; Kim 2010).

2.2.3.3 Patient/Carer Education

1. Knowledge and information concerning wound management.

   Patients must be provided with knowledge and information concerning wound management and methods to avoid recurrence.
2. Patients must be aware that controlling smoking, hypertension, diabetes, and hypercholesterolemia can improve wound healing capacity and decrease the risk of heart diseases and stroke.
3. During education, the level of terms used and the degree of patients' understanding must be checked.

4. Proper education and patient cooperation are vital because successful treatment depends on patients' understanding of their condition and their active participation (Society SEMS 2005).

Advices for Physical Therapists

❶ Evaluation of patients' skin condition is required to treat symptoms, and physical therapists need to pay attention on the changes of patients' skin.
❷ Even when causes of pruritus vary, physical therapists should be able to provide with standardized methods that can ease the symptoms or prevent further damages.
❸ Physical therapists should be able to provide patients with proper education concerning the ways to increase or decrease inflammation.
❹ Clinical infections through wounds may appear after a week. Concerning the management of the skin around the wound, sterilization is performed from the center outward so as to restrict bacterial infection.
❺ Physical therapists should know patients' hygienic conditions regardless of their age, social condition, and economic status so that possible infection can be prevented.

2.3 Problem Solving

2.3.1 Wounds

Choose the most suitable physical therapy intervention method for each question.

Question 1
Patient A is a 43-year-old worker whose hands and fingers were injured by compression of an extruder. After the surgery was done, physical therapy on irregular skin surface was requested. What is the most proper physical therapy intervention method in this case?

1. Interference current therapy
2. Resistance exercise to enhance muscular strength
3. Subaqueous application using ultrasound
4. Skin rolling to prevent adhesion
5. Active exercise to maintain range of motion

Question 2
Patient A is a 68-year-old man whose head of the femur was fractured when he fell down on the stairs. Physical therapy was requested after pin fixation. What is the most proper physical therapy intervention method in this case?

1. Paraffin bath
2. Ultrasound treatment
3. Ion therapy
4. Microwave treatment
5. Transcutaneous electrical nerve stimulation

Question 3
While patient A was carrying baggage, he was cut by a sharp object. This accident resulted in a penetrating injury to the fascial layer. The wound developed into purulent inflammation because it was not treated properly. What is the most proper physical therapy intervention method in this case?

1. Interference current therapy using negative pressure
2. Ultraviolet irradiation for sterilization
3. Deep tissue massage to break adhesion
4. Hot pack treatment to enhance circulation
5. Infrared irradiation after applying cream on the wound site

Question 4
Among the general wound treatment methods, what is the closure stage in which a wound tape is used for suturing because the wound is clean with the minimal contamination?

1. Primary closure
2. Secondary closure
3. Tertiary closure
4. Quaternary closure
5. Quinary closure

Question 5

While patient A was working as an excavator driver, he was hit by a piece of stone. This injury developed into a chronic ulcer because he did not receive a proper treatment. Later on, physical therapy was requested by the internal medicine department. What is the most proper physical therapy intervention method in this case?

1. Infrared therapy using thermal effect
2. Ion therapy using electric attraction
3. Whirlpool bath treatment with water temperature higher than 120°F
4. Neuromuscular microcurrent stimulation using low pulse frequency and low current
5. High-voltage pulsed current stimulation using cathode as an active electrode with the goal of bacterial growth inhibition

Answers

Question 1-③, Question 2-②, Question 3-②, Question 4-①, Question 5-⑤

References

Ahn S, Jang GH, Song JW, SH. C. Common skin disease of Koreans. Daijeon: Doctor's Book; 2009.

Alloju SM, Herndon DN, McEntire SJ, Suman OE. Assessment of muscle function in severely burned children. Burns : journal of the International Society for Burn Injuries. 2008;34(4):452–9. Epub 2008/02/05.

Chang CH, Kim KY, Kim SH, Kim YH, Kim HD, Park JH, et al. Principles & techniques of patient care. Seoul: Epublic Korea Co; 2008.

Fang JY, Sung KC, Wang JJ, Chu CC, Chen KT. The effects of iontophoresis and electroporation on transdermal delivery of buprenorphine from solutions and hydrogels. J Pharm Pharmacol. 2002;54(10):1329–37. Epub 2002/10/25.

Gong WT, Yun BC. Orthopedic physical therapy. Seoul: Daehak Publishing Co; 2009.

Guide to Physical Therapist Practice. Part 1: A description of patient/client management. Part 2: Preferred practice patterns. American Physical Therapy Association. Physical Ther. 1997;77(11):1160–656. Epub 1997/11/22.

Han SK. Management of diabetic wound. Paju: Koonja Publishing Co; 2008.

Hunt TK, Heppenstall RB, Pines E, Rovee D. Soft and hand tissue repair, biological and clinical aspects. New York: Praeger Scientifie; 1984.

Kang SH, Kwon MJ, Kim GJ, Kim MJ, Kim SY, Kim SJ, et al. O'Sullivan & Schmitz physical rehabilitation assessment and treatment. Seoul: Yeong Mun Publishing Inc; 2007.

Kim TY, Hwang SS. Fundamentals of manual therapy. Seoul: Yeong Mun Publishing Inc; 2002.

Kim JM. Physical rehabilitation. Seoul: Jungdam Media Inc.; 2010.

Kloth LC, McCulloch JM. Wound healing alternatives in management. Philadelphia: F.A. Davis Company; 2001.

Moffat M. Integumentary essentials: applying the preferred physical therapist practices patterns SM. Thorofare: SLACK Inc.; 2006.

Park RJ, Park CE, Han DU, Nam HC. Phototherapy. Seoul: Daehak Publishing Co; 2005.

Park RJ, Kim DH, Kim SH, Kim JH, Nam GW, Nam HC, et al. Saunders manual of physical therapy practice. Seoul: Daehak Publishing Co; 2006.

Park RJ, Kim YJ, Kim EY, Park GY, Song MY, Oh HJ, et al. Clinical electrophysiology: electrotherapy and electrophysiologic testing. ed r, editor. Seoul: Yeong Mun Publishing Inc.; 2009.

Pawar R, Sagar S, Kumar S. Evaluation and management of diabetic foot. J Surg Sci. 2010;1(1):41–5.

Pliquett UF, Martin GT, Weaver JC. Kinetics of the temperature rise within human stratum corneum during electroporation and pulsed high-voltage iontophoresis. Bioelectrochemistry. 2002;57(1):65–72. Epub 2002/06/07.

Society SEMS. Wounds and lacerations: emergency care and closure. Paju: Koonja Publishing Co; 2005.

Wound Therapy Research Group. Wound therapy. Seoul: Korea Medical Book Publisher; 2002.

Reference Sites

American Physical Therapy Association. http://www.apta.org.

European Wound Management Association. http://www.ewma.org.

Korean Wound Management Society. http://www.woundcare.or.kr.

National Pressure Ulcer Advisory Panel. http://www.npuap.org.

Decubitus Ulcer

3

Ji Whan Park

ICD-10 Code
L-89 Decubitus ulcer and pressure
L89.0 Stage I decubitus ulcer and pressure area
L89.1 Stage II decubitus ulcer
L89.2 Stage III decubitus ulcer
L89.3 Stage IV decubitus ulcer
L89.9 Decubitus ulcer and pressure area, unspecified

Learning Outcomes
After completing this chapter, you should be able to do the following:

- Understand the concept of decubitus ulcer.
- Describe the causes and symptoms of decubitus ulcer.
- Evaluate and record decubitus ulcer.
- Perform physical therapy interventions.
- Solve clinical case problems.

Key Terms
Braden scale
PUSH scale
Gauze dressing
Diabetic ulcer
Wet dressing
Pressure ulcer
Decubitus ulcer, bed sore
Management for decubitus ulcer
Scar tissue release

3.1 Decubitus Ulcer

3.1.1 Overview

A decubitus ulcer is a condition where soft tissue or underlying tissue over a bony prominence is injured by peripheral circulatory disturbance or unrelieved pressure over a localized area, resulting in ischemic necrosis by hypoxia and nutritional deficiency. A decubitus ulcer is a typical skin damage of long-term bed-rest patients and patients with vascular disease, sensory neuron lesion, diabetes, dementia, and spinal cord injury, frequently occurring in soft tissues (Charette 2012). Physical therapists, by mastering the physical therapy interventions according to the symptoms and diagnosis of decubitus ulcer, should prevent the secondary infections or complications not to mention curing decubitus ulcer.

J.W. Park
Daejeon Health Institute of Technology, Daejeon, South Korea
e-mail: jiwhan@hit.ac.kr

J.-W. Park, D.-I. Jung (eds.), *Integumentary Physical Therapy*, DOI 10.1007/978-3-662-47380-1_3

3.1.2 Causes

3.1.2.1 Pressure

A decubitus ulcer occurs frequently to long-term bed-rest patients or wheelchair users. Prolonged pressure over a bony prominence is the major cause of developing decubitus ulcer. Generally, pressure greater than 32 mmHg decreases tissue resistance and damages soft tissue by impeding capillary blood flow. The greater the pressure applied and the longer the time elapsed, the more severe the degree of decubitus ulcer. Distal parts of the body especially, when pressed over a period of time, are subject to developing decubitus ulcer even under less intense pressure. Unrelieved pressure causes capillary occlusion, thrombus formation, and regional tissue hypoxia, ultimately leading to pressure ulcer. In the case of lying supine, the predilection sites of pressure ulcers are the sacrum, occiput, scapular spine, and heel (Fig. 3.1).

3.1.2.2 Skin Trauma

Skin injury results in desquamation and hemorrhage. If not properly treated, subsequent bacterial infection and interstitial edema cause dermoepidermal necrosis, which leads to the development of decubitus ulcer.

3.1.2.3 Skin Friction

The friction of skin sliding against the contact surface, especially the skin friction by external forces or sharp objects, can be a cause of decubitus ulcer with abrasion.

3.1.2.4 Sense Deprivation

When cutaneous sensation is lost or decreased, the skin tissues are subject to damage. Because patients in such condition cannot sense that their skin is damaged, the secondary decubitus ulcer could develop. Tabes dorsalis, for example, impairs sensory neuron, resulting in loss of sensation (particularly nociperception and arthresthesia). A classic example is plantar perforating ulcer, which develops on the soles of patients with tabes dorsalis.

3.1.2.5 Impaired Vasomotor Response

Impaired regulation of vasomotion hinders blood flow, leading to the formation of decubitus ulcer. In the case of patients with spinal cord injuries, for instance, the vasomotion of both legs below the injured level is not regulated, consequently resulting in the development of decubitus ulcer (Fig. 3.2).

3.1.2.6 Body Temperature and Humidity

Because the moisture on the skin's surface acts as a medium for bacterial growth, the moist skin is subject to developing decubitus ulcer. Raised body temperature as well is a risk factor for decubitus ulcer. Higher body temperature results in higher metabolic needs (such as needs for oxygen and energy), and when the raised needs are not sufficiently provided, decubitus ulcer develops. Accordingly, relatively lower pressure or pressure with shorter duration can cause decubitus when body temperature is raised (http://www.ibestian.com/02_burn06_02.asp).

3.1.2.7 Malnutrition

Not only is poor nutrition associated with the failure of healing, but it leads to insufficient supply of oxygen and nutrition to epidermal tissues, making them vulnerable to decubitus ulcer.

3.1.3 Classification

Once an ulcer occurs, whether it is from pressure or diabetes should be determined. Physical therapists can distinguish ulcers to some degree by carefully observing their shapes and positions. For example, red ulcers on bony prominences and black ulcers with localized edema on lower ankles are likely to be pressure ulcers and diabetic ulcers, respectively.

3.1.3.1 Pressure Ulcer

A pressure ulcer is clinically called as a bed sore. It is caused by prolonged and unrelieved pressure over a bony prominence and eventually results in ischemic necrosis (Fig. 3.3). It often develops

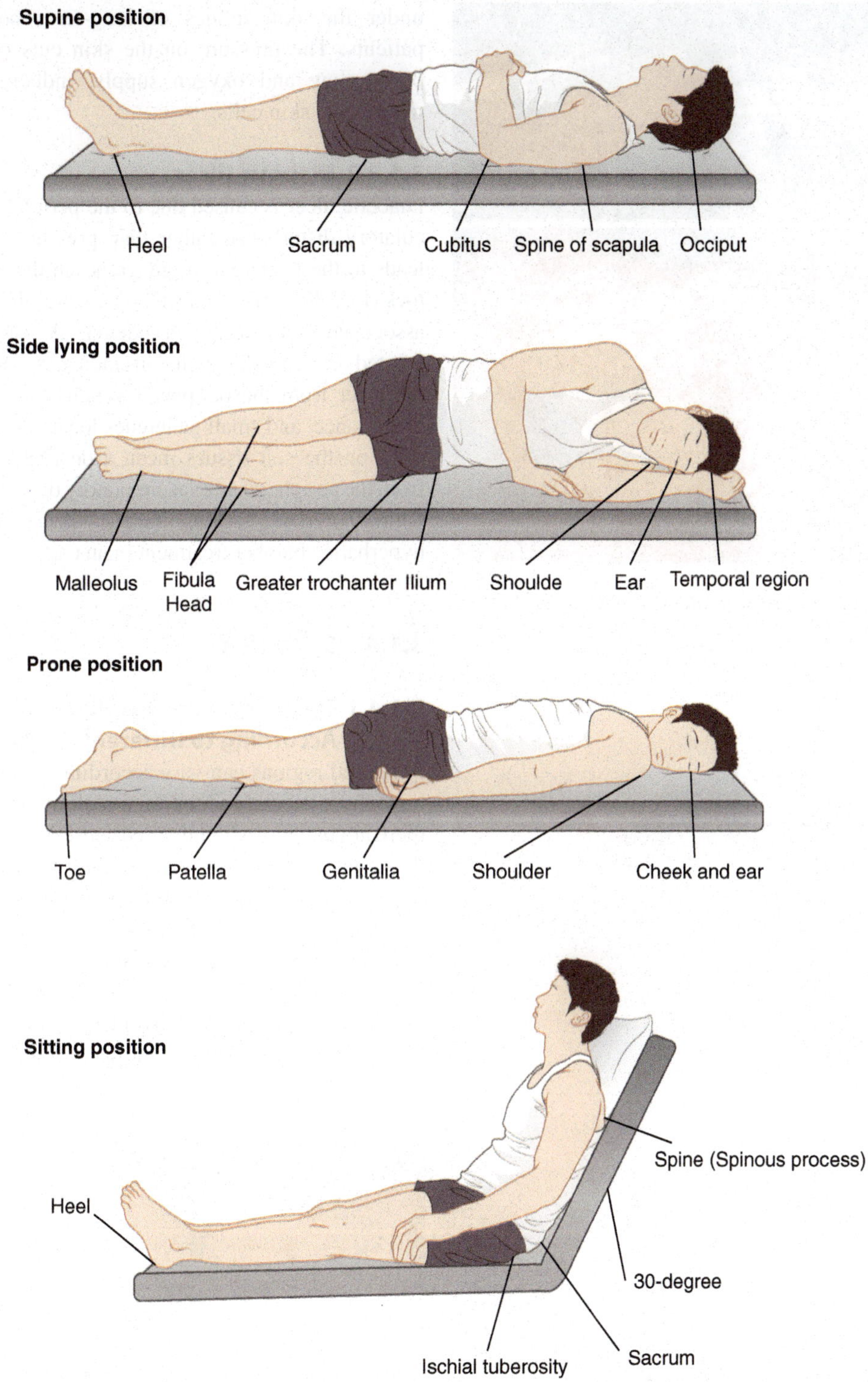

Fig. 3.1 Types of the decubitus ulcers caused by different positions

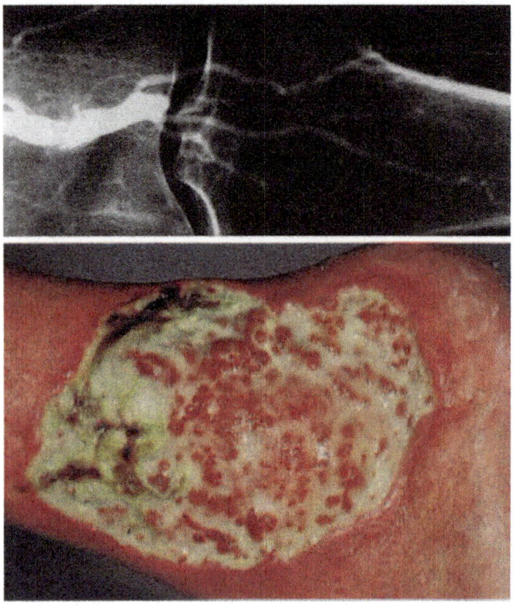

Fig. 3.2 Decubitus ulcer from vasomotor lose

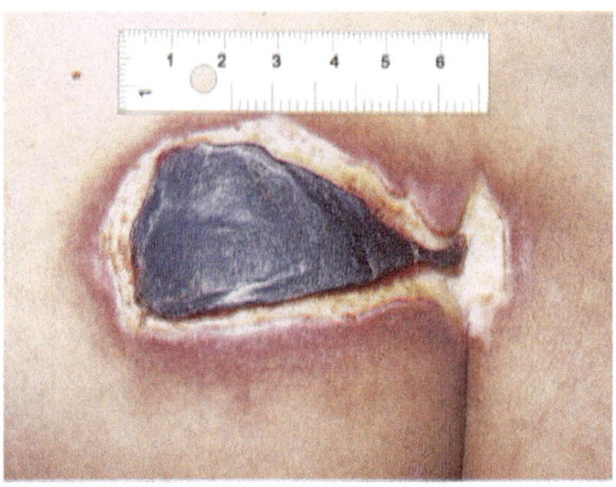

Fig. 3.3 Pressure ulcer

under the skin tissues of long-term bed-rest patients. The pressure on the skin cuts off the blood flow and oxygen supply, inducing the necrosis of skin cells.

3.1.3.2 Diabetic Ulcer

Diabetic ulcer is caused due to the peripheral circulatory disturbance rather than pressure, and it leads to the formation of gangrene on the feet or toes (Fig. 3.4). Most diabetic ulcers are black and associated with localized edema. A gangrene located on the medial malleolus indicates a decubitus ulcer from the peripheral venous circulatory disturbance, and small gangrenes located sporadically on the soft tissues mean a decubitus ulcer from the peripheral arterial circulatory disturbance. Unlike pressure ulcers, diabetic ulcers require hyperbaric chamber treatment in an early stage.

3.1.4 Symptom

3.1.4.1 Types of Decubitus Ulcers According to Different Postures

Pressured regions can vary according to the postures that patients tend to take for a long time, and there are patients with impaired sense of pressure, those who cannot alter their posture themselves, those who lack soft tissues on bony prominence, and those who have difficulties in communication. Therefore, physical therapists should carefully observe the condition of the skin. The predilection sites of decubitus ulcers according to the postures are as follows: the sacrum for supine

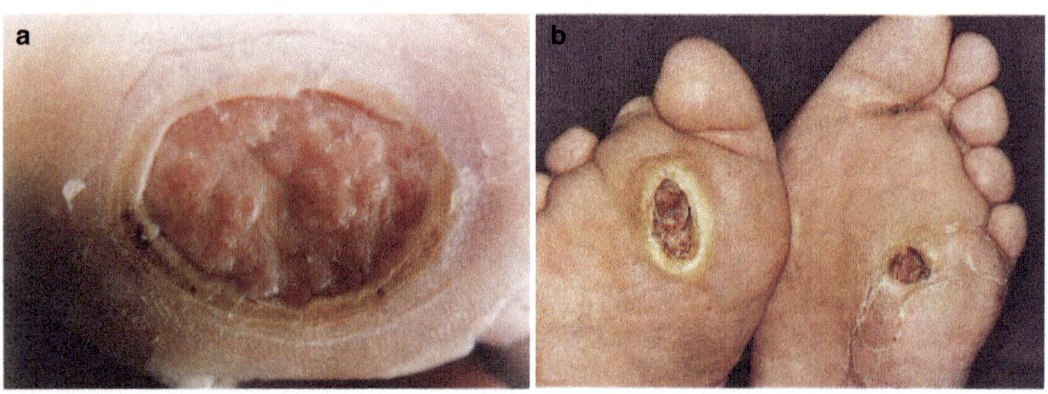

Fig. 3.4 Diabetic ulcer. (**a**) Gangrene of the foot (**b**) Gangrene of the sole

position, the patella for prone position, the fibular head for side-lying position, and the ischial tuberosity for sitting position (Fig. 3.1).

3.1.4.2 Progressive Stages of Decubitus Ulcers

The NPUAP (National Pressure Ulcer Advisory Panel) categorized pressure ulcers into four stages: stage (1) erythema on skin, stage (2) damage to the epidermis and dermis, stage (3) damage to subcutaneous tissue, and stage (4) damage to muscle tissue (Fig. 3.5) (http://www.expertlaw.com/library/mapractice/decubitus_ulcers.html).

3.1.5 Test and Assessment

3.1.5.1 Assessment of Decubitus Ulcer

When physical therapists assess decubitus ulcer, they should check the following ten evaluation factors:

1. After ocular inspection and palpation, record the result.
2. Observe the shape and the color of the tissues adjacent to the decubitus ulcer and record the result.
3. Record the kinds and the amount of the exudate.
4. If it smells, figure out the kinds and the degree of the smell.
5. Check if there are symptoms of inflammation or infection.
6. Examine if there is a trace of being pressured or stimulated.
7. If there is an edema, figure out the location and the degree of it.
8. After recording the location of the decubitus ulcer, measure the size and the depth of it.
9. Take a photograph of the site of the decubitus ulcer.
10. If the decubitus ulcer is caused by a wound (abrasion, penetrating injury, laceration), figure out the kind of it.

3.1.5.2 The Guidelines for Recording

After the assessment of decubitus ulcer is finished, record the result on a PT progress note according to the following ten guidelines:

1. Record the site of the decubitus ulcer.
2. Record the stage of the decubitus ulcer according to NPUAP categories.
3. Measure the size and the depth of the decubitus ulcer and record the result.
4. Assess the depth of the decubitus ulcer tunnel that is under the skin and invisible to the naked eye.
5. Examine the color of the decubitus ulcer (red, yellow, black) and assess the percentage of the decubitus ulcer that is covered on the skin.
6. Record the shape (concentration, viscosity, color) and the amount of the exudate.
7. After cleansing the decubitus ulcer with saline solution, record the smell associated with necrosis.
8. Observe the edema, inflammation, or sclerosis of the tissues adjacent to the decubitus ulcer and record it.
9. Observe the condition (dry, wet, loose, tense, warm) of the skin adjacent to the decubitus ulcer.
10. If there is a pain, record its relevance to the decubitus ulcer and the pain intensity in VAS (visual analog scale).

3.1.5.3 The Assessment Tools for Decubitus Ulcer

Braden Scale

Braden scale is a risk assessment tool made up of six indicators: sensory perception, moisture, activity, mobility, nutrition, and friction. Each indicator is scored 1–4 (1–3 for friction) with total score ranging 6–23. The lower the total score, the higher the risk for decubitus ulcer. As for inpatients, a score of 15–18, a score of 13–14, and a score of 13 or lower indicate low risk, middle risk, and high risk, respectively. In the case of non-patient elderly, a score of 17 or lower indicates high risk of pressure ulcer (Table 3.1).

PUSH Scale

PUSH scale (Pressure Ulcer Scale for Healing scale), developed by the NPUAP, sorts out the pressure ulcer with respect to surface area, exudate, and type of wound tissue, and each category

Stages	Skin changes	Treatment
Stage one	• Skin is in not damaged, but when pressure is removed, erythema does not disappear. • Usually half of the reactive hyperemia appears when circulatory disturbances occur by pressure. Reactive hyperemia must be distinguished from the stage one of a decubitus ulcer 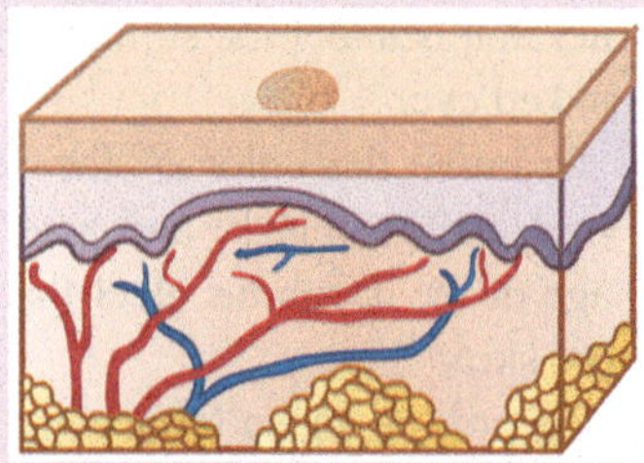	• Pressure relaxation methods Turn over frequently Use tools to relieve pressure Change positions 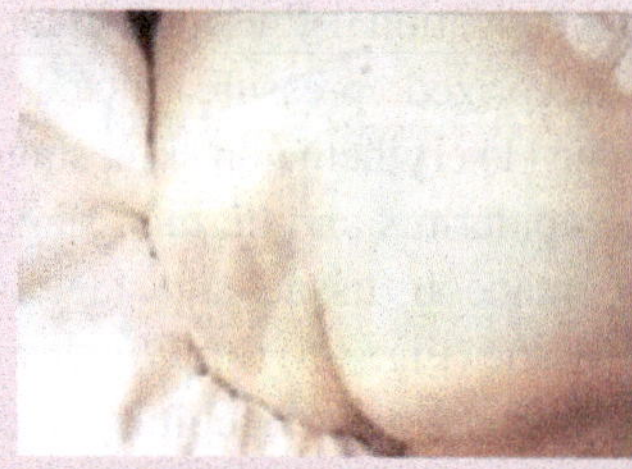
Stage two	• Loss of fragmentary thick skin invaded into the epidermis and dermis. • The Ulcer is superficial, and has abrasion, herpes, and shallow holes. 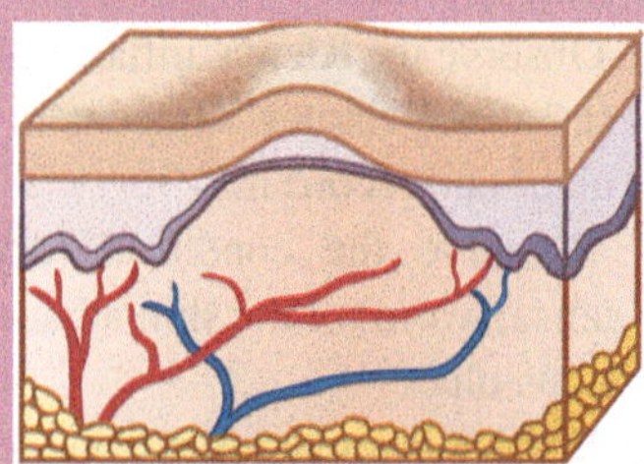	• Keep in a moist environment for treatment • Use normal saline • Gauze dressings (Improve natural therapy and interrupt scab formation) 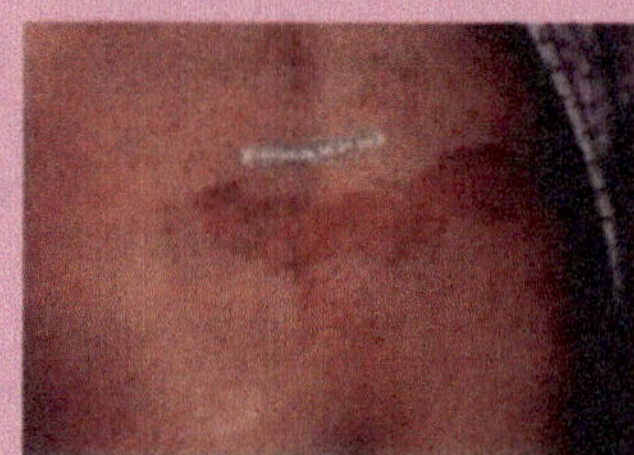
Stage three	• Loss of the fragmentary thick skin with necrotic tissues invaded into the subcutaneous tissue (not into the fascia). • Ulcers are holes in skin but it doesn't affect the central tissues. • Debridement (necrectomy) execution 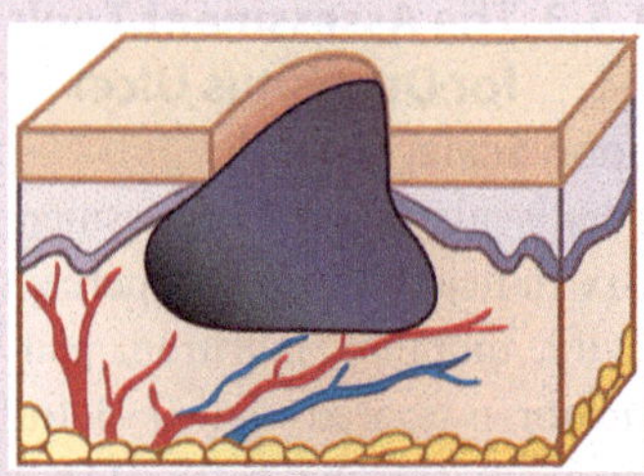	• Debridement (necrectomy) execution Wet dressing Surgical intervention Proteolytic enzyme 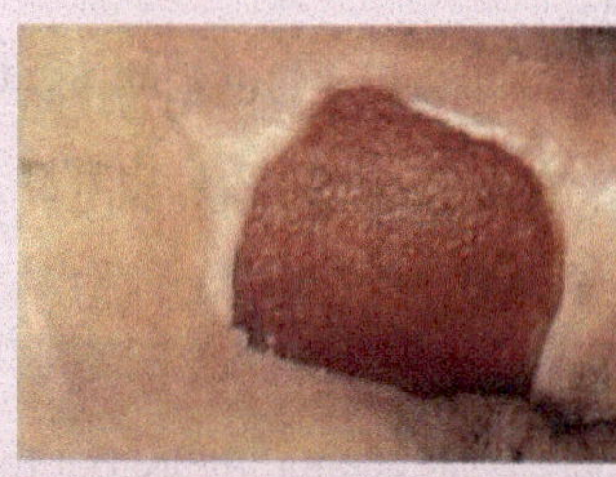
Stage four	• The complete loss of the skin including necrosis and damages muscles, bones, tendons, and joints. • Sinus tract (pupil tract) is a stage four decubitus ulcer 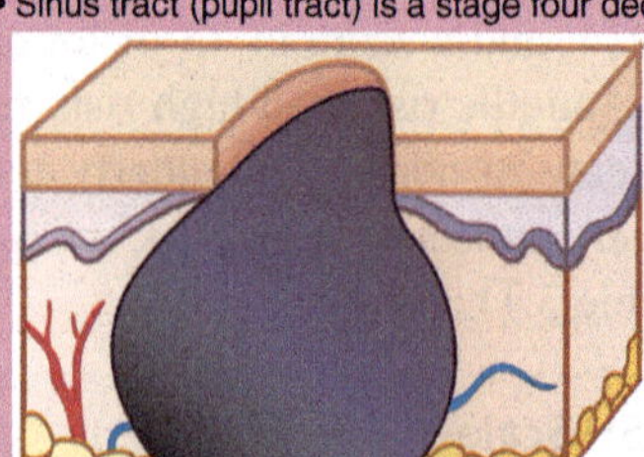	• Noncontact dressing (change every 8–12hours) • Skin graft if necessary 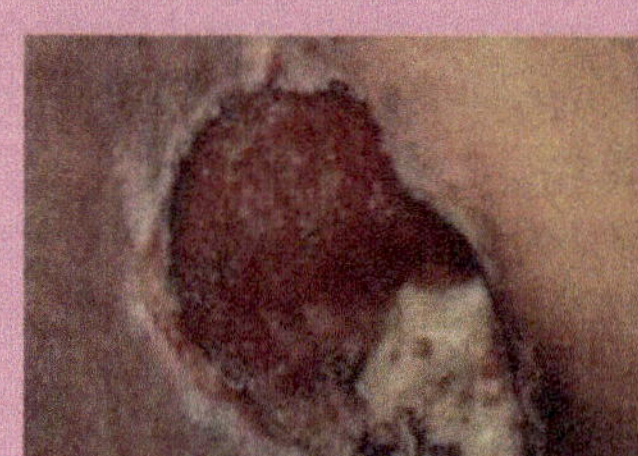

Fig. 3.5 Four stages of decubitus ulcer

Table 3.1 Braden scale (http://www.npuap.org/resources/educational-and-clinicalresources/pressure-ulcer-categorystagingillustrations/)

Braden scale
Patient name ____________________ Assessor name ____________________ Date ________________
Sensation sense
Reaction to discomfort associated with pressure
1. Fully limited
Patients are unable to change the position of the body, arms, and legs without help.
2. Very limited
Patients are able to change the body, arms, and legs slightly but not often and not on their own.
3. Slightly limited
Patients are able to slightly change the position of the body, arms, and legs often.
4. No obstacle
Patients are able to change and control their position.
Wetness
Level of wetness to which the skin is exposed
1. Always wet
The skin is always in wet condition due to sweating and urines. Such wetness can be found every time the patient moves or changes position.
2. Extremely wet
The skin is frequently in wet condition. Bedding should be replaced at least once when the patient changes position.
3. Occasionally wet
The skin is occasionally in wet condition. Bedding should be replaced at least once a day.
4. Rarely wet
The skin is usually in dry condition. Bedding can be replaced on a regular basis.
Activity
Level of physical activity
1. Stuck in the bed
The patient cannot leave the bed.
2. Stuck in the chair
The patient is severely restricted for walking or cannot walk. He/she cannot support his/her weight and/or needs support from the chair or wheelchair.
3. Occasional walk
The patient walks occasionally in a day, but it is possible for only a short distance with/without assistance. He/she spends most of the day in the bed or chair.
4. Frequent walk
The patient walks outside at least two times a day and walks inside at least once in every 2 h.
Mobility
Ability to change and control positions
1. Completely restricted
The patient cannot change positions of his/her body or arms and legs without assistance.
2. Highly restricted
The patient can move his/her upper body or arms and legs a little bit but not frequently or fully.
3. Somewhat restricted
The patient can frequently change his/her body or arms and legs slightly.
4. Not restricted
The patient can change his/her position without assistance.

(continued)

Table 3.1 (continued)

Nutrition
Types of food ingestion
1. Very poor
Patients are unable to finish provided food. Ingesting 1/3 of the provided food is rare. Ingest protein foods (dairy product or meats) less than twice a day. Lack of water. Unable to have liquid food.
2. Not enough
Completing a meal is rare and usually leaves 1/2 of the provided food. Ingest protein foods three times a day and have supplemental foods sometimes; eat less liquid food than the diet requires or take tube feeding.
3. Enough
Eating more than 1/2 of the provided food.
Ingest protein four times a day. Sometimes reject eating but usually eat provided supplemental food; take tube feeding or the total parenteral nutrition.
4. Excellent
Eat all of the provided food for them. Do not reject meals. Usually ingest protein foods more than four times a day; sometimes eat between meals.
Supplement food are not needed.
Frictional force and shearing force
1. Problem
Maximum help needed during the movements. Lifting the body without slips is impossible. Need help to get into the proper position because the patient slips very often. Stiffness, contracture, and swinging can cause a continuous frictional force.
2. Potential problem
Patient moves weakly or minimal help is needed. Skin slips against the seats, chairs, or other apparatus during the movements. Keeping the proper position on chairs and beds for the most part but the body slips sometimes.
3. No problem
Independently moves from a bed and chair and can lift their own body with enough muscular strength. Able to keep the proper position on a bed or chair.
Total: points/23 points

is scored accordingly. The progression of pressure ulcer can be assessed by comparing the total scores (Table 3.2).

Pressure Ulcer Healing Chart

Pressure ulcer healing chart, also developed by the NPUAP, allows to monitor and record trends in PUSH scores over time (Table 3.3).

3.1.5.4 Peripheral Vascular Examination

Decubitus ulcer is associated with gangrene formation by peripheral circulatory disturbance, so physical therapists, before stepping into physical therapy intervention, should examine the peripheral vascular (arterial/venous) circulation of the patients with diabetes.

Peripheral Arterial Examination

The rubor of dependency test evaluates the condition of peripheral arterial circulation. The test is performed by observing the color change of the patient's lower extremity after that is passively elevated and returned (Table 3.4):

① Note the color of the foot while the patient is in the supine position (normal, pink).
② Elevate the patient's leg to an angle of 60°, hold it for 1 min, and observe the color of the lower extremity (abnormal, pink color disappeared).
③ Return the leg to the original position and observe the color (normal, foot color returns to pink in seconds; abnormal, it takes more than 30 s for the color to return).

Table 3.2 PUSH scale pressure ulcer scale for healing, PUSH

PUSH Tool 3.0

Patient name ________________________ Patient number ____________________

Ulcer area ______________________________________ Date ________________________

Method of use

Observe and measure the decubitus ulcer. Describe the surface area, the types of exudates, and wound tissue. Record the sub-score and total score of each measurement. Compare the measured total scores with the decubitus ulcer's treatment period and provide records of the ulcer's state to observe whether it is improving or worsening.

Length × Width (in cm^2)	0 0	1 <0.3	2 0.3 ~ 0.6	3 0.7 ~ 1.0	4 1.1 ~ 2.0	5 2.1 ~ 3.0	Sub-score
		6 3.1 ~ 4.0	7 4.1 ~ 8.0	8 8.1 ~ 12.0	9 12.1 ~ 24.0	10 >24.0	
The amount of exudates	0 No exudate	1 Slight exudate	2 Severe exudate	3 High level of exudate			Sub-score
Type of wound tissue	0 Closed	1 Epithelial tissue	2 Granulation tissue	3 Slough	4 Necrotic tissue		
							Total score

Length × width: measure the longest length and widest width by using a centimeter ruler. Multiply two measured values (length × width) and record the area (cm^2).

Caution: do not estimate the value. Always use a centimeter ruler whenever measuring the size of an ulcer and use the same method at each time.

The amount of exudates: estimate the amount of exudates after removing the dressing and before applying local medicine on the ulcer.

Type of ulcer tissue: it is classified by tissue types on the wound bed. When necrotic tissues are present, the score is four, and when slough is observed without necrotic tissues, the score is three. When the wound is clean and has granulation tissues, the score is two and the reepithelializing shallow wound is a score of one. When the new skin has closed over the wound, its score is zero

4 – Necrotic tissue: black, brown, or yellow brown tissue is strongly attached and it is harder or softer than the surrounding skin.

3 – Slough: yellow and white tissues are thick and lumpy or mucinous if found at the bottom of the ulcer.

2 – Granulation tissue: it is shiny, moist, and granular in appearance. Pink or red tissue is seen.

1 – Epithelial tissue: new pink or moist tissue has grown from the surface of the tissue or the edges of the tissue to become a shallow ulcer.

0 – Closed: the skin covers the wound completely (new skin).

www.npuap.org

11 F

PUSH Tool Version 3.0: 9/15/98

Peripheral Venous Examination

The venous filling time test is used to examine the condition of peripheral venous circulation. It is proceeded by measuring the time taken to fill the emptied veins after the patient's extremity is elevated and returned (Table 3.5):

① While the patient is in the supine position, elevate the patient's lower extremity and hold it for a minute.
② Return the extremity and let it hang off the bed.
③ Note the time taken to fill the emptied veins (normal, filled within 15 s; venous insufficiency, filled within 5 s; arterial insufficiency, takes more than 20 s).

Peripheral Vascular CT Angiography

After injecting the contrast media into the blood vessels, make a visual measurement of the time taken for the intravascular concentration of

Table 3.3 Pressure ulcer healing chart

Pressure ulcer healing chart														
Monitoring PUSH scores of the continuous measurement														
Patient name ______________ Assessor name ______________														
Ulcer area ______________ Date ______________														
Method of use														
Observe and measure the decubitus ulcer with the tools of PUSH provided at regular intervals														
Record the date, the subtotal from the PUSH, and the total score on the pressure ulcer healing chart below														
Date	Ulcer healing record													
Length × Width														
The amount of exudates														
Type of tissue														
Total score of PUSH														
Record total score of PUSH on the pressure ulcer healing chart below														
Total score of PUSH	Ulcer healing graph													
17														
16														
15														
14														
13														
12														
11														
10														
9														
8														
7														
6														
5														

4														
3														
2														
1														
Heal = 0														
Date														
Result analysis														
Record the total score of PUSH on the pressure ulcer healing chart. Create a graph that follows the changing score of the ulcer. If the score is decreased, it means the decubitus ulcer is getting better, and if the score is increased, it means the decubitus ulcer is getting worse														
www.npuap.org														
11 F														
PUSH Tool Version 3.0: 9/15/98														
©National Pressure Ulcer Advisory Panel														

Table 3.4 Rubor of dependency test (http://www.worldburn.org/links.asp)

Test	Result
Pale for 45–60 s → pink recovered	Severe arterial insufficiency
Pale for 30–45 s → pink recovered	Moderate arterial insufficiency
Pale for 25 s → pink recovered	Slight arterial insufficiency

Table 3.5 Venous filling time test result of the venous filling time test

<5 s Venous insufficiency
5–15 s Normal
>20 s Arterial insufficiency

contrast media to reach the maximum peak. This enables the diagnosis of aneurysm or varix caused by decubitus ulcer and the three-dimensional assessment of patency and stenosis (Fig. 3.6).

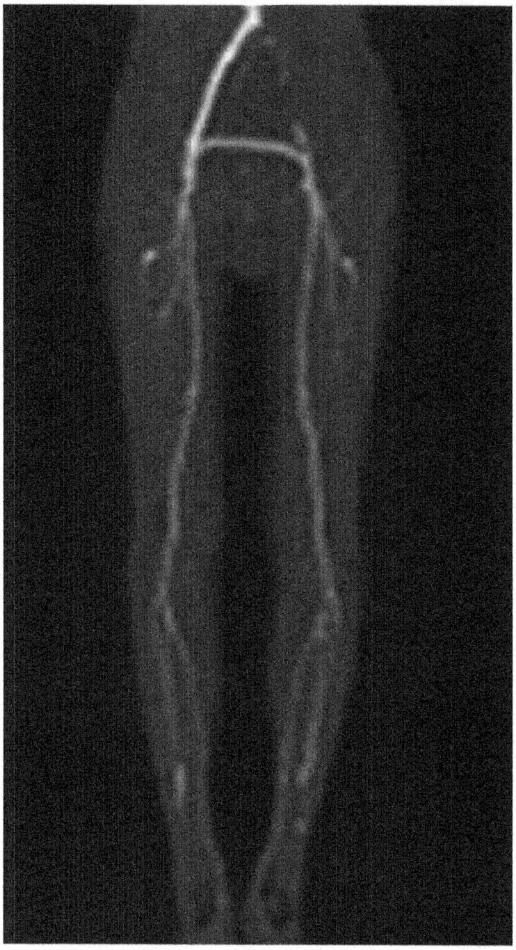

Fig. 3.6 Lower limb's angiography

3.2 Intervention

3.2.1 Intervention

3.2.1.1 Intervention Approach

Physical therapists need to check for the factors that can be signs of a decubitus ulcer (local compression, shearing force and friction, exercise and dysesthesia, deficiency of nutrition, old age, past medical history) and establish a physical therapy program to prevent them. A case at risk of decubitus ulcers requires a team approach between related fields – physical therapists, occupational therapists, dermatologists or surgeons, nurses, nutritionists, social workers, and caretakers. Effective intervention can be achieved through effective communication between team members. It is especially important to educate patients and request them to report to a physical therapist right away if possible symptoms of a decubitus ulcer appear (Kane et al. 2011).

Advices for Physical Therapists

Contact a therapist immediately if one of the following symptoms occurs:

① The ulcers grows.
② The region of decubitus ulcer releases bad odor.
③ The redness becomes worse.
④ Severe pain or edema.
⑤ New wounds.

3.2.1.2 Medical Treatment

The Goal of Decubitus Ulcer Management

Doctor's and physical therapists' goals of decubitus ulcer management are the following.

① Protect the decubitus ulcer and tissue surrounding it to prevent an additional injury.
② Relieve tissue tension surrounding the decubitus ulcer.
③ Protect the area around the decubitus ulcer from epidemiology stress from the patient's activities.
④ Decrease the virus microbes around the decubitus ulcer.
⑤ Improve the process of decubitus ulcer management.
⑥ Prevent new decubitus ulcer formation.

Treatment of Decubitus Ulcer According to Each Stage

1. Stage 1 decubitus ulcer (erythema exists which does not become pale by pressure)

   Remove the factors causing pressure and keep the skin clean. Take action to prevent friction and shear forces.
2. Stages 2 and 3 decubitus ulcer (granulation tissue has been formed without discharge secretion)

   Keep moisture around the decubitus ulcer and protect the tissue from the infection.
3. Stages 2 and 3 decubitus ulcer (granulation tissue has been formed with discharge secretion)

   Keep moisture around the decubitus ulcer, protect the tissue from the infection, and absorb the exudates.
4. Stage 4 decubitus ulcer (necrotic tissue has been formed without discharge secretion)

   Keep moisture around the decubitus ulcer and protect the tissue from the infection. Soften the tissue through debridement.
5. Stage 4 decubitus ulcer (necrotic tissue has been formed with discharge secretion)

   Keep moisture around the decubitus ulcer and protect the tissue from the infection after conducting debridement, and absorb the exudates.

Dressing

Dressing is a basic method treating decubitus ulcer. There are two types of decubitus ulcer dressing: gauze dressing and wet dressing.

① Gauze dressing

By placing dry gauze after sterilizing the ulcer area, the gauze dressing absorbs the exudates and protects the decubitus ulcer by keeping the ulcer area sterilized. However, the gauze dressing does not keep moisture for a long time and does not protect against the infection (Fig. 3.7).

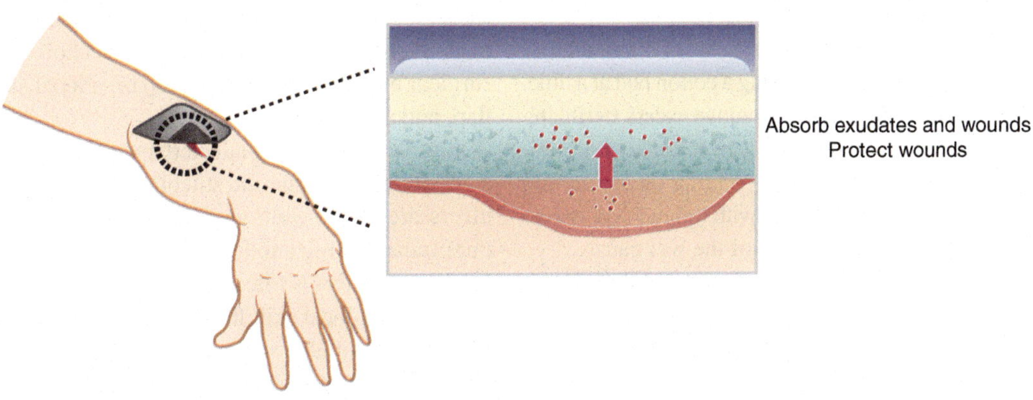

Fig. 3.7 Gauze dressing

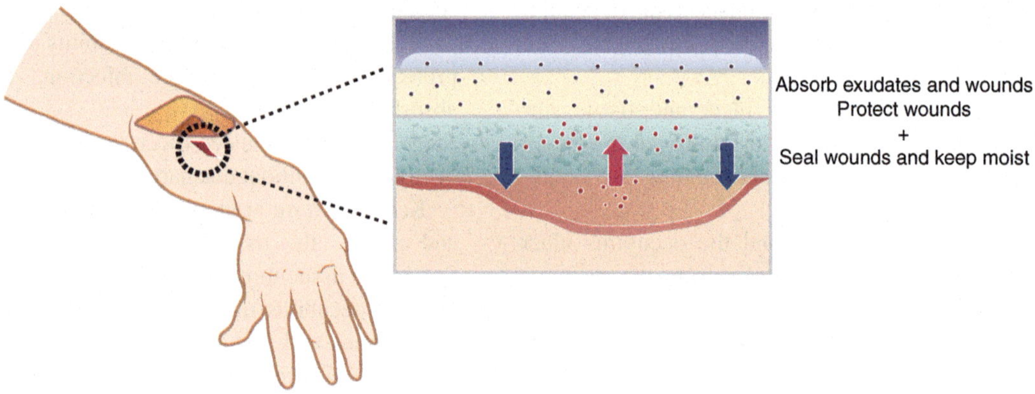

Fig. 3.8 Wet dressing

② Wet dressing

Keeping moisture of the decubitus ulcer area shortens the ulcer's and soft tissue's treatment times and it also helps to prevent scars. Choose a hydrocolloid, hydrogel, or polyurethane dressing depending on the decubitus ulcer's condition (Fig. 3.8).

③ Dressing process

- Prepare dressing materials. Put on disposable gloves and remove the dressing.
- Observe the wound shape as well as the amount and character of any secretions.
- Take off the disposable gloves and wash hands.
- Pour sterilizing solution.
- Soak the 434 gauze with the sterilizing solution.
- Sterilize the ulcer starting from the middle of the decubitus ulcer using a cotton bud at a time.
- Squeeze the gauze to remove excess sterilizing solution, and then put it on the area of decubitus ulcer followed by pressing the gauze into the center of the ulcer with tongue depressors.
- Put 434 gauze on top of the wet gauze.
- Prevent the contamination of decubitus ulcer by using surgical pads or abdomen pads.
- Take off the gloves and fix the dressing with tape or a bandage.

Medicine Treatment

Injecting antibiotics (bacitracin, polysporin, neomycin, etc.) is effective to prevent local infection of the decubitus ulcer. Antiseptic drugs are not recommended for a decubitus ulcer patient because the drugs remain in the body. To use neomycin, it has to be checked if the decubitus ulcer patient has an allergic reaction to it.

Surgical Treatment

If the decubitus ulcer's necrotic tissue is big or treatment is impossible through dressing, then surgery is needed (skin graft, flap). Surgery for decubitus ulcer involves in removing ulcers and infected bone, trimming the protrusion bone, and suturing the skin with healthy tissues. Transplantable tissue should be able to provide an enough bearing capacity and durability. The surgery method is decided by the decubitus ulcer's location, size, and depth. Some choices of surgical methods are a simple repair, a local skin flap, and a free skin flap.

Simple repair is conducted by pulling both sides of normal tissue and stitching them up when ulcers are small. Skin graft is a surgical procedure transplanting another part of the skin to the lesion if the ulcer is filled with granulation tissues (Fig. 3.9). A local skin flap is used to restore the ulcer area through a surgical procedure that takes a healthy flap of the skin tissue from around the decubitus ulcer. A free skin flap is a surgical procedure that takes a healthy flap of the skin from another area of the body and uses it to restore the ulcer area.

3.2.2 Physical Therapy Intervention

3.2.2.1 Postures Preventing Decubitus Ulcers

Posturing

The posturing of decubitus ulcer patients can prevent deformities and complications of decubitus ulcer. As shown in Figs. 3.10, 3.11, 3.12, and 3.13, when a patient is standing in one position for a long time, a pillow or a cushion is used to prevent aggravating the decubitus ulcer by dispersing pressure on the protrusion bones:

① Supine position

Supine position is lying down with shoulders parallel to the hips and straight backbones. Placing a small pillow or a cervical roll under the patient's head is necessary. The height of the pillow should not make the neck and body bend too much or round shoulders.

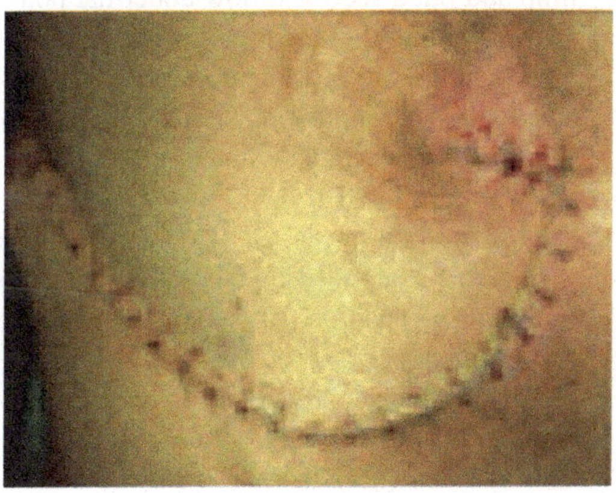

Fig. 3.9 Decubitus ulcer's skin graft

Placing a small cushion under the knees helps to make the patient comfortable and prevent lumbar lordosis. If a cushion is too big, it may cause contracture on the iliopsoas and hamstring so the long time used should be avoided. To disperse the pressure on the heel, a small towel can be used, but it should be used carefully to avoid hyperextension. Don't let the patient's arms fall outside of the bed; put them next to the body or on the chest.

② Prone position

The prone position makes a patient's shoulder and backbone parallel to each other. Patients, who have feelings in their arms or don't have any problem communicating, put their arms next to the body or head. But physical therapists should ask the patents if their arms feel numbness or become insensitive when they are in the prone position for a long period of time. Decubitus ulcer can occur or become worse because of the nerve compression and poor circulation.

When a patient is in prone position, put a small pillow under their head and turn the patient's head to one side or put on table with a hole (table with a head hole; Fig. 3.11). Armrests and face control tables help patients to have a comfortable position because patients can have enough spaces and supports for their heads. This table is used to keep a patient's neck balanced (Fig. 3.12).

Putting a pillow under a patient's stomach can reduce lumbar lordosis. Putting towels under the shoulder increases scapular adduction

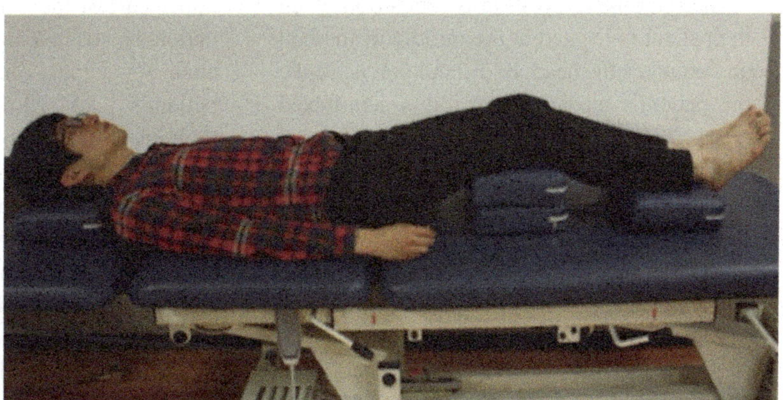

Fig. 3.10 Supine position

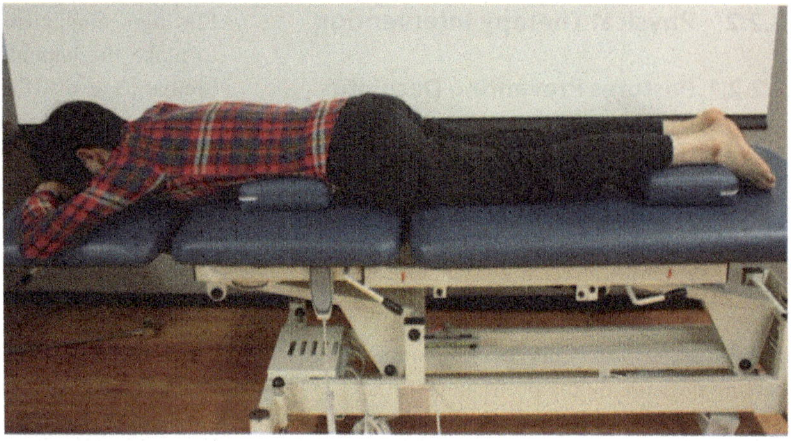

Fig. 3.11 Prone position

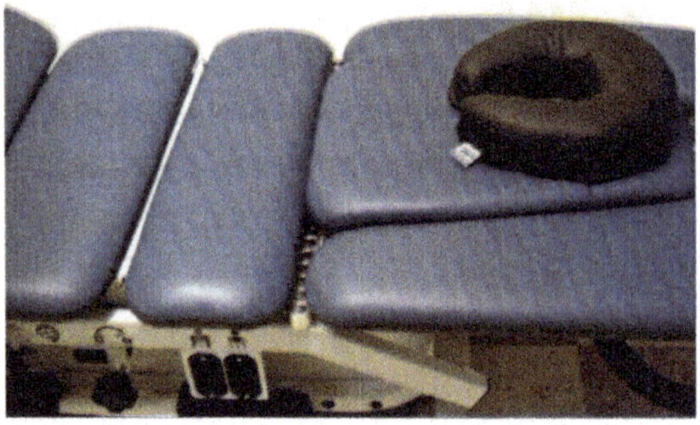

Fig. 3.12 Armrests and face control tables

and protect the humerus head by reducing tension on the adductor canal between the scapulas. Relax the pelvis and lumbar and reduce the hamstring muscle tension by putting a small pillow or a roll under the patient's ankle. But a big pillow may cause the hamstring muscles to contract by bending the knees.

③ Side-lying position

The side-lying position is a position when the patient is located at the middle of the bed and arranges the head, body, and pelvis. Make the patient's hip and knee joints semiflexed (Fig. 3.13). Support the upper legs with a couple of pillows and locate lower legs a little bit to the back. Let the lower part of the legs support the patient's pelvis and lower half of the body. Prevent a patient's upper body from inclining through supporting the brachial with a pillow in front of patient's chest.

Use a safety belt and a thick pillow when the patient can't lie on his side by himself. Increase the body's comfort and safety with the patients arm. If protection is needed under the bony spur concerned with the decubitus ulcer development due to the compression, put a pillow at the distal end of the limb and put a second pillow under the bony spur. Avoiding the direct compression to the bony spur is the most important in a long-term side-lying position. Therefore, side-lying position against something should be considered.

④ Sitting position

A stable chair needs to be used for patients in the sitting position. A patient's foot should rest on the floor or a prop of a wheelchair. The femoral buttocks tissue and deep tissue shouldn't be compressed from the edge of chairs or the wheelchairs. Use more than one pillow when a patient sits against the treatment table and let the patient support the upper part of the body (Fig. 3.14). When the patient has been leaned against the back of the chair for a long time, put a cushion on the patient's back. Move the patient's arms to their knees or onto the armrests. When patients are sitting for a long period of time, make them do push-ups holding the armrests and lifting their hips, move their upper body to the left and right, or bend their upper body every 15 min to relieve hip compression. Using a special wheelchair with a tilt-in-space or a reclining back will be more comfortable (Fig. 3.15).

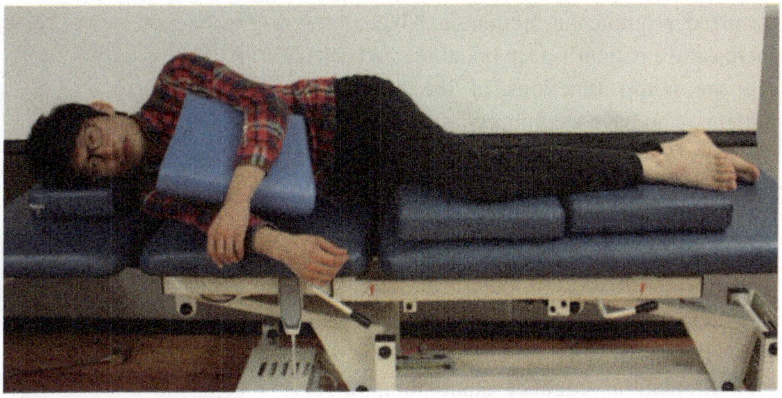

Fig. 3.13 Side-lying position

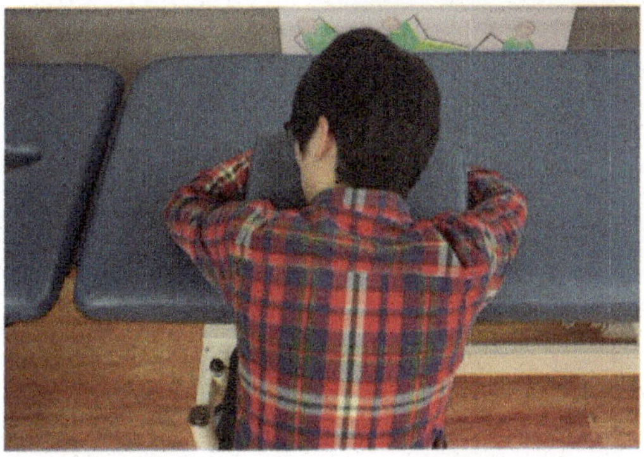

Fig. 3.14 Sitting position that supports the body forward

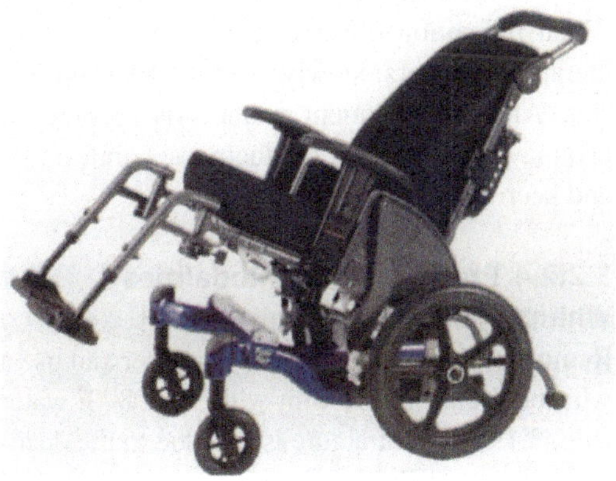

Fig. 3.15 Angle controllable wheelchairs

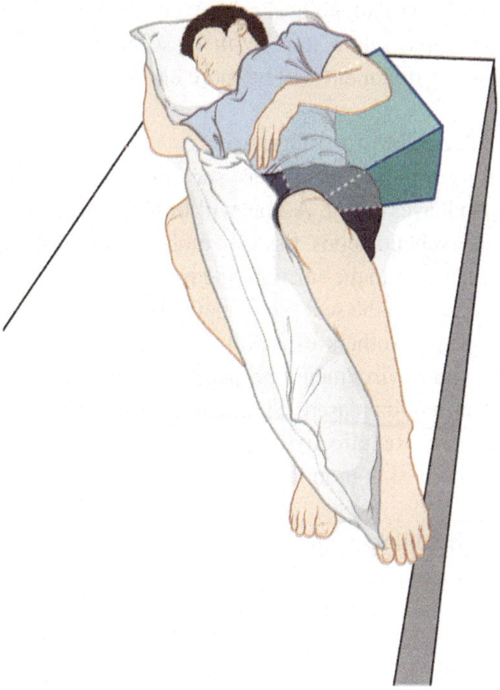

Fig. 3.16 30° angle law

Changing Position

Because the continuous compression is the reason of decubitus ulcers, change position at least every 2 h when a patient is lying down and every 15 min when a patient is sitting. When a patient is lying down on their side (e.g., watching TV), lay down making the body 30° to the floor in any direction following the 30° angle law (Fig. 3.16). Keep a 30° angle of the patient's arms, legs, and even head by using pillows (O'Sullivan and Schmitz 2010).

3.2.2.2 Exercise Therapy

Exercise therapy for decubitus ulcer focuses on aerobic exercise and enhancing peripheral circulation. When a compression decubitus ulcer has occurred, promote the circulation of ulcer through increasing a patient's deep breathing and enhancing the pump functions of the calf muscle. Patients who have a compression decubitus ulcer on their legs should do aerobic exercise, for example, increasing the amount of time they spend exercising by walking on the treadmill or the ground or riding a stationary bicycle for 15 to 40 min. They should do these exercises three or five times a week with the intensity at 60–80 % of their HRmax. When trying to enhance the peripheral circulation, conduct ankle-pumping exercises 20 times a set, and do two or three sets per day. After that, do heel raise exercises ten times a set, three sets a day. With these exercises, the dietary treatment will be more effective.

3.2.2.3 Manual Therapy

A decubitus ulcer surgery such as a skin graft or flap leaves a scar. A scar will limit the epidermis and subcutaneous tissue's mobility through its adherence to the surrounding tissues. It can cause pain inside the scar. Some patients can have more pain than others especially on rainy days or in humid environments because their sensitivity to pain has increased. Skin rolling and scar tissue release are effective ways to relieve pain and increase skin mobility.

Skin Rolling

Physical therapists hold the wounded skin softly with their thumb and index finger and roll it up, down, and diagonally (Fig. 3.17). When a sutured wound is too thick for rolling, hold the skin farthest away from the wound and roll the skin by moving toward the center. Conduct skin rolling in a variety of ways. However, before conducting the skin rolling, remove the skin's oil from the skin of therapist and patient, and keep the area clean.

Scar Tissue Release

Ask the patient which sutured wound is the most sensitive, and press it with the tip of an index finger. The therapists' fingers should turn clockwise and the therapists should continue to ask a patient which sutured wound is the most sensitive. At this point, repeat the scar tissue release to induce a loosening of the tissue through light compression and retrogression of the tissue (Fig. 3.18). Pain and bleeding may occur during this process. When relaxation doesn't occur near the tip of therapists' fingers, slowly remove the compression. After the treatment, patients may feel loose and may want to sleep. Let them rest comfortably and keep them warm with sheets.

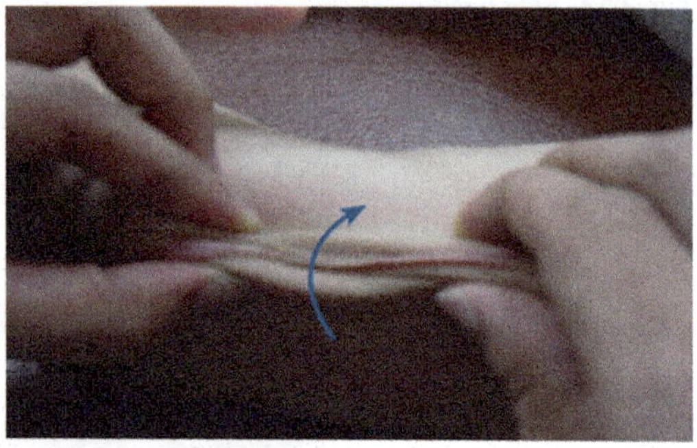

Fig. 3.17 Skin rolling along the stitches of a decubitus ulcer

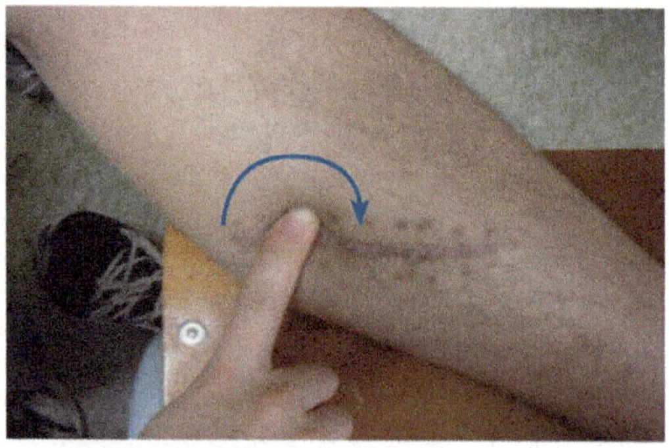

Fig. 3.18 Wounds mobilization

3.2.2.4 Physical Agent Modalities

Whirlpool Bath Treatment

Remove the dressing of decubitus ulcer and use a whirlpool bath for 10 min with 92 ~ 98 °F water (Fig. 3.19). If contracture is bad due to the decubitus ulcer, do light extensional movements and joint motion exercises while in the whirlpool. After the whirlpool bath, clean the ulcer with a physiologic salt solution. The whirlpool bath removes dirty ulcer fragments, bacteria, exudates, and blood residue, reduces pain, and stimulates the decubitus ulcer healing through hydrating the ulcer areas with water. The therapists should wear gloves, a mask, a head cover, and a clean robe to

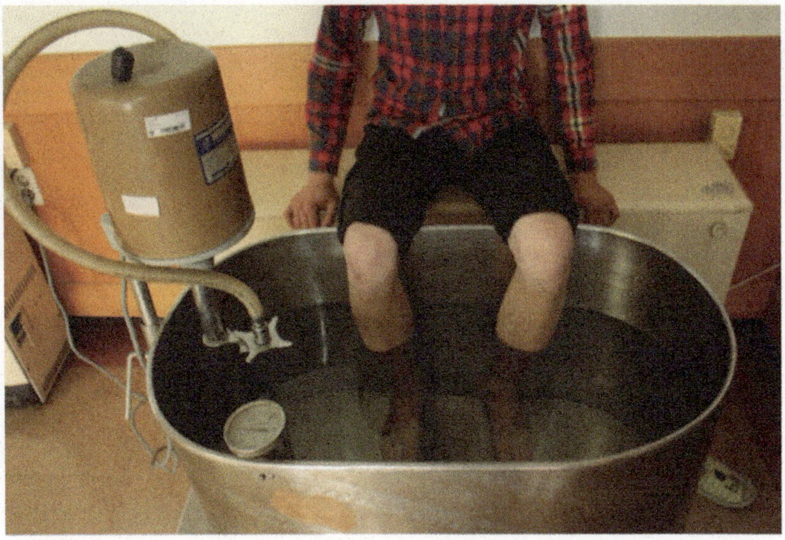

Fig. 3.19 Whirlpool bath for decubitus ulcers on legs

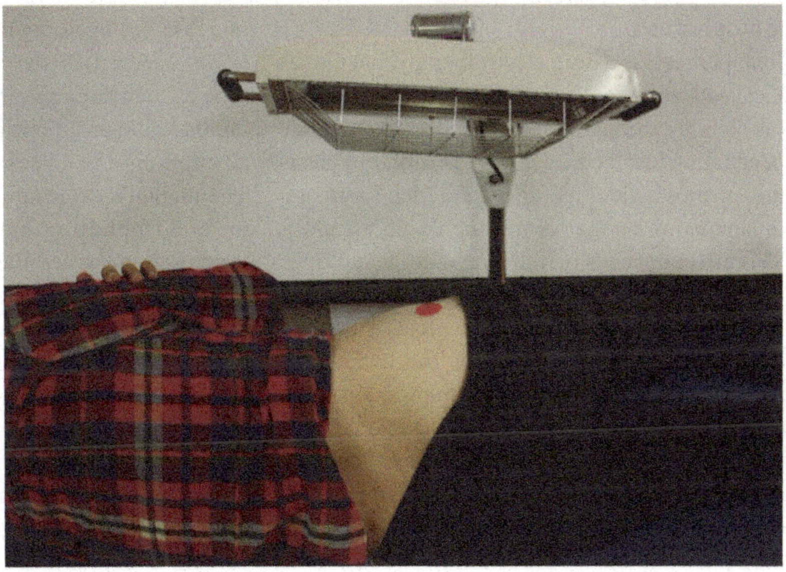

Fig. 3.20 Ultraviolet therapy for a decubitus ulcer

prevent the secondary infection when conducting a whirlpool bath treatment.

Ultraviolet Therapy

Ultraviolet radiation is effective to improve immunity by creating vitamin D while sterilizing the area around the decubitus ulcer (http://www.vitaminmd.co.kr/). Ultraviolet therapy destroys decrepit cells, improve regrowth of cells, and boost treatment for the decubitus ulcer by causing a crust to form on the necrotic tissues. Ultraviolet radiation has three different forms, which are UVA, UVB, and UVC (Fig. 3.20). The shortest wavelength UVC is used in the therapy because UVC stimulates the fibroblast which creates collagen, kills bacteria and viruses, and boosts the transfer of oxygen to the ulcer tissues through expanding the veins. Use an ultraviolet lamp 2 ~ 4 in. away from the area of the decubitus ulcer and start with a 1° erythemal dose for a level 1 ~ 2 ulcer and 2° erythemal for a level 3 ~ 4 ulcer, and gradually increase the dose. The treatment time is determined by the intensity with the distance of the ultraviolet lamp.

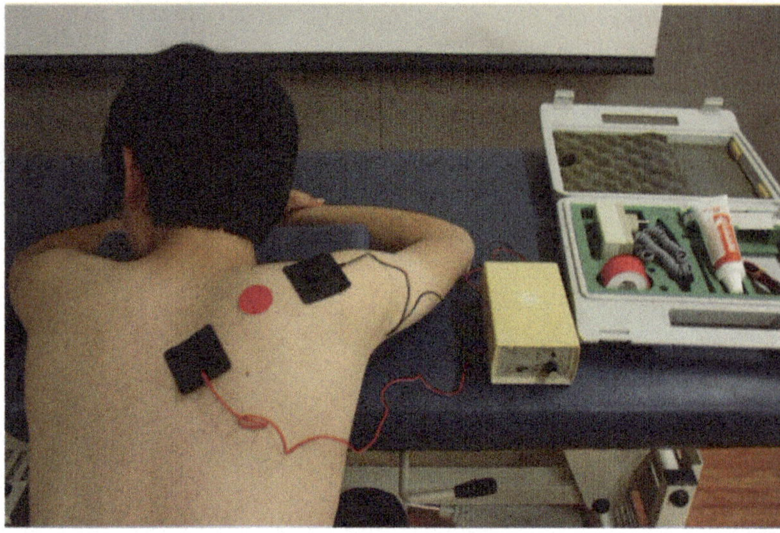

Fig. 3.21 Iontophoresis for a decubitus ulcer

Iontophoresis

Iontophoresis is a drug electrotherapy that passes local activating ions to scar tissues of the decubitus ulcer by using continuous anode and cathode penetrating into the skin (Fig. 3.21). Iontophoresis has an anesthetic effect that can reduce pain and inflammation on the area of the decubitus ulcer. This effect depends on the type of drugs used for the electrode. Using copper for the positive and negative poles has a sterilizing effect, and using dexamethasone and Xylocaine for both poles reduces inflammation. Magnesium boosts the relaxation of the muscles and salicylate reduces the edema. Using an acetate acid cathode degrades calcium deposits, and using a chloride cathode increases skin adhesion. Arrange the drug electrode and the reduction electrode 4–6 in. apart from each other, and determine the treatment time depending on the amount of the drugs and the intensity of the therapy. Usually, it is conducted every other day for 3 weeks. Do not use iontophoresis on insensitive part of the skin or on granulation tissue. Stop immediately if signs of an allergic reaction are shown.

Laser Therapy

Low-strength lasers are effectively demonstrated by animal experiments and clinical trials that they reduce inflammation, increase prostaglandins' concentration, boost ATP creation, increase collagen, and increase fibroblast cells. It also increases the phagocytosis of macrophages, activates the immune system, and promotes cell proliferations by stimulating the absorption of exudates and a diffusion reaction. The methods determining the time and doses of the laser application are as follows. Two types of laser treatment are the contact probe and the noncontact probe application. The contact probe can cause compression on the decubitus ulcer. Therefore, the noncontact probe is used in clinical trials. Using the He-Ne laser (632.8 nm) and infrared laser (904 nm) at the same time showed positive effects. The energy density of 4 J/cm^2 placed about 15 ~ 20 cm away from the decubitus ulcer with the right angle is applied for 15 min every day, for 4–6 weeks (Fig. 3.22). After the laser treatment, dress the wound and sterilize the ulcer to prevent the secondary infections.

3.2.3 Prevention and Management

3.2.3.1 Diabetic Ulcer

① Prevent a decubitus ulcer through clean foot care.

② Wear customized shoes to prevent toe pressure and deformity.

③ Wear layered socks to reduce frictional force.

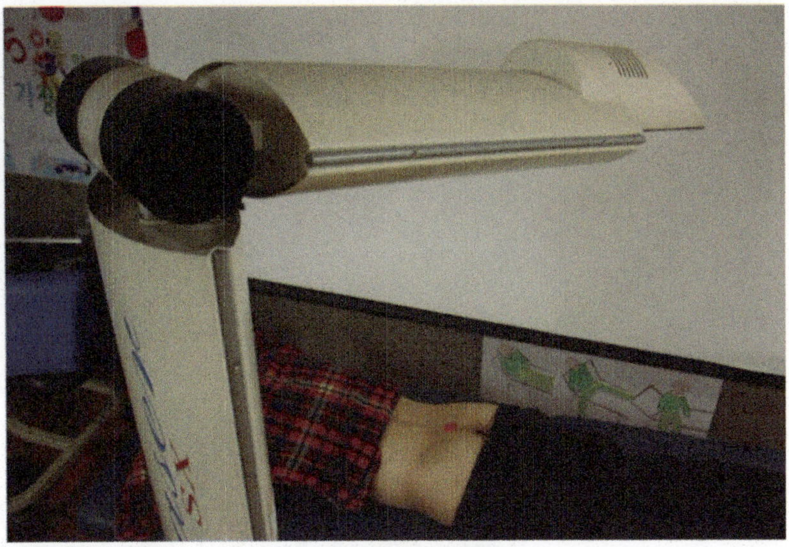

Fig. 3.22 Laser treatment for a decubitus ulcer (He-Ne laser)

④ Educate the patients so they can prevent peripheral neuropathy through controlling their blood glucose.

⑤ Increase muscular strength and bloodstream flow through regular exercise (aerobic exercise, endurance training, and progressive resistance exercise) to improve their balance and ability to walk.

⑥ Lose weight by dietary treatment to remove weight from the patient's legs.

3.2.3.2 Pressure Ulcer

① Remove the pressure of the protruding bones through the use of a pillow or a cushion.

② Educate the patient to change positions every 2 h [e.g., position change, lift their bottom on a wheelchair, lift their pelvis in a supine position, or lift their body from a sitting position (Fig. 3.23)].

③ Disperse the pressure through the use of an air mattress or a water mattress.

④ Protect the area of bone protrusions by using joint guards and bandages.

⑤ Take care to not make abrasions on a patient's skins when changing the mattress sheets or a patient's position.

⑥ Establish the early mobilization programs and practices.

3.2.3.3 Management (Maki and Mallroy 2000)

① Reduce the pressure on the areas of bone protrusion which can easily form a decubitus ulcer.

② Establish a program to change the patient's position and practices.

③ Provide enough nutrients and liquids.

④ Practice movements and an exercise program at an early stage.

⑤ Boost the new tissue regeneration through debridement.

⑥ Keep the skin clean.

⑦ Maintain the urogenital organs clean after urination and defecation when a patient has a urinary incontinence or fecal incontinence.

⑧ Sterilize and dress the ulcer area regularly.

⑨ Educate the patients and caretakers on how to manage decubitus ulcer.

⑩ Establish a decubitus ulcer prevention program.

3.2.3.4 Patient/Carer Education

Communication (Myers 2011)

① The cure for decubitus ulcer requires a team approach and the communication among patients/carers, dermatologists, surgeons, physical therapists, occupational therapists, nurses, and dietitians.

Fig. 3.23 Lifting the body from a sitting position

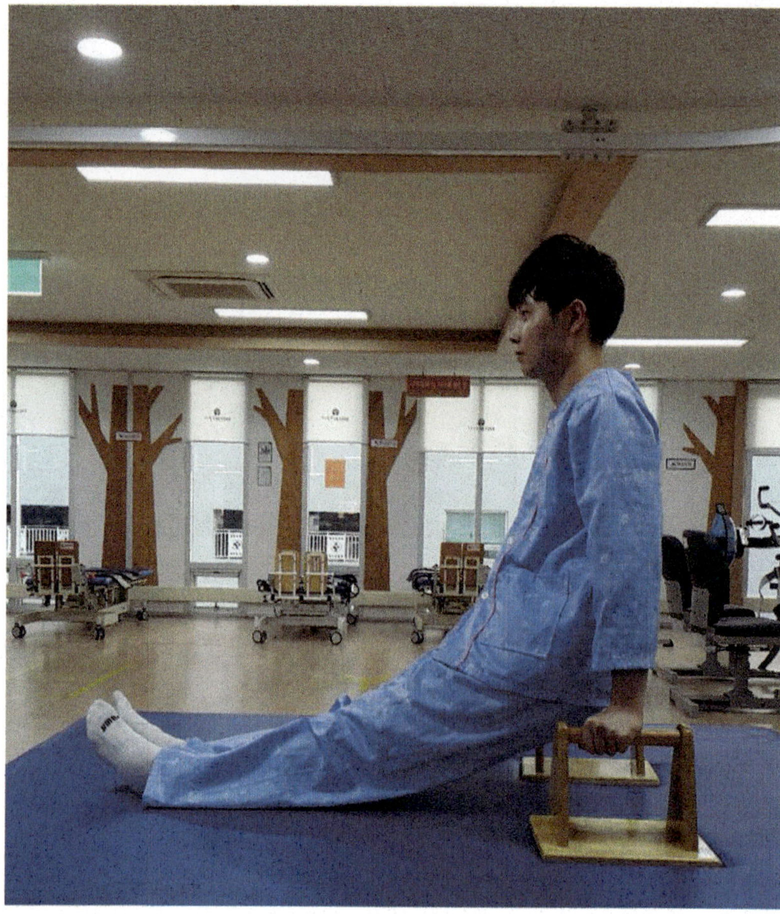

Table 3.6 How to prevent frictional and shearing force

① Prevent the skin from pulling along when moving the body.
② Do not let the head (pillow) lifted.
③ Avoid pressure on protruded bones.
④ Place a cushion under the heel.
⑤ Do not lie with bedsores or rebufaction parts facing the bed.
⑥ Lift up the body once in every 15 min in a sitting position.

② The contents of the communication include altering the posture of patients, moving manners, factors of pressure, dressing, removing methods of necrotic tissues, skin care, and prevention.

③ Patients/carers should be provided with the information concerning medical supplies from the government and social workers.

④ Patients/carers should be aware of the importance of early mobilization in curing decubitus ulcer.

The Items of the Training

① The systematic methods for the skin checkup (particularly insensitive regions and protruding bone regions)

② The observation of erythema with a mirror

③ The appropriate manners of moving and altering the postures

④ The ways to avoid friction and shear (Table 3.6)

⑤ The ways to manage urinary/fecal incontinence

⑥ The skin care methods (sanitizer/diaper/moisturizer/dressing)

Advices for Physical Therapists

❶ Physical therapists hold an important role because they provide professional advices about therapy intervention, a decubitus ulcer's management, proper positioning, and early mobility.

❷ Record the assessment of the decubitus ulcer using the Braden scale which was referred to earlier, and be sensitive with the ulcer's changes and evaluate the decubitus ulcer at least every month. The therapists must observe the patient for risk factors that lead to the occurrence of a decubitus ulcer, whether a patient can change their position, and also check around the patient for anything stopping them from changing positions.

❸ Advise patients to keep their skin clean and dry especially those that are suffering from urinary incontinence, diarrhea, or constipation. Check for possibility of skin contact with excretions. Recommend patients to use urine and feces' collector to prevent skin maceration which can be caused by urinary reflux.

❹ Pressure and frictional forces should be minimized against the skin while washing or showering. Checking the soaps' ingredient is important because some soaps have alcoholic ingredients that can cause festering or pain.

❺ Physical therapists must clean their hands after a physical therapy intervention and wear protective equipment (masks, gloves, etc.) to protect patients they have direct contact with. All treatment equipment must be sterilized after use and disposable equipment must be thrown away.

3.3 Problem Solving

3.3.1 Decubitus Ulcer

Choose the best method for a physical therapy intervention.

Question 1

Patient A is 55-year-old man who suffers from obesity and was diagnosed with diabetes 8 years ago. He had the tip of his right big toe amputated 2 years ago. Blisters and infections have appeared under his amputated toe 6 days ago. What test must be used before using a physical therapy intervention?

1. Blood sugar test
2. Blood pressure test
3. Pulse test
4. Vital capacity test
5. Peripheral vascular vessel test

Question 2

Patient A is a 53-year-old overweight woman who was diagnosed with diabetes. A decubitus ulcer has appeared on the tip of her left big toe 6 months ago. She was recommended physical therapy 2 weeks ago due to fragments of the ulcer and exudates having a heavy odor from the putrefaction of germs and blood. What physical therapy intervention is needed to remove this ulcer?

1. Iontophoresis
2. Ultraviolet therapy
3. Scar tissue release
4. Aerobic exercise
5. Whirlpool bath

Question 3

Patient A is 36-year-old man who has paraplegia and spends a lot of time sitting in a wheelchair. His hips are in pain, and blister and erythema have occurred on his ischial tuberosity. What management method is right to reduce this skin wound?

1. Change positions
2. Using a water bed
3. Wearing joint guards
4. Lifting pelvis from a lying down position
5. Lifting hips with spread elbows.

Question 4

A decubitus ulcer has occurred on both of person A's heels. The therapist removed the gauze and put person A in a whirlpool bath for 10 min. What is the purpose of the whirlpool bath?

1. Strengthen muscles
2. Expedite muscle relaxation
3. Anti-amyotrophia
4. Remove necrotic tissue
5. Improve joint range

Question 5

Person A is suffering from a diabetic ulcer on his foot. What physical therapy intervention should be used to prevent the ulcer?

1. Warm foot bath
2. Strengthen foot muscles
3. Increase pressure on the foot
4. Apply slight pressure to the foot
5. Disperse pressure on the foot by using cushions

Answers

Question 1-⑤, Question 2-⑤, Question 3-⑤, Question 4-④, Question 5-⑤

References

Charette SI et al. Muscle hypertrophy responses to resistance training in older women. J Appl Physio. 6th ed. 2012.

Kane RI, Ouslander JS, Abrass IB. Essentials of clinical geriatrics. 3rd ed. New York: McGraw-Hill; 2011.

Maki BE, Mcllroy WE. Tailoring teaching to the elderly in home care. Worcester: Home Health Q. Clin Geriatr Med; 2000.

Myers BA. Wound management: principles and practice. New Jersey: Pearson Education, Inc; 2011.

O'Sullivan SB, Schmitz TJ. Physical rehabilitation. 4th ed. Postural control in the adult, Philadelphia: FA Davis; 2010.

Reference Sites

Hansol Hearth Care (Vitaminmd). http://www.vitaminmd.co.kr/.

International Society for Burn Injuries. http://www.worldburn.org/links.asp.

Medical data for burns (Seoul Bestian Medical Center specialized in burn treatment). http://www.ibestian.com/02_burn/burn06_02.asp.

National Pressure Ulcer Advisory Panel. http://www.npuap.org/resources/educational-and-clinical-resources/pressure-ulcer-categorystaging-illustrations/.

Pressure ulcer information and related sites. http://www.expertlaw.com/library/malpractice/decubitus_ulcers.html.

Burn

4

Han Shin Jeong

> **ICD-10 Code**
> *T20-T32 Burns and corrosions*
> T20-T25 Burns and corrosions of external body surface, specified by site
> T26-T28 Burns and corrosions confined to the eye and internal organs
> T29-T32 Burns and corrosions of multiple and unspecified body regions

Learning Outcomes
After completing this chapter, you should be able to do the following:

- Explain the definition and causes of burn.
- Estimate the depth and range of burn.
- Describe the clinical symptoms of burn.
- Perform prevention and first aid.
- Perform physical therapy intervention.

Key Terms
Eschar
Pressure garment
% total body surface area, % TBSA
Intensive care unit
Skin graft
Scar tissue
Inhalation burn

H.S. Jeong
Professor, Department of Physical Therapy, Kunjang University College, Gunsan, South Korea
e-mail: hsjung@kunjang.ac.kr

4.1 Burn Injuries

4.1.1 Overview

Burn is the phenomenon that skin cells are destructed or necrotized by heat sources. In addition to the burns caused by heat sources, hot water, friction by hot objects, high-voltage electricity, various chemicals, the toxic gases, carbon monoxide, and even the damage of the airway caused by exhaust fumes fall into the category of burns in a broad sense.

In the United States, approximately more than 2 million of burn victims are reported every year, and approximately 6000 people among those 2 million of burn victims die of burn and burn complications (Delisa 1998).

As the appropriate medical treatment is provided to the burn victims at an early stage and the medical science has been developed, the treatment for burn victims has improved, and it contributes for steady improvement of survival rate and quality of life.

For these improvements, the therapeutic team approach, by a variety of medical fields for the recovery of burn victims' medical, functional, and sociopsychological functions, is needed (Braddom 2000).

J.-W. Park, D.-I. Jung (eds.), *Integumentary Physical Therapy*, DOI 10.1007/978-3-662-47380-1_4

4.1.2 Causes

4.1.2.1 Hot Fluid Burn

Hot fluid burn is caused by hot liquids (water, oil, etc.) or hot steam. Hot fluid burns are mainly second-degree burns and often occur in young children or elder people.

The course of the treatment varies depending on the contamination range of the fluid.

4.1.2.2 Flame Burn

Flame burn is caused by fire or gas explosion. It mainly breaks out in confined areas in industrial sites or at home. And the burn victims are mostly damaged by the flame, and the depth of the damage is severe. In flame burns, serious damage to the respiratory system is caused by inhalation of the gas accompanying the flame.

4.1.2.3 Electrical Burn

Electrical burn is caused by exposure to high-voltage electricity. It is mostly caused by electrical shock in the industrial sites, and electrical burn induces serious damage to internal organs.

4.1.2.4 Chemical Burn

Chemical burn is caused by the contact with acid, alkali, and other toxins. The severity of damage varies depending on the nature of the chemical, concentration, and the duration of the contact.

4.1.2.5 Contact Burn

Contact burn is caused by the direct contact with a hot grill, cooking utensils, electric iron, electric blanket, or play equipment exposed to the sunlight for a long time.

The damaged area is topical but most of the contact burns lead to the second-degree deep lamella burn.

4.1.2.6 Inhalation Burn

Inhalation burn is caused by breathing in high-temperature heat directly or inhaling carbon monoxide or harmful combustion substances directly.

When inhaling toxic gases produced from harmful combustion substances, airway resistance increases due to bronchoconstriction.

As a function of the cilia in the airway mucosa is degraded, and alveoli are necrotized, the series of respiratory failure symptom that air ventilation is declined, namely, the pulmonary edema, is induced. Also, the mortality rate of inhalation burn is very high due to respiratory failure and high risk of secondary infection (Ko and Kang 2009).

4.1.3 Classification

4.1.3.1 First-Degree Burn

First-degree burn or superficial burn refers to the burn that only the epidermis is damaged, and it is commonly caused by sunburn. First-degree burn does not involve blisters but the skin is rubified and inflamed, and it is accompanied with pain after the skin damage. It is then accompanied with a slight headache, but it will be healed in 3–10 days without leaving a scar unless there's inflammation (Fig. 4.1).

4.1.3.2 Second-Degree Burn

Second-degree burn or partial-thickness burn is classified into second-degree superficial burn (or partial-thickness superficial burn) and second-degree deep burn (or partial-thickness deep burn) depending on whether the entire epidermis and dermis are damaged or some part of the epidermis and dermis are damaged.

Second-degree superficial burn refers to the burn that the epidermis and the papillary layer of the dermis are damaged, and it involves blisters, erythema, edema, and pain, and it takes about 1–3 weeks to be healed, whereas second-degree deep burn refers to the burn which the entire epidermis and dermis are damaged, in other words, even the reticular layer is damaged as well as the papillary layer.

In the case of second-degree deep burn, formed blisters are destroyed and the burnt area is red or white. Hypoesthesia and pain may be accompanied and it takes about 3–5 weeks to be healed (Fig. 4.2).

4.1.3.3 Third-Degree Burn

Third-degree burn or full-thickness burn refers to the burn that the damage reaches to full thickness of the skin, i.e., epidermis, dermis, and subcutaneous tissue.

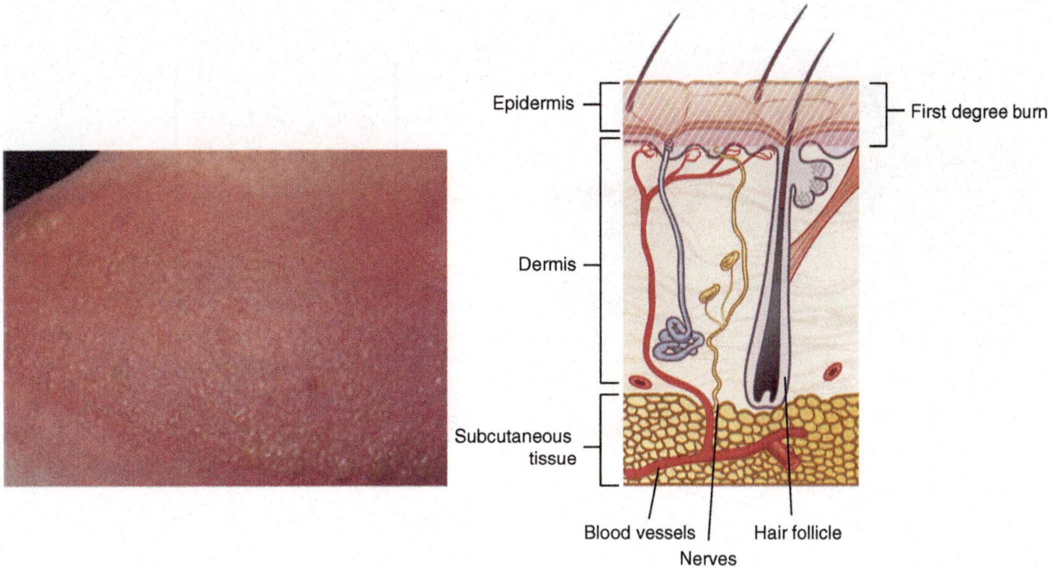

Fig. 4.1 First-degree burn

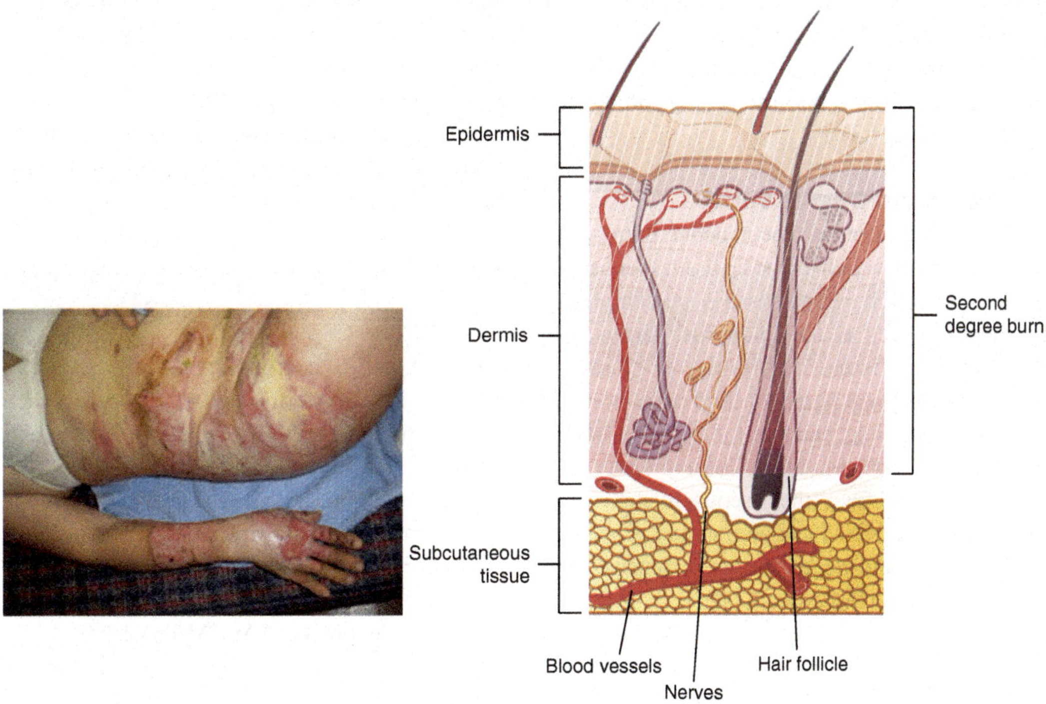

Fig. 4.2 Second-degree burn

The burnt area is white or brown due to the blood clot and becomes hard and dry like dried leather. As nerves are damaged, the patient cannot feel any pain and the skin becomes insensible. In addition, eschar is formed due to necrotic skin tissues, and necrotic skin tissues are naturally eliminated after 2–3 weeks.

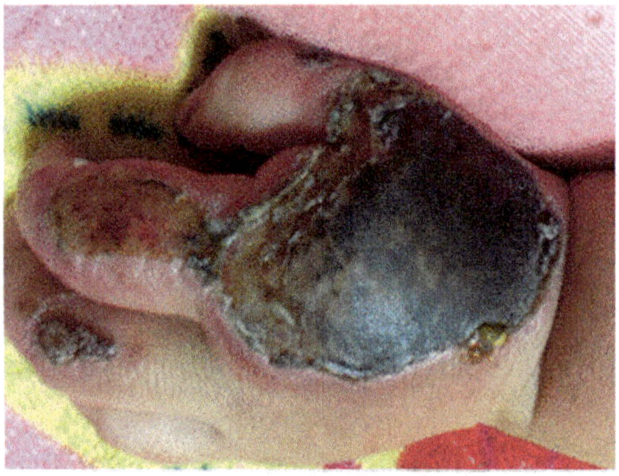

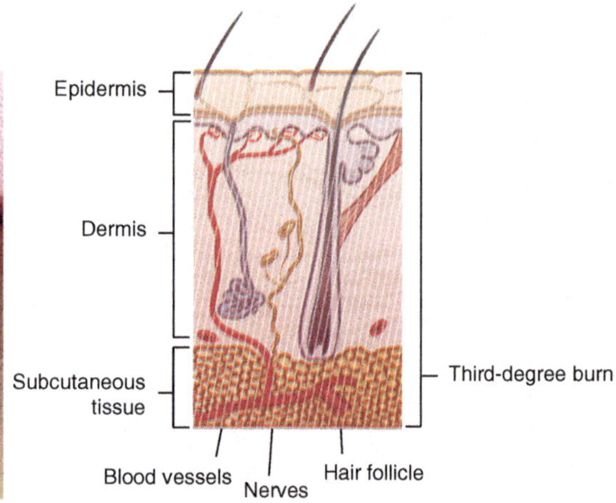

Fig. 4.3 Third-degree burn

If the treatment is appropriate, skin tissues will be regenerated; thereby, the wound can be healed. However, since skin regeneration function has been destroyed, skin graft is required for extensive wound treatment.

For third-degree burn patients, shock is the most important issue because of large amount of water loss (Fig. 4.3).

4.1.3.4 Fourth-Degree Burn

Fourth-degree burn or subcutaneous burn refers to the burn in which adipose tissues, muscles, tendons, and even osseous tissues are completely destroyed as well as the epidermis, dermis, and subcutaneous tissue. Fourth-degree burn is caused by electrical burn, hot fluid burn, or flame burn for a long time, and the skin becomes barren and dry as it gets burnt black like a mummy.

The damage affects the osseous, so sometimes the bones are exposed and amputation is needed.

To treat fourth-degree burns, extensive skin graft is required (Braddom 2000).

4.1.4 Test and Assessment

The assessment of the extent of the body damage caused by burn is very important in the treatment and prognosis, and it is determined by the percentage of total body surface area (% total body surface area, % TBSA) (Ahn et al. 2009; Braddom 2000).

4.1.4.1 Rule of Nines

It is general to assess the damaged skin area caused by burns according to the rule of nines which is designed by Pulaski and Tennison. This method is preferred to assess the damaged skin area for adult patients, and the method expresses skin area as 9 % or multiple of 9.

In this assessment method, damaged body surface area is assessed by calculating 9 % for the head and neck, 18 % for the front body, 18 % for the back side of the body, 9 % for each arm, 18 % for each leg, and 1 % for the genitals (Fig. 4.4).

4.1.4.2 Lund-Browder Chart

Assessing the damaged skin area in accordance with the rule of nines is simple and convenient, but there is a problem on its accuracy.

The rule of nines is not proper to apply to children for assessment of damaged skin area because children's skin distribution is different from the adults and also skin development state is behind the adults (Feldman and MacMillan 1980).

The Lund-Browder chart is a method of assessing damaged skin surface area in consideration of the growth and development state of the body from children to adults.

Particularly, they are subdivided into the upper limb and lower limb to assess damaged skin surface areas, so the upper limb is subdivided into the arm, forearm, and hand and the lower limb is

Fig. 4.4 Rule of nines

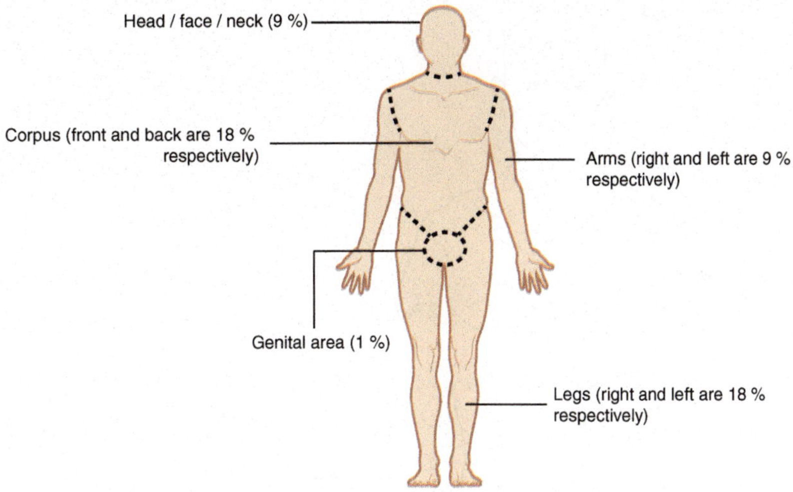

Table 4.1 Lund and Browder chart

Region	0–1 year old	1–4 year old	5–9 year old	10–14 year old	15 year old	Adult
Head	19	17	13	11	9	7
Neck	2	2	2	2	2	2
Corpus (front)	13	13	13	13	13	13
Corpus (back)	13	13	13	13	13	13
Buttock (right)	2.5	2.5	2.5	2.5	2.5	2.5
Buttock (left)	2.5	2.5	2.5	2.5	2.5	2.5
Genitals	1	1	1	1	1	1
Upper arm (right)	4	4	4	4	4	4
Upper arm (left)	4	4	4	4	4	4
Forearm (right)	3	3	3	3	3	3
Forearm (left)	3	3	3	3	3	3
Hand (right)	2.5	2.5	2.5	2.5	2.5	2.5
Hand (left)	2.5	2.5	2.5	2.5	2.5	2.5
Thigh (right)	5.5	6.5	8	8.5	9	9.5
Thigh (left)	5.5	6.5	8	8.5	9	9.5
Lower leg (right)	5	5	5.5	6	6.5	7
Lower leg (left)	5	5	5.5	6	6.5	7
Foot (right)	3.5	3.5	3.5	3.5	3.5	3.5
Foot (left)	3.5	3.5	3.5	3.5	3.5	3.5

subdivided into the thigh, lower leg, and foot (Table 4.1, Fig. 4.5).

4.1.4.3 American Burn Association Classification

When assessing a burn patient, age of the patient, burn area, and the cause of the burn should be fully considered as well as the depth and the area of the burn. The American Burn Association has classified burns into minor burn, moderate burn, and major burn depending on severity of the burn (area, depth, and site of the burn), the type of the burn, and the age and also has provided treatment plans accordingly (Table 4.2).

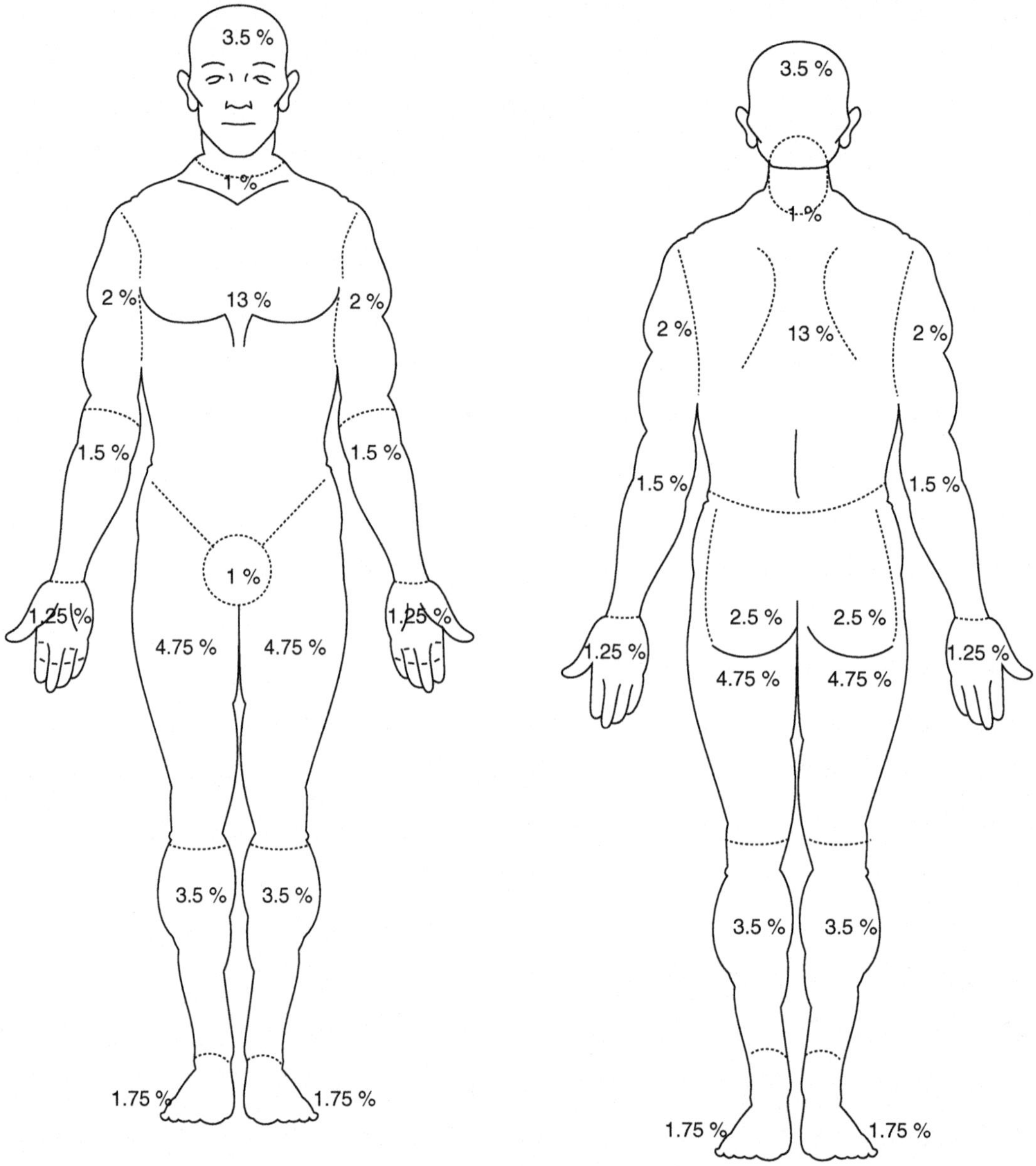

Fig. 4.5 Body surface area caused by burn according to Lund and Browder chart (for adults)

4.1.5 Symptoms

The severity of symptoms may vary depending on the temperature of heat source, duration of the application of heat, and thermal conductivity of the tissue.

The higher the temperature of heat source and the longer the duration of the application of heat, the more severe the symptoms are. With regard to thermal conductivity of the tissue, the symptoms vary depending on the thermolysis abilities such as water content of the tissue, with or without natural secretion, the extent of pigmentation, thickness of the skin, and blood flow of the regional tissue.

Table 4.2 Burn treatment criteria classified by the American Burn Association

Extent of the burn	Classification	Treatment guidelines
Mild	The burn less than 10 % of the total body surface area (adult) The burn less than 5 % of the total body surface area (children, elderly) Full-thickness burn of less than 2 % of the total body surface area	Out-patient care
Moderate	The burn with 10–20 % of the total body surface area (adult) The burn with 5–10 % of the total body surface area (children, elderly) Full-thickness burn with 2–5 % of the total body surface area Electrical burn Inhalation burn is suspected The burns enclosing the entire body or limbs and legs Hospitalizing when accompanying with susceptible diseases (such as diabetes)	In-patient care
Severe	The burn more than 20 % of the total body surface area (adult) The burn more than 20 % of the total body surface area (children, elderly) Full-thickness burns with more than 5 % of the total body surface area Electrical burn Inhalation burn Burns on the face, eyes, ears, and genitals If the major injuries such as fracture are being accompanied	Intensive care unit

4.1.5.1 Pathophysiological Symptoms During Different Recovery Stages

Shock Phase

Burn victims may fall on shock over 2 to 3 days after a burn. As the symptoms in this phase, the ratio of blood cells including red blood cells is increased, whereas plasma volume is decreased. Therefore, blood becomes more viscous, and it leads to decreased blood circulation and cardiac output and increased heart rate (Harden and Luster 1991).

Eschar Detachment Phase

The skin of the burn is replaced with eschar and it begins to be detached after 3–4 weeks. In case of first-degree burn or second-degree superficial burn, the burn begins to be healed from the bottom layers of the skin naturally, but second-degree deep burn or third- to fourth-degree burn requires surgical treatment such as skin graft.

Healing Phase

First-degree burn or second-degree superficial burn is healed to normal without any burnt mark, but scar tissues can be formed in some cases.

However, second-degree deep burn or third- to fourth-degree burn requires skin graft or surgical treatment which might take over several weeks or several years.

4.1.5.2 Systematic Symptoms

Symptoms on the Skin

The skin functions as a barrier to prevent loss of heat and water from the body and also has defensive mechanisms to prevent pathogen invasion from outside of the body. However, such functions of the skin will be destroyed as a result of burns.

Whereas the normal person's water loss through the skin is approximately 15 mL/m^2 a day, the amount of water loss from full-thickness burn patient reaches up to 200 mL/m^2 a day. In addition, pathogen invasion through the burnt wound occurs easily; in particular, the eschar which is formed in full-thickness burn is the pathway of the pathogenic bacterial invasion.

Symptoms on the Blood and Cardiovascular System

Capillary permeability is sharply increased due to the damage caused by the burn, and as a result, the blood flow rate is significantly reduced, whereas the amount of interstitial fluid is increased.

Only a small amount of intercellular fluid comes out from the body through the burn wound, but due to a large amount of water and protein lost from the blood vessels around the burn, edema caused by interstitial fluid is resulted.

In case of the major burns, plasma loss is increased compared to loss of red blood cells immediately after a burn, and hemoconcentration consequently takes a place. Due to the hemoconcentration, blood circulation is declined, and it leads to a failure of oxygen supply to tissue. Therefore, cardiac output drops in the early days of the burn because of increased resistance in the peripheral blood vessels, decreased blood flow, and increased blood viscosity. Furthermore, decreased blood flow and declined cardiac output cause hypovolemia and urinary frequency in severe burns. If it is more developed in an untreated state, it leads to acute renal failure.

Symptoms on the Circulatory and Immune Systems

The initial shock phase of the burn typically lasts about 48 h. After the shock phase, it is turning into catabolism state in which the tissue breaks down until the wound caused by burn is completely covered. A lot of energy is consumed because of the tissue catabolism. This results in a large amount of water evaporation through the wound on the burn and the heat loss accordingly. For protein, in addition to the loss of protein through the wound and the loss of protein due to increased capillary permeability of the tissue around the wound, nitrogen emission through the urine is increased. For carbohydrates, glycogenolysis in the liver is increased due to epinephrine secretion, and glycogenesis is also increased due to the increased glucocorticoid, and hyperglycemia and acidosis appear. In addition, there is change in immunologic function; therefore, the frequency of infection and extent of hypofunction vary depending on the degree and the depth of the burn. However, in the case of severe burn in which TBSA is over 50 %, the risk is very high.

4.1.5.3 Systemic Symptoms

Symptoms in Shock Phase

For the burn patients, preventing the shock caused by the burn is more important than anything else. Systemic symptoms in the shock phase are restlessness, paleness, coldness, sweating, and thirst. And symptoms in cardiac and respiratory systems include decrease in blood pressure, tachycardia, cyanosis, and respiratory failure.

Symptoms After the Shock Phase

After the shock phase, the symptoms such as pain, decrease in range of motion, and failure appear because eschar is detached and wound tissue is formed. In addition, amputation of the arm or leg may be needed in some cases due to the burn. Also the patient may suffer from dysfunction of the hands, severe trauma, or being placed in the state of socially handicapped.

4.1.6 Prognosis and Complication

4.1.6.1 Prognosis

The age of the patient, percentage of total burn surface area (% TBSA), and inhalation burn influence the prognosis of burn patients. The prognosis of the elders over 70 years old and children below 10 years old is poorer than others. And the burn patients who are over 20 % of TBSA must be treated in the intensive care unit. In the case of inhalation burn patients caused by the burn on the face, their morality rate is higher.

The survival rate of the burn patients can be estimated with the following formula:

The probability of survival (%) 5 100 2 (age, 1, % of the total damaged skin surface).

However, this formula does not apply to children below 10 years old.

4.1.6.2 Complication

Hypertrophic scars, joint contracture, amputation, photosensitivity, and pruritus are the complications that occur secondarily to the burn patient. These complications cause serious dysfunction and social and psychological problems to the burn patients; therefore, a lot of difficulties are incurred to the patient, family, and even to the community.

Hypertrophic Scar

Hypertrophic scar commonly occurs to the burn patients who have second-degree deep burn or severe burns, and it refers that the scar becomes thicker and projected in the process the wound is being recovered.

This is aesthetically ugly and very itchy, and it causes severe discomfort due to pain. It is red in an early stage but it turns into blackish red and hard as it develops.

Burn patients start to have a hypertrophic scar from 1 to 2 weeks later as the wound becomes healed and lasts up to 2 years, and if left untreated, it can last permanently so the secondary skin contracture or joint contracture can be caused.

To soften the hypertrophic scar which is incurred during the recovery of the wounds, ultrasound treatment is effective.

Contracture

As hypertrophic scar develops, it may cause skin or joint contracture secondary to the burn patients who suffer from the second-degree deep burn or severe burns.

At this time, stretching should be applied to maintain or extend the range of motion, and it is effective to perform the heat treatments such as paraffin bath or infrared before stretching.

Amputation

Amputation is often implemented to the burn patients who get severe burn such as third-degree burn or high-voltage electrical burn because nerves, blood vessels, and even osseous tissues including the skin are damaged and the recovery is impossible.

Amputation to the burn patients often incurs the problems if the patients are with prosthetics because skin condition of the patients is not good. Skin peeled off can be caused easily even with low friction, and heterotrophic ossification can occur at the distal joint and near the cut end.

Photosensitivity

Second-degree deep burn patients have an abnormal skin reaction to sunlight. Melanogenesis continues over 6 months after the burn, and melanization lasts up to 2–3 years after the burn. At this time, the burn can be discolored due to the exposure to sunlight; thus, it is important to block the sunlight so that the burn is not exposed through wearing long sleeves or a hat.

4.1.6.3 Pruritus

Pruritus is the complication that appears to most burn patients; it lasts about 6 month to 2 years after the burn. The burn site becomes dry due to destroyed sebaceous glands, and it causes pruritus. But the more serious problem is that the patients scratch the wound severely because of itchiness, and it badly deteriorates the wound and prolongs the recovery period. In order to minimize the complications, applying oil regularly to prevent skin from drying and constant skin care such as taking antihistamine agents or implementing desensitization treatments are needed.

4.2 Intervention

4.2.1 Intervention

4.2.1.1 Intervention Approach

According to the extent of the damage caused by the burn, the patients who can be cured through ambulatory care normally have mild symptoms. In the case of an adult, patients who have the burn which depth of the burn is partial thick and area of the burn is below 10 % of TBSA fall into this category. In the case of full-thickness burns, the patients who have below 2 % of TBSA burn can have ambulatory care for both adults and children. However, burn patients who have more severe than the cases above (moderate or severe burn patients) must have a professional medical care in the hospital (Helm et al. 1982).

4.2.1.2 Medical Treatment

Emergency Care

① Remove the cause of the burn and isolate the patient from the cause. If the burn area is wide or if the patient has the burn on the face, hand, and foot or around the anus, ask for help from a medical team.

② Cut out the clothes on the burn; however, if the clothes are stuck on the burn, do not remove the clothes by force. Especially when removing the metallic stuffs such as wristwatch or ring, one should care not to cause secondary damages.

③ Cover the burn with sterile gauze or a clean cloth. Damp gauze or cloth also can be used depending on the state of the burn.

④ Do not apply unascertained medicine (creams, ointments, or any other similar medicines). This may cause the secondary infection and can make the recovery process difficult.

⑤ In case of chemical burns, dilute the chemical by applying running water sufficiently. At this time, be careful that the chemical is not transferred to other parts of the body.

⑥ While being prepared to carry the patient to the hospital where manages the burn patients professionally, observe carefully whether the symptoms such as shock, respiratory disorder, or trauma occur to the patient or not.

Fluid Therapy

Fluid therapy is absolutely necessary to prevent the shock because water loss is sharply increased in the early days of the burn. Fluid therapy must be started if damaged area is over 20 % of TBSA.

Wound Treatment

The purpose of wound treatment caused by the burn is to prevent infections and to have less secondary damages so that the treatment duration can be shortened by helping the healing of the wound and also dysfunction and deformity can be lessen as much as possible. In case of first-degree burns and second-degree burns, clean and dress the wounded areas to prevent infection. And in case of third-degree burns and fourth-degree burns, the early excision of necrotized tissues and skin graft are needed to cover the wounds.

Nutrition Supply

For burn patients, nutrition supply is very important. Nutritional imbalance may arise due to an excessive amount of nitric acid loss and declined nitrogen intakes. Resistance to infection of malnourished patients becomes weak, and their crust separation and wound healing period are prolonged. In case of severe burn patients who cannot swallow the food, feed them protein and high-calorie food mainly using the Levin tube.

4.2.1.3 Surgical Treatment

Burn Plastic Surgery

Primarily, burn plastic surgery prevents hypertrophic scars caused by the burn which is formed as a burn injury becomes larger in order to make the scars smaller as much as possible. Secondarily, it is performed to recover the appearance and to eliminate the dysfunction by eliminating contracture scars caused by hypertrophic scars (Fig. 4.6).

Necrotized Tissue Debridement

The treatment that can effectively heal the burn by removing the necrotized tissue on the wound caused by a burn is the necrotized tissue debridement.

There are three ways in necrotized tissue debridement. The first way is the surgical way that removes adhesive tissue directly using surgical knives or scissors. The second way is mechanical method that removes necrotized tissue through pressure irrigation, water therapy, and stimulation of electrical therapy. The third method is autolysis that efficiently removes the wound of a small area using an enzyme. In order to remove the necrotic tissue more effectively to improve the skin condition of the patient, a nutritional support such as albumin or protein helps in healing of the wound.

Skin Graft

Skin graft is implemented to cure the area where burns, torn wounds, ulceration, and pressure sore occur. It is the only medical treatment method that can close the open wounds. For major burn

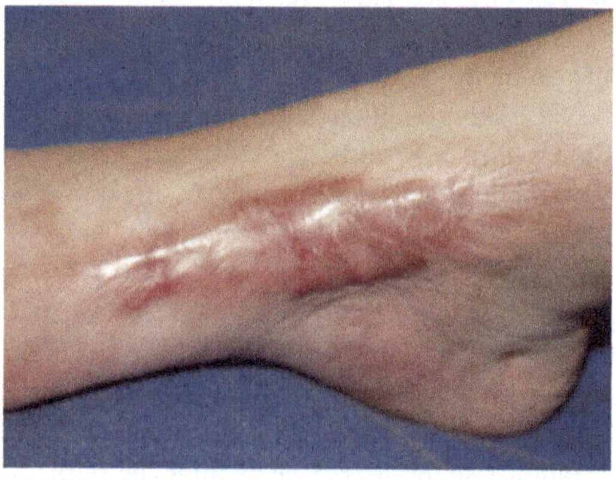

Fig. 4.6 Hypertrophic scars caused by burns

patients who are suffering from third- or fourth-degree burns, it is better to implement skin graft as early as the eschar is separated, and it is essential for full-thickness burn patients whose wound's diameter is larger than 2 cm. However, the skin graft is needed in some cases if the wound is on the face, neck, armpit, knees, hands, or feet even though the damaged area is small.

4.2.2 Physical Therapy Intervention

The purpose of physical therapy for burn patients is to restore the lost function and to help them to return to a normal life. To achieve these purposes, preventing the infections by keeping the wound clean for the recovery of the wounds and skin graft and controlling edema and pains should be prioritized. In addition, it should help the patients to obtain independency in their daily activities such as walking by promoting improvement of joint movable range, strength, and endurance and by preventing the complications of the respiratory system. An active intervention is required for the physical therapy after discharged from the hospital and the surgery as well as the physical therapy for the hospitalized patients.

4.2.2.1 Wound Treatment

Damaged skin due to the burn is treated using the sterilized sponge or gauze. For regeneration of epithelial cells, place the dry sterilized gauze on the burn for 7–10 days. At this time, bland soap can be used if necessary to clean effusion or used medicines, but the most effective way is the mechanical method contacting the burn with running water. And the burn area must be wrapped with sterilized dry net clothes, which stimulates the growth of granulation tissue and also helps to make the new granulation tissue area flat.

4.2.2.2 Edema Treatment

Locate the burn higher than the heart in order to reduce edema. It helps to make the injured burn area soft and flexible and also to be kept in a leveled state. Applying the heat, massage, or pressure on the injured area using the elastic bandage or a face mask during healing period can mitigate the edema.

4.2.2.3 Positioning

In order to prevent contracture and maintain the functional posture, it is very important to adopt a correct posture from the beginning. The patients who have the burn on the face should adopt half-lying position to prevent edema; the patients who have the burn on the front part of the neck should assume the supine position and maintain extension state by placing the pillows under the neck and shoulder joints to prevent contracture of the head and the trunk (Fig. 4.7) (Fader 1985). In case of the patients who have burns on the shoulder joints, assume the positions and maintain those positions such as abduction, flexion, and lateral rotation. The patients who have burns on elbow joint areas should maintain the positions of extension and supination (Fig. 4.8) (Hurlin et al. 2002). And the burn patients who have burns around the wrist joint and hand areas should assume the functional hand position by doing wrist joint extension, MP joint flexion, IP joint extension, and thumb abduction and then wrap each finger in a gauze individually (Figs. 4.9 and 4.10) (Fess and Philips 1987). Also the patients who have a burn on knee joint area maintain the position of extension, and the patients who have a burn on the ankle joint and foot area raise the entire leg by maintaining mid-position or dorsiflexion position (Table 4.3).

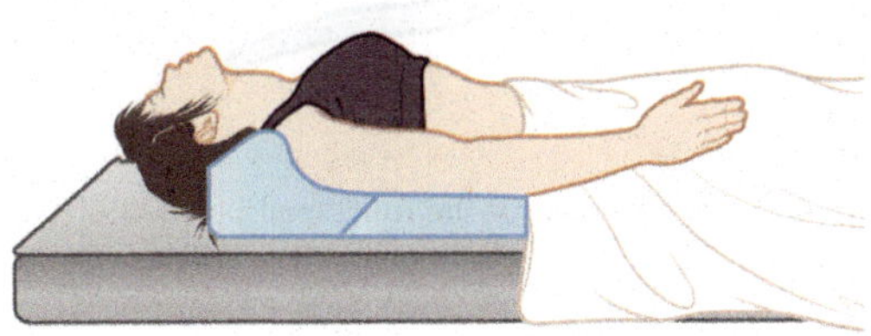

Fig. 4.7 The position for the burn patients on the neck

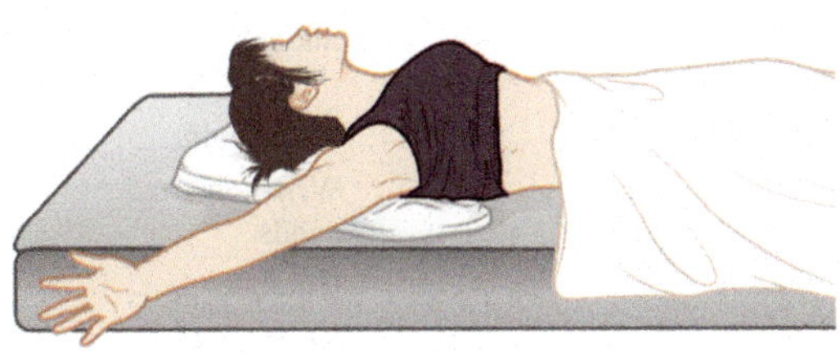

Fig. 4.8 The position for the burn patients on shoulder joint area

4.2.2.4 Physical Agent Modalities

Hydrotherapy is often used because it has the burn wound healing, pain control, and tissue releasing and calming effects.

Whirlpool bath is a partial immersion bath and is applied to the patients who have the burn on the arm or the leg. It is applied for 20 min in 40 °C water, and the mechanical pressure generated from the stirrer of whirlpool bath helps in healing wounds (Fig. 4.11).

Hubbard tank is a full-immersion bath and is applied to the patients who suffer from extensive burn including the corpus. It is applied for 15 min in 38 °C water, and in addition to the effects of whirlpool bath, a strength exercise and the joint motion exercise utilizing the buoyancy of water are effective (Fig. 4.12).

Contrast bath is effective for healing the wound, and boosting metabolism due to the mobility of blood vessels on the arms and legs is boosted as immersing the burn area in the hot and cold water alternately. For the application of contrast bath, use hot and cold water by spells which is about 45 °C and 15 °C, respectively, and start and finish the treatment in hot water (Fig. 4.13).

Paraffin bath (paraffin bath) is the treatment agency that facilitates heat application of the stereoscopic injured area such as the hand and foot. Apply the paraffin mixture in which paraffin and oil are mixed in the ratio of 7:3 and be maintained to be 50 to 52 °C to the injured area

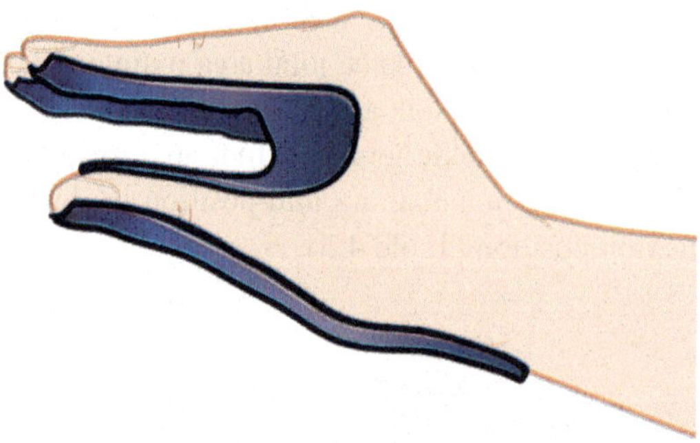

Fig. 4.9 The position for the functional position of the hands

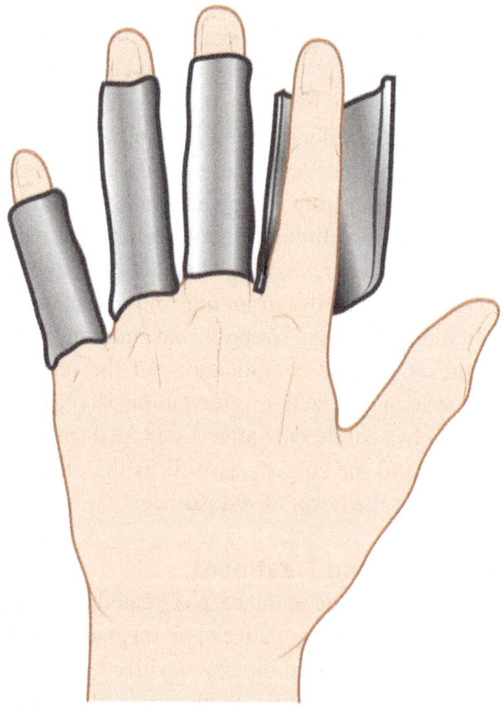

Fig. 4.10 The position for the burn patients on the finger

Table 4.3 Assuming the position for contracture prevention

Site of the burn	Proper position	Orthosis
Neck	Extension	Maintaining extension by using a pillow
Shoulder joint	Flexion, abduction, and lateral rotation	Airplane splint
Elbow joint	Extension, supination	Elbow extension orthosis
Wrist joint and hands	Functional position of the hands, finger abduction	Resting pan splint
Hip joint	Extension, abduction	Hip abduction orthosis
Knee joint	Extension	Knee extension orthosis
Ankle joint and foot	Dorsiflexion, raising leg at a neutral position	Plastic AFO

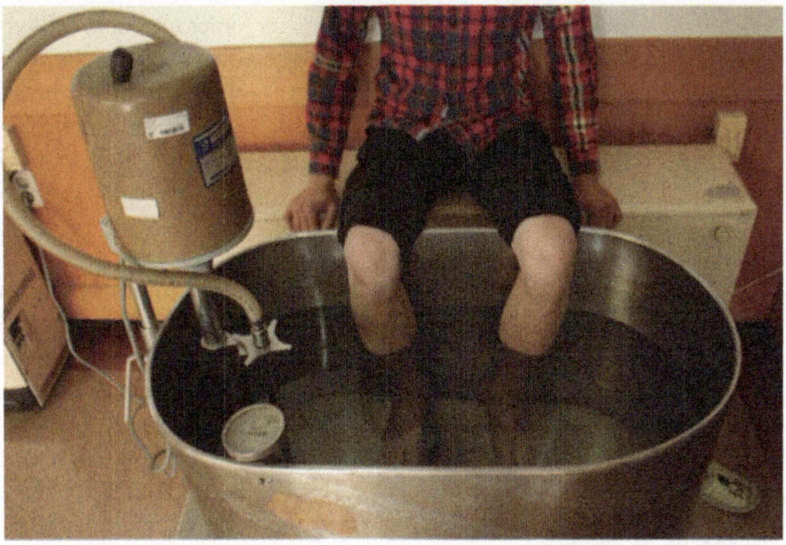

Fig. 4.11 Whirlpool bath

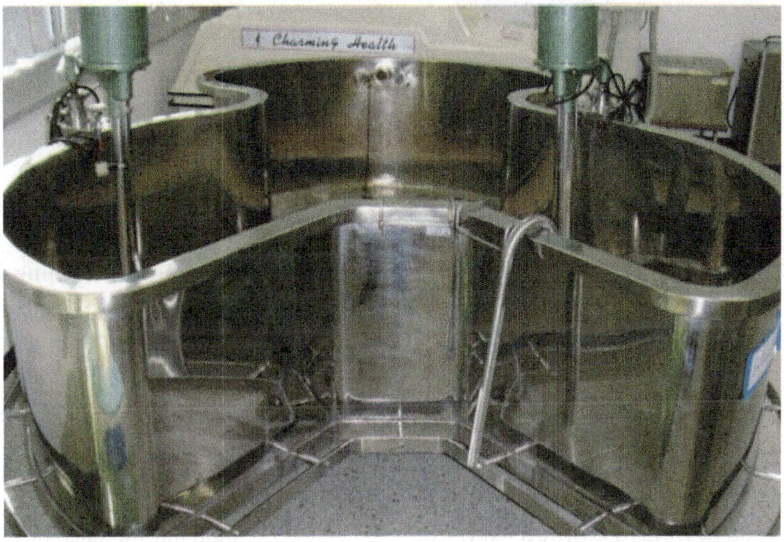

Fig. 4.12 Hubbard tank

for five to seven times. In particular, massaging the hands or feet after the paraffin bath promotes flexibility of the joint and prevents spasmodermia.

However, deep massage to the subcutaneous tissue should be avoided because it may rather form blisters. Start paraffin bath 5 days after the skin grafting surgery, and implement paraffin bath in one operation for both sites where provided and received grafted skin (Fig. 4.14).

4.2.2.5 Exercise Therapy

Start to implement exercise therapy within 48 to 72 h after the burn, and carry out two to four times a day. For all the joints which have burns, enforce an active or active-assistive exercise. Also enforce the exercise equally for the limbs and legs which are not burnt to prevent congestion and to prevent joint contracture or myoatrophy that may occur due to not being used so that the patient is not physiologically declined.

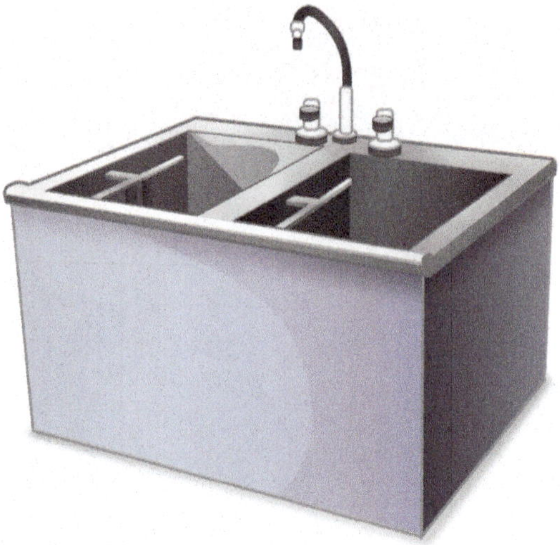

Fig. 4.13 Contrast bath

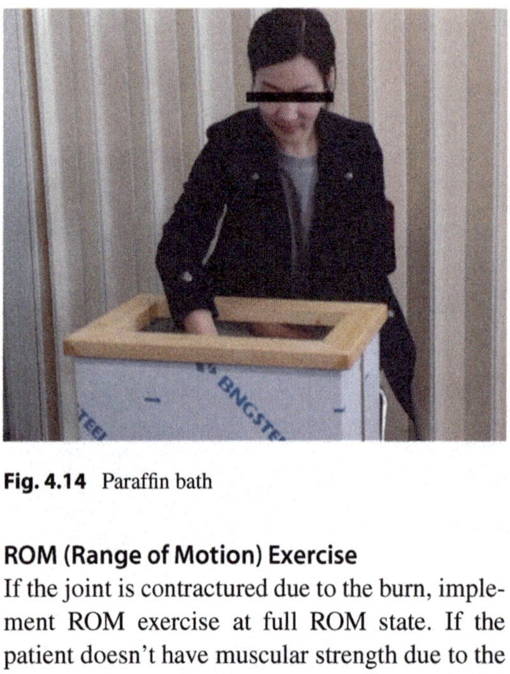

Fig. 4.14 Paraffin bath

ROM (Range of Motion) Exercise

If the joint is contractured due to the burn, implement ROM exercise at full ROM state. If the patient doesn't have muscular strength due to the damaged nerves, implement passive ROM exercise in order to prevent contracture, to maintain and promote the ROM, and to prevent edema. Also proceed gradually to the active-assistive ROM exercise and the active ROM exercise depending on the patient's muscular strength. These ROM exercises should be enforced 2–5 days after having the burn.

In addition, restoring the functions of the hand is the most important than any other things in order to enable skilled movement of the patient. Implementing the ROM exercise for the hands should be constant and gentle, because doing exercise too rapidly may cause the damage on the joint or tendon. Particularly, one should focus on that the patient can maintain the functional hand position.

Strengthening Exercise

Strengthening exercise is essential to enhance the strength for weakened muscles.

Enforce isometric exercise even with wearing the orthosis or in the state of being fixed in order to prevent disuse atrophy. And furthermore, proceed to the isotonic exercise in the full ROM to enhance the strength efficiently, if possible.

Stretching

Scars caused by burns tend to lose elasticity as the scars become enlarged and contracted. At this time, pains, dysfunction, and restrictions on joint movement are resulted. These are caused because collagen synthesis, joint capsule, and ligament are degraded rapidly. Therefore, joint mobility must be retained, and stretch and retain the scar tissue through the continuous stretching is the most effective way. To prevent dry skin, skin lubricant is being used during the stretching.

Applying the heat to the injured area has a variety of effects such as enhancing the stretching, reforming the scar on the connective tissue, increasing blood circulation, releasing the pain, and mitigating the muscle cramp; therefore, applying the heat sufficiently prior to stretching is needed. Sometimes, hydrotherapy is also recommended but controlling the water temperature for a long time is not easy, and it is not convenient to use high-temperature hot water because it is hard to bear. Because flexion contracture occurs to the patients who have a burn on the neck area, pursue the extension naturally using the gravity and the head weight by putting a pillow under the head and the shoulder joint in a supine position (Fig. 4.8). Adduction and medial rotation contracture break out to shoulder joints, so enforce the stretching of abductor and lateral rotation muscle, and because flexion and pronation con-

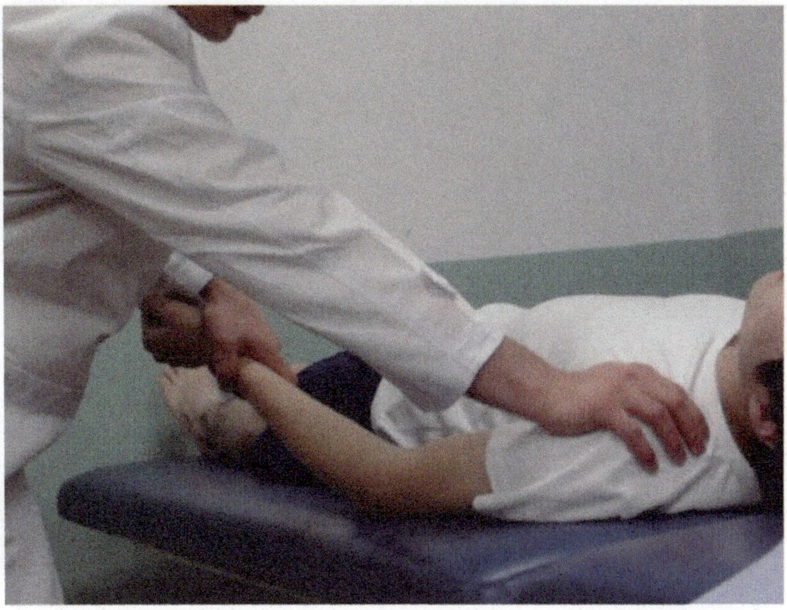

Fig. 4.15 Stretching for the elbow joint burn patients

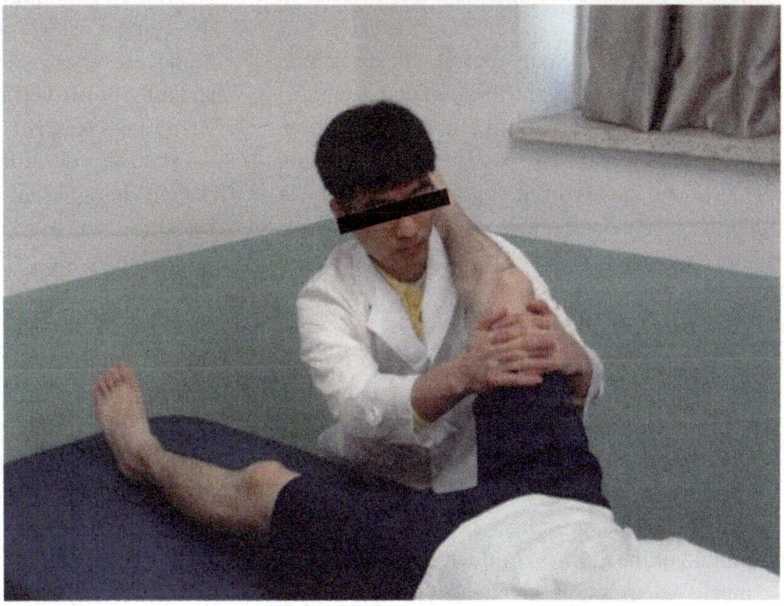

Fig. 4.16 Stretching for the burn patients on the hip joint and knee joint

tracture easily break out to elbow joint, stretching to extensor muscle and supinator muscle is needed (Fig. 4.15). And also implement stretching for plantar flexor on the wrist joint and adductor.

For hip joint, implement stretching of the flexor and adductor, and enforce the stretching of the flexor for knee joint. Also implement the stretching of plantar flexor for ankle joint (Fig. 4.16).

Breathing Exercise

Both breathing exercise and coughing training are very important exercises for the burn patients for smooth ventilation and secretion discharge especially in case of the burn patients who have a burn on the face so inhalation burn is accompanied, breathing exercise is more needed. But the individual should approach very carefully because edema commonly breaks out to the patients and it

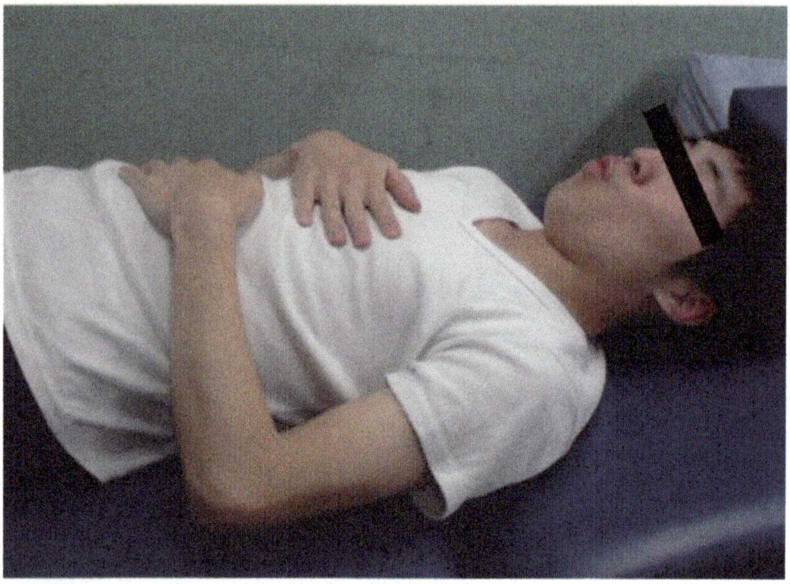

Fig. 4.17 Diaphragmatic breathing exercises

is the most desirable to implement this exercise in half-lying position.

Clean the nasal cavity before the breathing exercise, and maintain air filtration and humidification by inhaling through the nose. In addition, full exhalation can be possible by breathing regularly and slowly in the relaxed state and can minimize residual volume as well. But the patients should abstain from doing sudden activities or

① Diaphragmatic Breathing Exercise

The purpose of the diaphragmatic breathing exercise is to decrease the contracture of the accessory respiratory muscle by increasing the movement of the diaphragm which is the main respiratory muscle. Place one hand right below the ribs and place another hand in the middle of the thorax. Hold out the abdomen as much as possible while inhaling deeply through the nose, and then exhale while contracting the abdominal muscles. At this moment, the patient should purse the lips at most so that the exhalation can be made.

The ratio of inhalation and exhalation should be 1:2, and repeat doing the exercise for 1 min and take a rest for 2 min at the beginning, and increase gradually up to doing exercise for 10 min twice a day.

At the beginning, enforce doing exercise in the lying position and gradually implement doing exercise in a seated position and in a standing position (Fig. 4.17).

② Breathing Exercise through Pursed Lips

The purpose of breathing exercise through pursed lips is to slow down the frequency of breathing and to reduce the airway resistance through extending the exhalation.

Inhale through the nose and purse the lips at most while exhale making use of muscles of the abdomen, so that exhale through the mouth slowly at most.

The ratio of inhalation and exhalation should be 1:2. As pursing the lips at most while exhaling, air increases bronchoalveolar pressure, and consequentially airway resistance is reduced; thus, the ventilation rate can be increased.

Initially implement this exercise in a supine position and later implement gradually in the seated position and stand position and while walking.

③ Coughing Training

The purpose of the coughing training is to discharge mucus and other materials from the trachea and bronchus. After taking a deep breath slowly through the nose in the position of bending and lowering the upper body slightly, breathe out through the mouth without moving it. And after breathing in deeply, hold the breath for a few seconds, and then cough quickly using the muscles of the abdomen, thigh, and buttocks while lowering and bending the upper body forward. At this time, coughing should be done at the beginning of exhalation.

4.2.2.6 Physical Therapy for Skin Graft

In severe burns such as third-degree or fourth-degree burns that have very severe damage, surgical skin graft operation is required. Approximately 2–3 weeks has been taken until the grafted skin is formed properly. During this period, massage around the grafted skin gently enhances the fluidity and promotes the improvement of circulation or nutritional condition.

For donor site, promote skin recovery after the surgery through ultraviolet treatment and should help in epithelialization through the effect of disinfection.

4.2.2.7 Management of Burn Scar

The scars caused by second-degree deep burn or by major burns become solid and swell, when 6 months have passed, and the hypertrophic scars are developed in the process of healing these scars which are very vulnerable to frictional forces and shearing forces. Especially, skin-grafted area requires more intensive cares. Apply elastic wraps to control the edema and the scar on the grafted skin area when the wound fails to withstand shearing force, and start to wear a pressure garment on the wound when the wound can withstand well against shearing force. Pressure garment that can be worn for various areas should be applied in the beginning, because it has effects of minimizing the scar tissue formation and mitigating pruritus and desensitization as the scar becomes flat and soft, as well as it helps the circulation or controls edema

Pressure garment should be prescribed well so that it fits properly to each patient on the face, body, limbs, or legs depending on the burnt areas (Fig. 4.18).

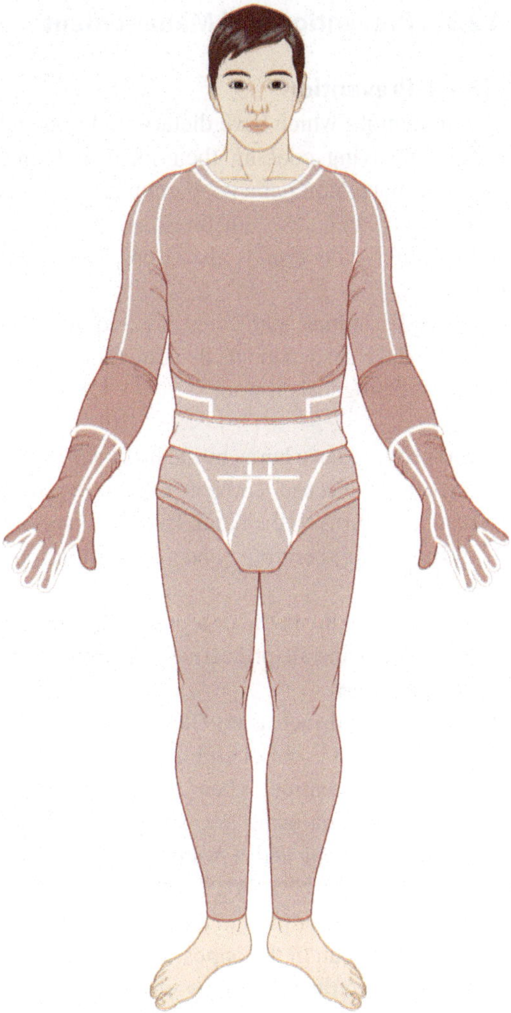

Fig. 4.18 Pressure garment

4.2.2.8 Orthosis

Prescribing orthosis to the burn patients is essential. Static orthosis is helpful until the patient starts to exercise, and it is prescribed to the patients to hold the functional position (Cho 1998).

Orthosis must be designed depending on the patient's needs and recovery stages, and it should allow the movement in the extent to which soft tissue is not tightened while sleeping.

On the other hand, dynamic orthosis, in addition to the indication of static orthosis, has advantages of enhancing muscular strength and maintaining the range of motion (Hicks et al. 1989; Conine et al. 1989).

4.2.3 Prevention and Management

4.2.3.1 Prevention

In communities which have dietary tradition and culture involving cooking their meal at home, there are many burn patients, particularly in children due to carelessness of their parent, and the lack of safety concerns is also a problem to the elders.

Special cautions and cares are required for children and elderly patients because their further course and prognosis is poor.

① It is prone to have burns by steam of a pressure cooker or electric cooker. Especially, if it results in burns to the hand, it leads to serious dysfunction; therefore, special cautions are required.
② Do not place the kettle or a pot on the electric heater, and install protective net around the electric heater.
③ Cook hot food such as noodles or coffee in the place where it is out of children's reach.
④ Pay extra attention when using hot water, especially when using hot water in a bathtub in the bathroom and a water purifier in the kitchen.
⑤ If you use pots or pans in the kitchen, turn the knob of the pan in the opposite direction.
⑥ Prevent electrical burns by installing safety equipment such as placing the caps on electrical outlets.
⑦ Make sure that there is no gas leakage through daily examination, and be sure to lock gas valve after use.
⑧ High-voltage electricity exposure must be avoided in the working places dealing with electricity.

4.2.3.2 Patient/Caregiver Education

After receiving proper hospital treatments, care for the patient after the discharge must be continued. Scar tissues that commonly appear in burn patients may induce restrictions to the daily activities due to the joint contraction and failure; therefore, education on self-stretching and strengthening exercise should be provided so that the patients can implement them regularly in their daily living. In particular, the burn patients who have burns on the hands, armpit, or front part of the neck require more intensive care and management because the range of joint contracture and failure in those patients is more severe. Those patients who have burns on the chest area have severe respiratory function disability, so education on breathing exercise and coughing training should be provided. For those patients who have burns on their face or hands, education regarding the utensil usage and chewing/swallowing food exercise should be provided.

Careful consideration and encouragement from family members and colleagues are needed for burn patients because sociopsychological aspect management for burn patient is also a very important factor as well as caring for their physical failures. Thereby, burn patients can have independent daily living and return to their previous way of life completely (http://www.burnwelfare.net).

Advices for Physical Therapists

❶ Education for burn patients is required. Especially, it is important for the elderly burn patients over 70 years old, because they have poor safety awareness and poor prognosis.
❷ Provide healing of the wounds caused by burns.
❸ Minimize scars and deformities caused by burns.
❹ Enforce active ROM exercise more than 2 h a day in order to minimize contracture.
❺ Wear proper orthosis in association with stretching.
❻ Provide enhancement of strength and endurance.
❼ Encourage to have independent activities of daily living.
❽ Relieve psychological instability such as depression.

4.3 Problem Solving

4.3.1 Burn

Choose the correct examination or physical therapy intervention that has greater possibility in each item.

Question 1
Mr. A is a 35-year-old worker, and he suffered from a second-degree full-thickness burn on the entire right side arm. He had a surgery to remove damaged skin and had skin graft in the specialized hospital for the burns. Which is the necessary initial physical treatment intervention for him?

1. Resistive exercise
2. Breathing exercise
3. Electrotherapy
4. Stretching
5. ROM exercise

Question 2
A is a 45-year-old male and he had a third-degree burn on the back of his hand during work. After having the surgery of skin grafting, physical therapy for his hand is supposed to be implemented. Which is the necessary physical therapy intervention can be performed independently?

1. Stretching
2. Paraffin bath
3. Resistive exercise
4. Whirlpool bath
5. Ultrasonic therapy

Question 3
Mr. A is the employee of the electric power company, and he had a burn on his arm including his shoulder while he was replacing the transformer, so he has been hospitalized for the treatment. Physical therapy is suggested by the department in charge because of the limited mobility of his shoulder. Which is the necessary physical therapy intervention currently for this patient?

1. Paraffin bath
2. Sling exercise
3. Resistive exercise
4. Iontophoresis
5. Aerobic exercise

Question 4
In which burn vesicles break out?

1. First-degree burn
2. Second-degree burn
3. Third-degree burn
4. Superficial burn
5. Full-thickness burn

Question 5
What is the purpose of implementing Hubbard tank for third-degree burn patients?

1. To enhance the muscular strength
2. To prevent infections
3. To intensify respiratory muscles
4. To remove necrotic tissue
5. To increase the range of motion (ROM)

Answers
Question 1-⑤, Question 2-①, Question 3-②, Question 4-②, Question 5-④

References

Ahn S, Jang GH, Song JW. Diagnosis and treatment of Korean's common skin disease. Daijeon: Doctors book; 2009.

Braddom RL. Physical medicine and rehabilitation. 2nd ed. Philadelphia: WB Saunders; 2000. p. 1329–36.

Cho KJ. Fiberglass reinforced plastic orthotic appliances. Yonsei Med J. 1998;29(4):350–6.

Conine TA, Carlow DL, Stevenson-Moore P. The vancouver microstomia orthosis. J Prosthet Dent. 1989;61(4):476–83.

Delisa JA. Rehabilitation medicine: burn injury rehabilitation. 3rd ed. Philadelphia: Lippincott-Raven; 1998. p. 1580–5.

Fader P. A self-instructional package: neck conformer. J Burn Care Rehabil. 1985;6:124–7.

Feldman AE, MacMillan BG. Burn injury in children: declining need for reconstructive surgery as related to use of neck orthoses. Arch Phys Med Rehabil. 1980;61(10):441–9.

Fess EE, Philips CA. Hand splinting, principles and methods. 2nd ed. St Louis: CV Mosby; 1987.
Harden NG, Luster SH. Rehabilitation consideration in the care of the acute burn patient. Crit Care Nurs Clin North Am. 1991;3(2):245–53.
Helm PA, Kevorkian CG, Lushbaugh M. Burn injury rehabilitation management in 1982. Arch Phys Med Rehabil. 1982;63:6–16.
Hicks JE, Leonard JA, Nelson VS, Fisher SV, Esquenazi A. Prosthetics, orthotics, and assistive devices. Orthotic management of selected disorders. Arch Phys Med Rehabil. 1989;70(5-s):s210–7.
Hurlin Foley K, Doyle B, Paradise P, Parry I, Palmieri T, Greenhalgh DC. Use of an improved watusi collar to manage pediatric neck burn contractures. J Burn Care Rehabil. 2002;23(3):221–6.
Ko YJ, Kang SY. Physical medicine and rehabilitation. Seoul: Jung MoonGak; 2009.

Reference Site

http://www.burnwelfare.net

Frostbite 5

Keun-Jo Kim

ICD-10 Code
T33-35 Frostbite
T33 Superficial frostbite
T34 Frostbite with tissue necrosis
T35 Frostbite involving multiple body regions
T69 Other effects of reduced temperature
T69.0 Immersion hand and foot
T69.1 Chilblains
P80 Hypothermia
P80.0 Cold injury syndromes

Learning Outcomes
After completing this chapter, you should be able to do the following:

- Describe the disease types of cold injury.
- Describe clinical symptoms of frostbite.
- Explain General classification of frostbite.
- Prevent and manage frostbite.
- Perform physical therapy intervention for frostbite.

Key Terms
Frostbite
Chilblain
Trench foot
Immersion foot
Cold injury

5.1 Frostbite

5.1.1 Overview

Various physiological changes and direct tissue damages from hypothermia occur when the human body is exposed to external cold environment. Damages caused by cold are generally referred to as cold injuries. And failure of thermoregulation, physiological compensatory mechanisms can lead body parts exposed to freezing ambient to cold injuries. The primary cause of this skin ailment is inadequate blood circulation due to capillary freeze. Exposure to cold air or water for a long time can contribute to partial damage such as frostbite or systemic damage such as hypothermia. The term frostbite refers to the partial body damage caused by reduction of blood circulation in peripheral body parts. In extreme cold, or when the body is exposed to cold for long periods, body's protective strategy can reduce blood flow in some areas of the body to dangerously low levels. This lack of blood leads to the eventual freezing and death of skin

K.-J. Kim
Department of Physical Therapy, Gimcheon University, 214, Daehak-ro, Gimcheon-si, Gyeongsangbuk-do, South Korea
e-mail: kmjb042@gimcheon.ac.kr

J.-W. Park, D.-I. Jung (eds.), *Integumentary Physical Therapy*, DOI 10.1007/978-3-662-47380-1_5

tissue of the affected areas to preserve core temper and fight hypothermia. This can cause tissue damage onto the skin of the hands, feet, and ears and eventually cause necrosis and amputation.

5.1.2 Causes

Frostbite can be caused by fat shortage, old age, living on streets, drug or alcohol addiction, heart diseases, smoke, or being exposed to cold weather with inadequate clothing. And body parts such as the hands, feet, ears, and noses being exposed in extreme cold, circumjacent humidity, ventilation, clothing, medical state, personal emotion can also lead to frostbite. In general, the human body fails to control body temperature after being exposed to cold environment where the temperature is lower than 41 °F (5 °C), the body temperature, for a long time (Imray et al. 2009). Soft tissues get frozen causing inadequate blood circulation after being in extreme cold environment, which is below 32 °F (0 °C) or 35.6~50 °F (2~10 °C). Damage degrees depend on sensory temperature and altitude as well as temperature and exposure time.

For example, when the body temperature becomes lower than 95 °F (35 °C) due to long-term heat loss, a person experiences fatigue, weariness, and failure of proper thinking. Below 86 °F (30 °C), an individual experiences awareness ambiguity and arrhythmia, and he or she eventually dies when their body temperature becomes lower than 78.8 °F (26 °C).

5.1.3 Classification

Cold injuries can be classified into nonfrozen damage and frozen damage. Frostbite can be classified into stage 1–4 (Kim et al. 2012).

5.1.3.1 Nonfreezing Damage

Nonfrozen damage refers to injuries taken place above freezing point and high humidity. It takes place when there is whole body hypothermia, which means central temperature being below 95 °F (35 °C) when measured in the rectum. Trench foot is an example of such nonfreezing damage. During World War I, soldiers' feet were exposed to cold, wet trench for a long time, which resulted in trench foot with numb, whitened, softened, cracked, and swollen foot as its symptom (Fig. 5.1). There is another symptom called immersion foot. It is not as severe as frostbite, and it arises when marine crews stay in relatively cold ocean water for a long time. Their cutaneous blood vessels get paralyzed and resulted in circulatory insufficiency and tissue damage. Also, among nonfrozen damages, there is chilblain which frequently occurs in people who stay in cold environment for a long time such as market sellers (Fig. 5.2).

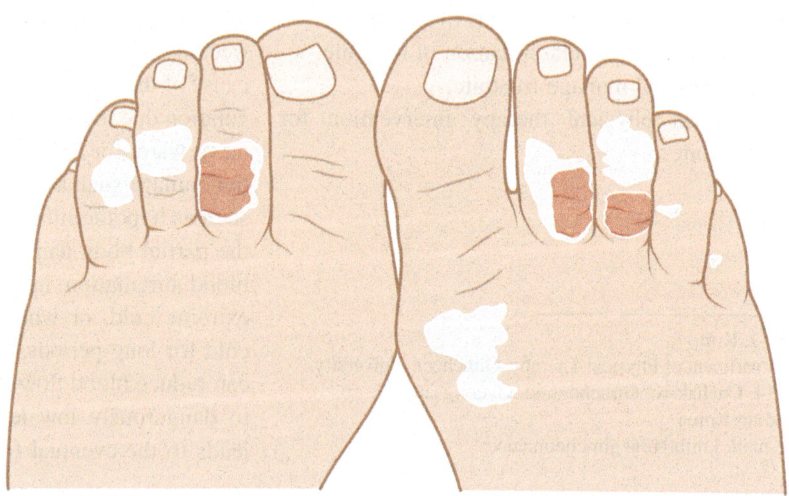

Fig. 5.1 Trench foot

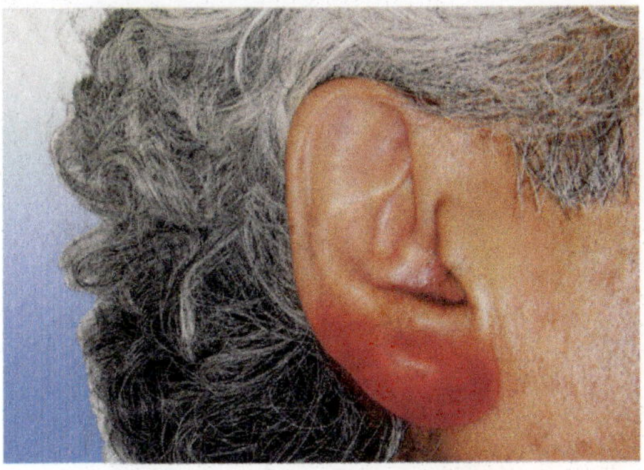

Fig. 5.2 Chilblain

Tip

① Trench foot is a medical condition caused by prolonged exposure of the feet to damp, unsanitary, and cold conditions. The use of the word *trench* in the name of this condition is a reference to, or mainly associated with, trench during World War I.

② Chilblain is a medical condition that occurs when a predisposed individual is exposed to cold and humidity, causing tissue damage.

③ Immersion foot refers to foot skin damage taken place when one's feet stays in 71.6 °F (22 °C) water or mud for 2–10 days (Reference: www.ko.wikipedia.org, http://en.wikipedia.org/wiki/Immersion_foot_syndromes).

5.1.3.2 Freezing Damage

Damage caused by prolonged neglect of physical body under freezing point or low humidity. Frostbite is one of them, and it can be divided into slight and deep frostbite by its symptoms.

5.1.3.3 Classification by Damage Severity

First-Degree Frostbite

Means damage on the outer skin. There are no symptoms of blisters, but you can see congested blood and edema, and there could be drop off skin within 5–10 days after the damage. One may feel pain from burning paresthesia or poking feelings (Fig. 5.3).

Second-Degree Frostbite

It refers to damage on all layers of the skin and has characteristics of congested blood and creating blisters over affected areas. Blisters form black crust, and after the crust gets removed, the new skin is reproduced. Symptoms include decreased sensitivity and sharp pain (Fig. 5.4).

Third-Degree Frostbite

The whole subcutaneous layers are damaged. Purple or congestive blisters are formed and black dried crust is formed after affected skin dies. The symptoms include numb skin and sharp pain (Fig. 5.5).

Fourth-Degree Frostbite

The whole hypodermic layers, muscle, and bones are frostbitten and show few or no edema, severe insensibility, mummification necrosis, and need to amputate. Patients feel sore joints (Fig. 5.6).

5.1.4 Symptoms and Complications

5.1.4.1 Clinical Symptoms

Frostbite brings pain on the ears, nose, and limb. The more one is exposed to cold or the colder it gets, the more one feels pin and needle pain and eventually loses skin sensitivity by 80 %. Skin looks red in the initial state of coldness, but it becomes pale or blue when it becomes more severe. From blisters and when it gets worse, one might get frostbite and partial necrosis and mummification (Fig. 5.7). General medical symptoms of frostbite are cold skin, pale skin, paresthesia, numb feelings, rubefaction, edema, blisters, and necrosis.

Superficial Frostbite

Mainly occurs on the face, ears, or fingers and toes. It is a freezing injury which does not form ice crystal or tissue loss. The skin gets pale due to vasoconstriction, and patients complain of hypesthesia around

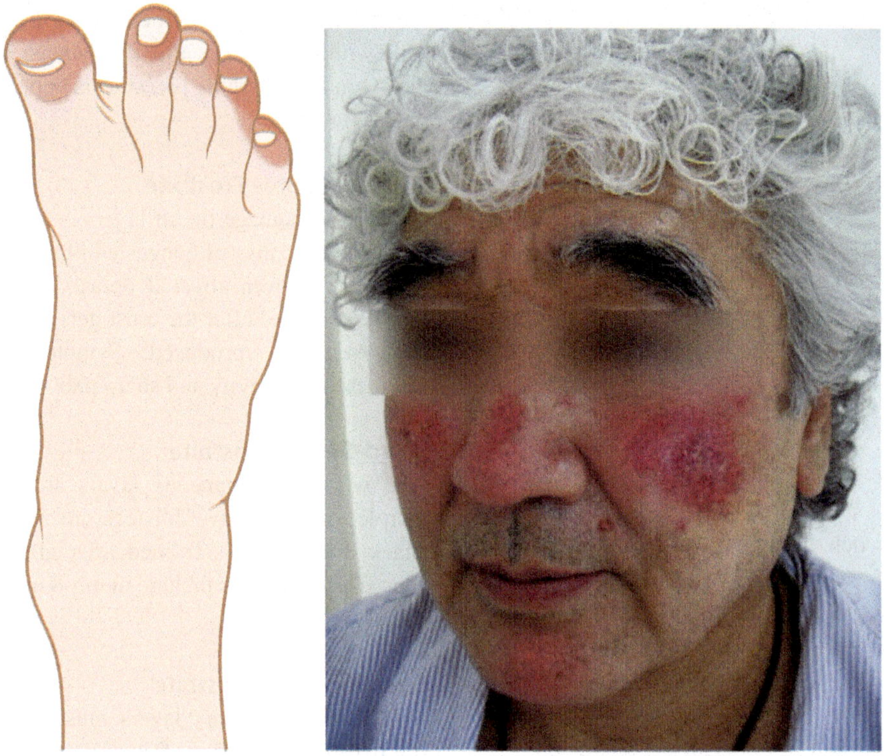

Fig. 5.3 Stage 1 frostbitten toe and face

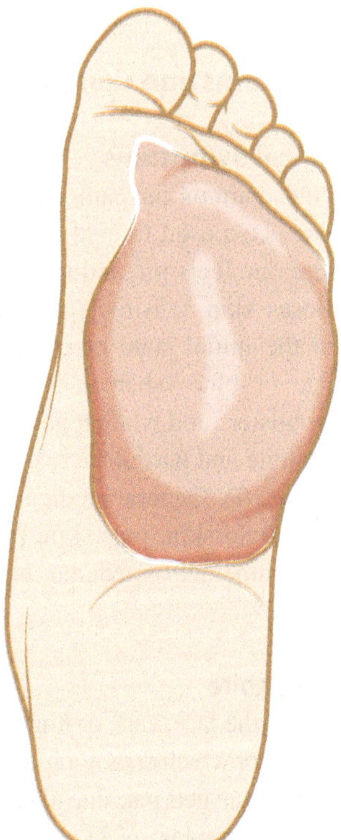

Fig. 5.4 Stage 2 frostbitten toe

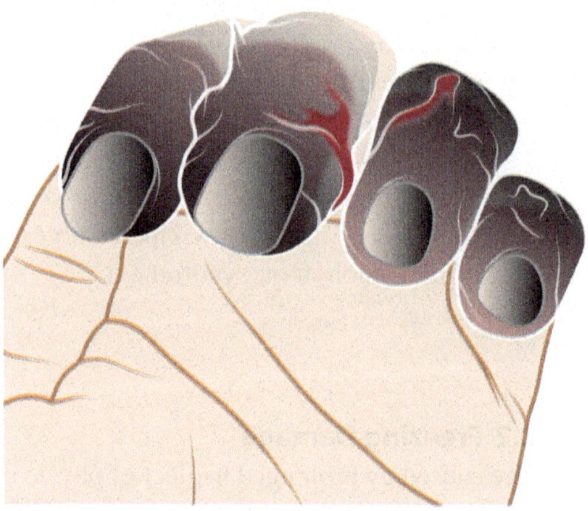

Fig. 5.5 Stage 3 frostbitten finger

impaired areas. In this case, symptoms go away and no tissues are lost as their body gets reheated, but there could be burning feeling, sting, or edema.

Deep Frostbite

Severe pain with blisters and necrosis on the whole skin layer. The necrotized area becomes dark and mummificated, so it eventually needs to be amputated.

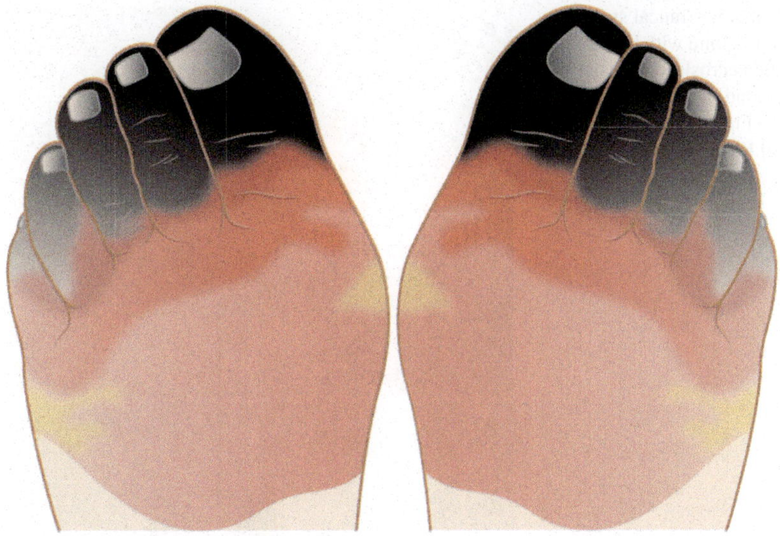

Fig. 5.6 Stage 4 frostbitten toe

Chilblain

It is a medical condition that occurs when a predisposed individual is exposed to cold and humidity, causing tissue damage. Women and children are main victims of chilblains. After being exposed to long time, it causes partial edema, rubefaction, and cyanoderma, and after being exposed to heat, the skin feels itchy with burning sensation. Chilblain fades away within 2–3 weeks generally. It has a tendency of reoccurrence, and when it gets worsened, there could be blisters and bacterial infection by blisters, later forming ulcers. For females, chilblains can get worse by irregular menstruation and hormonal and nutritional disorders.

Trench Foot

Trench foot occurs when the body part is exposed to humid and cold environment for a prolonged period. Loss of sensitivity due to damaged peripheral nerve and ischemic injury of tissues due to fine convulsion of blood vessel occurs.

5.1.4.2 Pathological Stages of Frostbite

Pathology stage of frostbite can be classified into two stages: before and after frostbite.

1. Before frostbite, skin surface temperature is dropped due to the exposure to cold, and loss of skin sensitivity after tissue temperature drops below 50 °F (10 °C). Also, blood plasma outflows blood vessels, resulting in increased blood viscosity. Due to the body temperature homeostatic mechanisms, blood vessel under exposed area gets shrunk, and plasma outflows, resulting in tissue edema.
2. Freezing level is when the surrounding temperature drops and the tissue's fluid freeze and form ice crystal (Fig. 5.8). At this time, the tissue's osmotic pressure increases and moves the cells' inside moisture to the outside causing cell dehydration (Korean Dermatological Association 2008). Cell dehydration continuously increases the cells' interior osmotic pressure, and it causes necrosis and devascularization. Blood begins to clot forming blood clots that lead to necrosis by ischemic injuries. Damaged skin becomes black and forms a dry eschar. Also when the area of the cold injury's temperature is raised, additional damage occurs, which is called a reperfusion injury. Therefore when the tissue, which was damaged, is reheated, the blood flow increases. At this point, the tissue edema becomes worse due to injured blood vessel's endothelial cells. Edema causes the ischemic injury through cell dehydration which leads to the generation of active oxygen causing the endothelial cell injury to become aggravated. Consequently, vasoconstriction factors create more tissue injuries through inflammation leading the tissues' ischemic injury become worse.

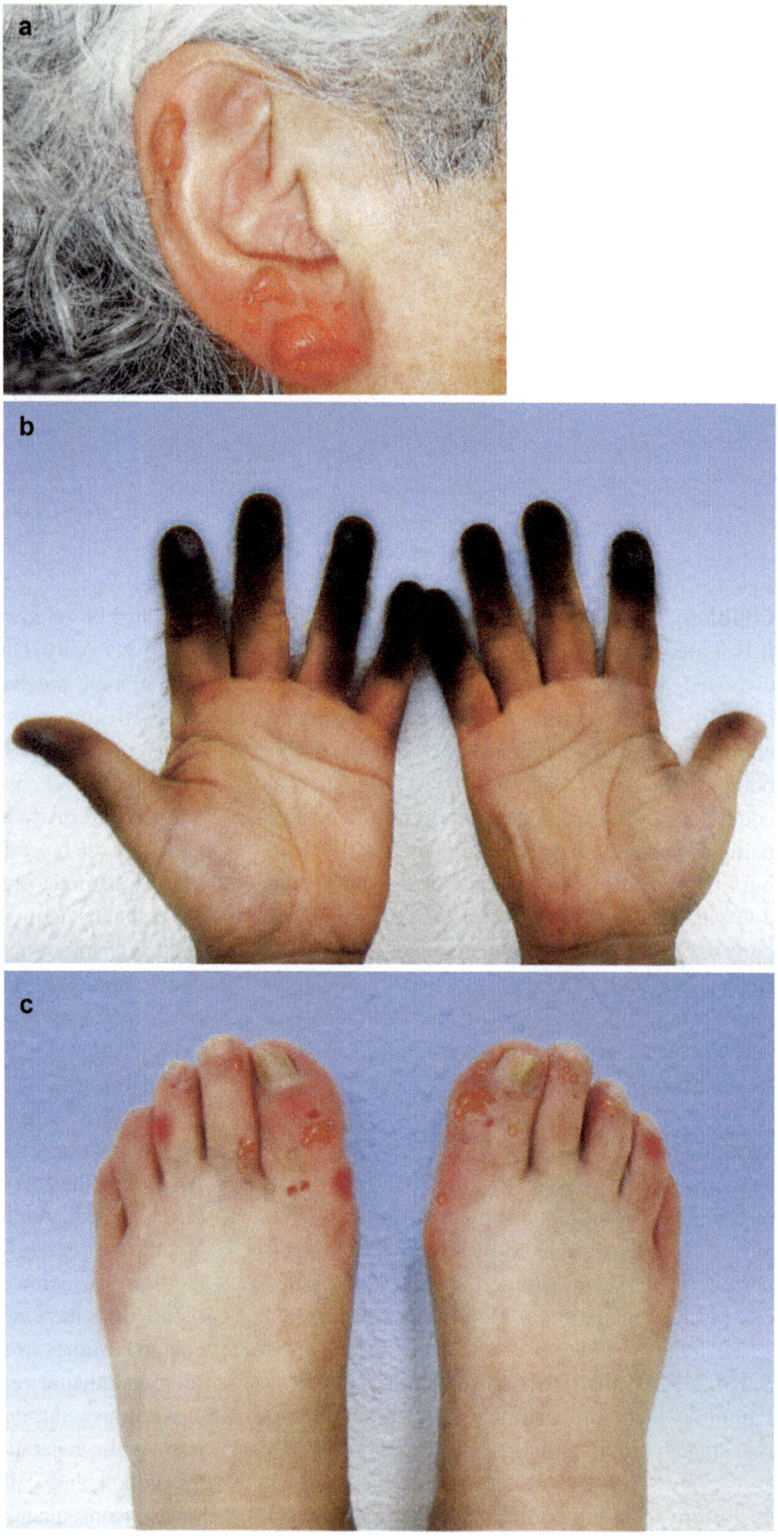

Fig. 5.7 Clinical symptoms of frostbite with blisters and necrosis. (**a**) Blisters around the auricle. (**b**) Finger necrosis. (**c**) Blisters around the toes

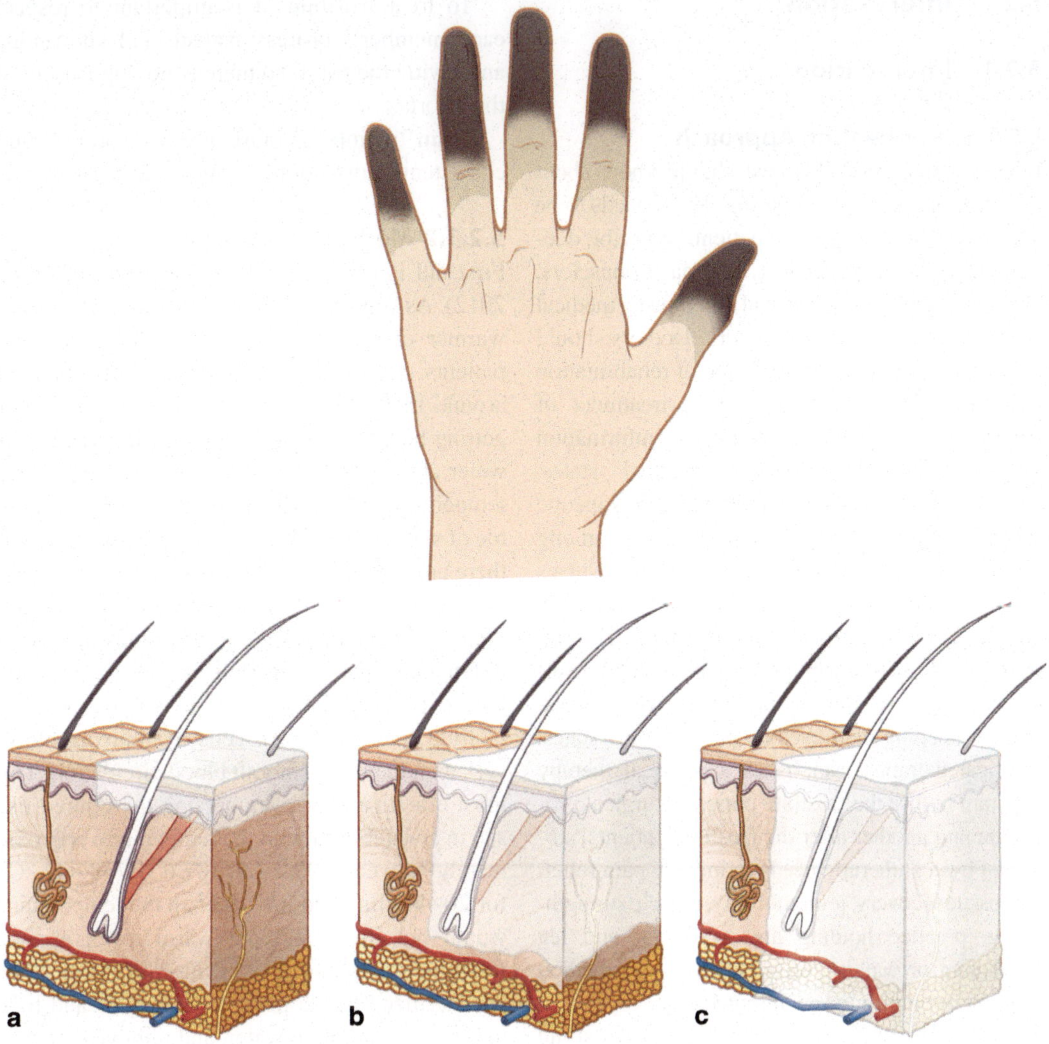

Fig. 5.8 Progress of frostbite. (**a**) Epidermis freeze. (**b**) Derma freeze. (**c**) Subcutaneous freeze

5.1.5 Test and Assessment

There are two ways to evaluate frostbite: subjective and objective ways. First, listen to the patient's medical history as a subjective evaluation, and then conduct inspection with the naked eyes and palpation of the skin as an objective evaluation.

When inspecting, observe color changes on the skin due to circulatory disturbances such as cyanoderma. Check humidity and temperature of the skin and whether there are sensitivity damage, blisters, ecchymosis, and skin necrosis. When conducting palpation, check if there is paresthesia and the range of affected area, and check skin temperature. Check range of necrosis and find survivable tissue by using 3D bone scan as a radiation evaluation (Barker et al. 1997). Lastly, there is a clinicopathologic evaluation such as general blood test, autoimmune antibody test, cryoglobulin test, cold agglutinin test, and blood vessel test especially for elders.

5.2 Intervention

5.2.1 Intervention

5.2.1.1 Intervention Approach

Protector and physiotherapist should know about the stage of patient's symptoms. There needs to be a team approach among the patient, protector, doctor, pharmacist, nutritionist, clinical counselors, physiotherapist, occupational therapist, medical social worker, nurses, and others. Doctors should provide explanation and guidance of rehabilitation treatment after providing surgical treatment of frostbite and provide protectors with information about the patient's overall medical states. Pharmacists should explain and inspect therapeutic dosage and possible interaction or toxicity among different drugs to patients and protectors. Nurses should be the frontline channel of communication among patient and experts including medical team, follow doctors' prescription, check patients' medical state, and conduct nursing tasks such as dressing and keeping their eyes on patients' scar states. Physical therapist establishes a physical therapy program before the frostbite patients' surgical procedure and another after the frostbite patients' surgery. Physical therapy needs to include pain relief, soft tissue recovery, joint mobility, muscle strengthening, practice holding and grabbing, and leg movement or walking recovery. Also use method of brace appliance for an amputee case.

Clinical counselors must help frostbite patients who are under stress by educating them on the phantom pain and methods of managing stress which helps blood circulation and accelerates the treatment for frostbite.

Dieticians can provide the necessary information to patients and caretakers about the methods to improve the patient's nutritive condition and dietary methods to increase blood pressure and blood sugar. Nutrition is especially important to frostbite patients for tissue treatment and regenerative strength. Medical social workers provide information on medical devices and medical supplies that frostbite patients might need when they have become handicapped due to frostbite and counsel the frostbite patient on their discharge planning and help them to return back into their local community by considering the patient's social situation.

To treat frostbite, it is important to respect each member's professionalism and knowledge and divide the roles, so there is no duplication of the efforts.

Team members must provide proper and consistent information to patients and caretakers.

5.2.1.2 Medical Treatment

First aid is crucial for frostbite (Tintinalli et al 2012). As soon as possible, bring the patients to a warmer environment, take wet clothes off the patients, dry their body, and put a warm blanket around their body (Fig. 5.9). There is a risk of getting burns if you put the damaged area in hot water abov 109.4 °F (43 °C). Conversely, water temperature below 100.4 °F (38 °C) is not capable of warming frostbitten parts effectively. When there are blisters, do not pop them. Put a bandage around blisters so they can be absorbed into the body (Zafren 2013). Do not rub or massage frostbitten area since ice crystals can destroy circumjacent plastid. The treatment of frostbite is melting freeze between cells by relaxing blood vessel and leading smooth blood circulation. The most effective way is immersing the injured tissue in a water bath with the temperature approximately between 100.4 and 107.6 °F (38 ~ 42 °C) for 20–40 min. Add hot water so the temperature would not drop, and put warm towel around frostbitten ears and face (Britt et al. 1991). Put dry sterilized gauze in between fingers and toes to remove remaining water, and remove pain and edema by putting frostbitten parts in high position. Do not walk right after having chilblains around legs.

Put humectant cream on frostbitten area, and form dressing to absorb humidity and protect the area. When there is compartment syndrome, conduct fasciotomy to remove pressure and promote blood circulation. For medical treatment, there are vasodilators and clot buster.

5.2.2 Physical Therapy Intervention

5.2.2.1 Positioning

After warming patients up, make the patient stay comfortable. The hands and feet are the most frequent frostbitten parts of the body. Put the

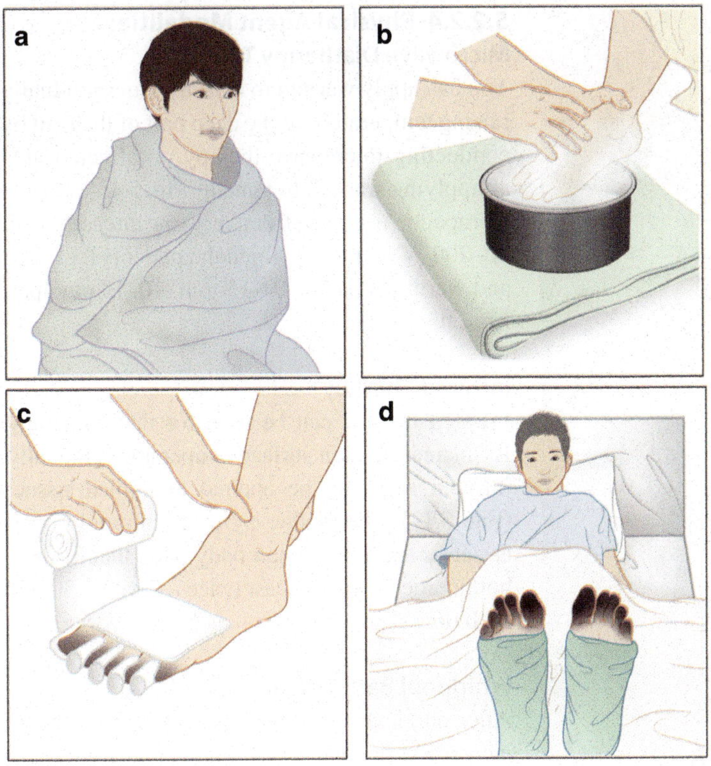

Fig. 5.9 Initial management for acute frostbite. (**a**) Wrapping up with a blanket. (**b**) Warm bath for feet. (**c**) Wrapping up with a bandage. (**d**) Leg elevation

hands and feet higher than the heart in order to decrease edema.

5.2.2.2 Exercise Therapy

Use kinesiatrics according to the patient's frostbite stage. Isometric and isotonic exercise, passive and active exercise, and resistance and extensional exercises can be used in accordance with the condition of each patient. Consider method, frequency, strength, and time, and use kinesiatrics at least twice a day, 30 min each time (Fig. 5.10). In case of the first-degree frostbite, joint motion is limited by factors such as edema, so isometric exercises or active exercises are performed with the purpose of improving joint mobility and heat production of the skin. For the second-degree frostbite, intense exercise should be avoided since blisters and crust form during this stage. Tender passive movements and gradual active movements are recommended. Check sensitivity first since there is a risk of damaging cutaneous sense. There could be dermolysis on third- and fourth-degree frostbites, so conduct kinesiatrics after the surgical and operational treatment. Especially patients who eliminated callus should have an active exercise in order to prevent adhesion. After amputation due to the tissue necrosis, recover joint mobility and motor sensation by conducting passive and active treatment in the initial state, and maintain muscle strength by conducting intervention treatment in the later state (Figs. 5.11 and 5.12).

5.2.2.3 Manual Therapy

Therapeutic Massage

Do not massage the affected area in the initial state of frostbite since it can damage circumjacent soft tissue with frozen fractals.

However, in the postface, after amputation, or after affected area is healed, therapeutic massage can be applied (Fig. 5.13). Massage is used to prevent synechia of soft tissues around affected area and also to improve peripheral blood

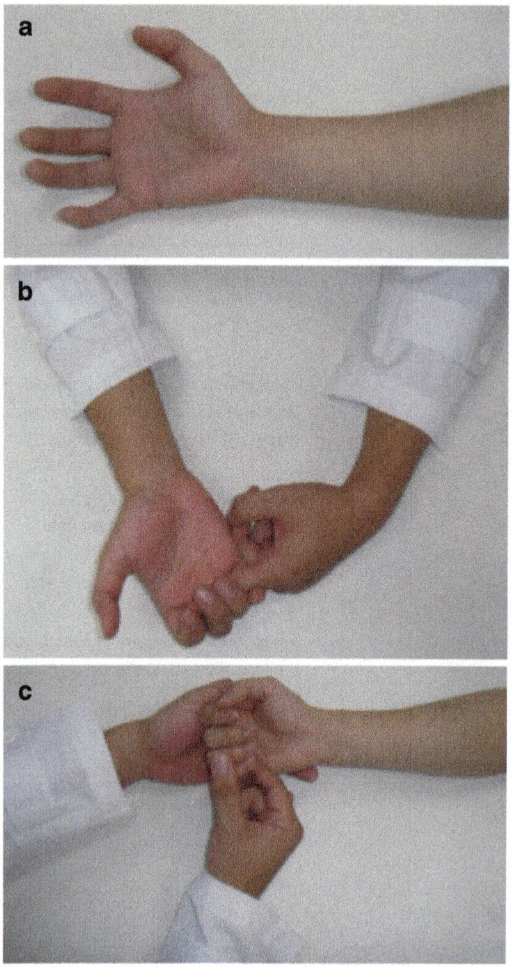

Fig. 5.10 Exercise for frostbitten fingers. (**a**) Active movement for fingers. (**b**) Passive movement for fingers. (**c**) Resistive movement for fingers

circulation, reduce edema, and protect skin flap on a cutting part. Massage can lead to thermogenesis as well. It includes effleurage, kneading, and stroking and is advised to be conducted at least twice a day, 30 min at a time (Fig. 5.14).

Joint Mobilization

Mobilize proximal joints of amputated parts for the sake of reducing pain and increasing mobility after limb amputation. Traction, gliding, rolling, and spin methods are used for joint mobilization. For reducing pain, conduct grade I ~ II joint mobilization, and for recovering mobility, conduct grade III to IV, at least twice a day, 30 min at a time (Fig. 5.15).

5.2.2.4 Physical Agent Modalities

Microwave Diathermy Therapy

You can apply warmth to frozen tissues gradually raising temperature of the deep part of the skin by conducting microwave therapy on affected area as applying warmth treatment (Fig. 5.16). For the therapeutic use, start from very low intensity with 50–200 W output, in which the patients feel cozy and warm, for about 10–15 min, 10–15 cm apart from the patient.

Infrared Therapy

Infrared therapy can be used for thermotherapy. By increasing skin surface temperature gradually, infrared rays can be applied to chilled tissues (Fig. 5.17). Thermotherapy using infrared rays is easier to apply to human body parts than using a hot poultice. Do it at least twice a day, 20–30 min each time.

Whirlpool Bath Therapy

After surgical treatment, take whirlpool bath to increase peripheral blood circulation. And it can be used to escharotomy by removing necrosis with sterilized water. Also, it can be applied before therapeutic exercise for joint and skin flap cutting parts (Fig. 5.18). For therapeutic use, the water temperature should remain between 100.4 and 104 °F (38 ~ 40 °C), and disinfection fluid like butadiene and saline solution should be used. Do it at least twice a day, 20–30 min each time.

Warm Bath Therapy

As an applying warmth treatment, frozen tissues can recover by gradually increasing skin surface temperature with warm bath (Choi et al. 2015). For therapeutic method, take a bath with water temperature approximately between 100.4 and 104 °F (38 ~ 40 °C) at least twice a day, 20–30 min at a time.

5.2.3 Prevention and Management

5.2.3.1 Prevention

The most important thing is to protect the body from cold outer environment. Always maintain exposed body parts warm and dry, and move your

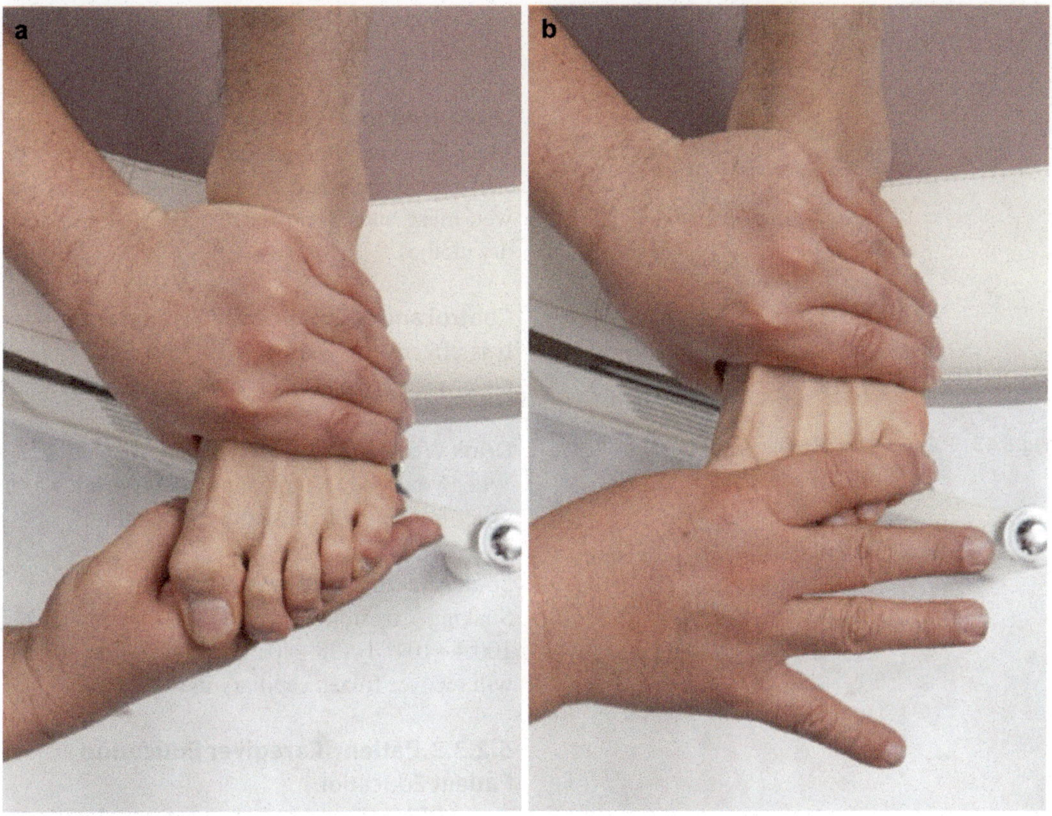

Fig. 5.11 Manual resistance exercise for toes. (**a**) Bending toe resistance exercise. (**b**) Stretching toe resistance exercise

Fig. 5.12 Ankle muscle strengthening exercise using resistance bend

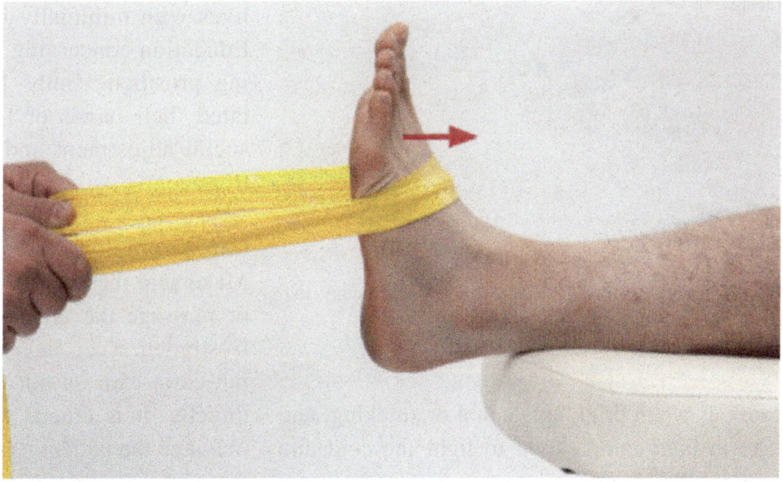

body parts. Putting on wind-breaking clothing or wearing as many clothes as possible helps. Change your wet clothing and shoes into dry ones as soon as possible (Shin et al. 2011). When doing outdoor activities in winter time, bring extra socks, gloves, shoes, and soles, and avoid long-time standing positions and tight clothing which prevent proper blood circulation. Be

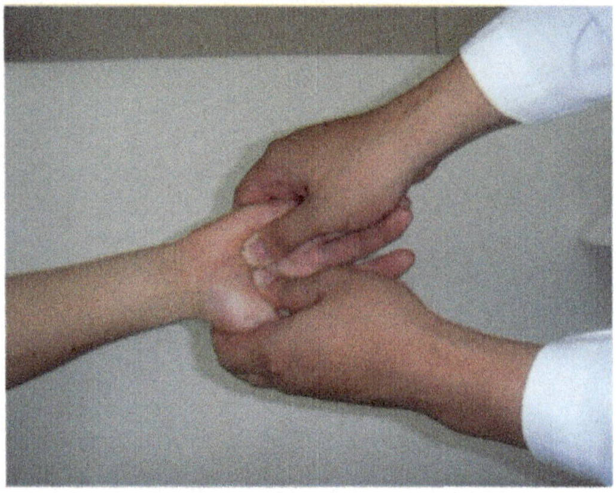

Fig. 5.13 Palm rubbing massage

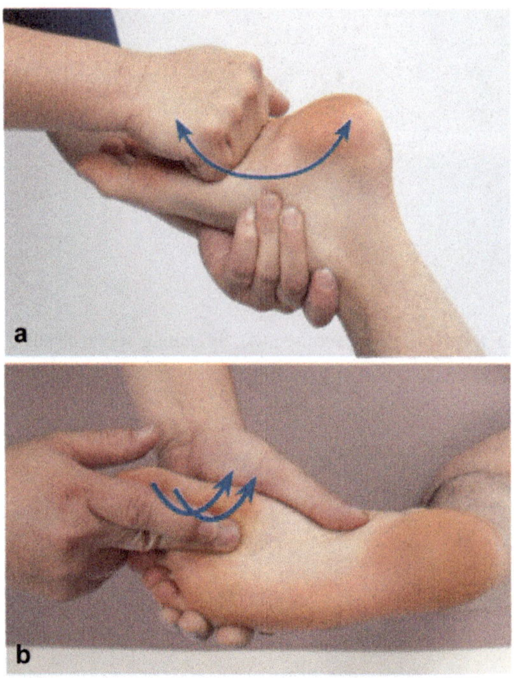

Fig. 5.14 Sole massage. (**a**) Stroking sole with fist. (**b**) Rubbing between bones with fingers

cautious when drinking alcohol or smoking, and take in high-calorie food to fight the cold and drink enough water.

5.2.3.2 Management

Never Stimulate Directly

It is not proper to give hot or cold stimulation when there are symptoms of frostbite. When you see the signs of frostbite, do not give direct tribe stimulation or massage.

Use Dried Cloth

Make sure your clothing such as gloves, shoes, or socks are dried when staying outside. If they get wet, make sure to protect the affected part with dry clothes.

Control and Maintain Body Temperature

It is effective if you put your frostbitten fingers under your armpits or in between your thighs.

Drink Warm Water

When your body temperature is low, drink warm water frequently to raise the temperature.

Soak Affected Area In Warm Water

Soaking frostbitten area in warm water 100.4 ~ 104 °F (38 ~ 40 °C) roughly for 20 min will recover frozen capillary in time.

5.2.3.3 Patient/Caregiver Education

Patient Education

Patient education should be performed with the purpose of protecting the wound sites of the patients and preventing soft tissue adhesion, which helps patients to maintain their daily lives with minimally restricted joint mobility. Education concerning phantom pain and wearing prosthetic limbs for patients who amputated their hands or feet is needed. Consider social adjustment and career choice after the treatment.

Caregiver Education

Make sure they do not pop the patient's blisters or massage the affected area soon after it has frostbitten. Keep indoor temperature warm, and put extra care on not to apply heat to the area directly. It is crucial that the protector do not massage the patient's affected area on the initial stage of the treatment. Patients should not drink since drinking alcohol leads to hypothermia by releasing body heat due to the blood vessel extension. Patients should not smoke either, since smoking arouses vasoconstriction and disturb blood circulation.

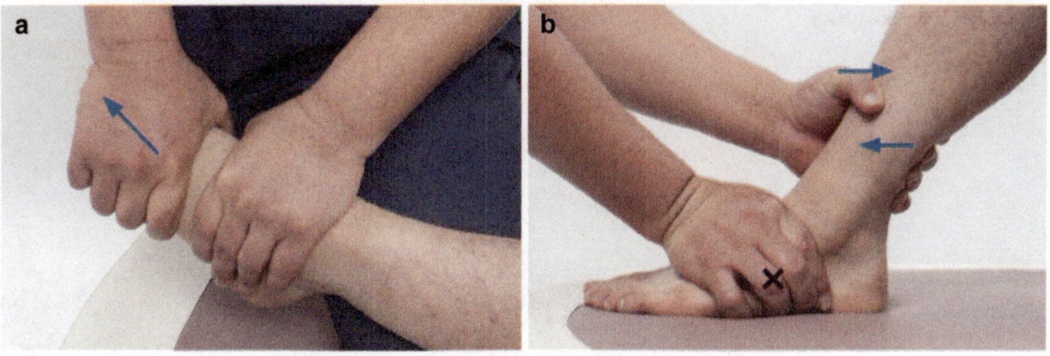

Fig. 5.15 Foot joint mobilization. (**a**) Lisfranc's joint mobilization. (**b**) Ankle joint mobilization

Fig. 5.16 Microwave therapy for hands

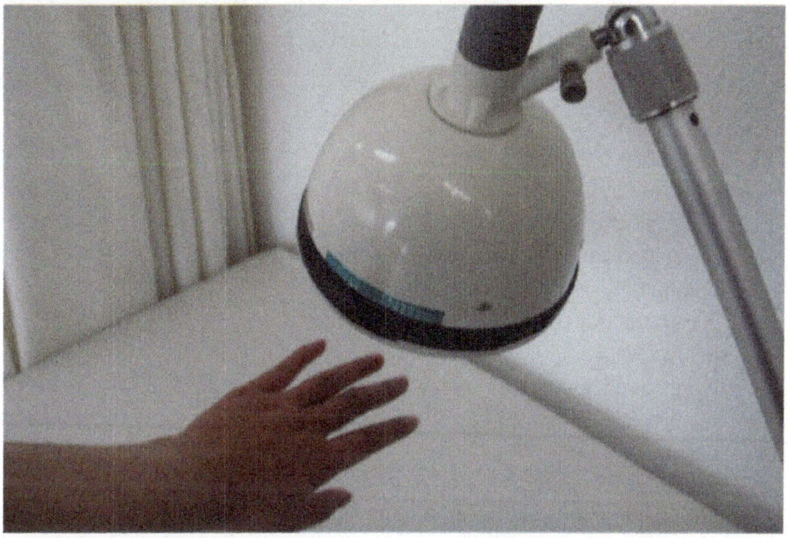

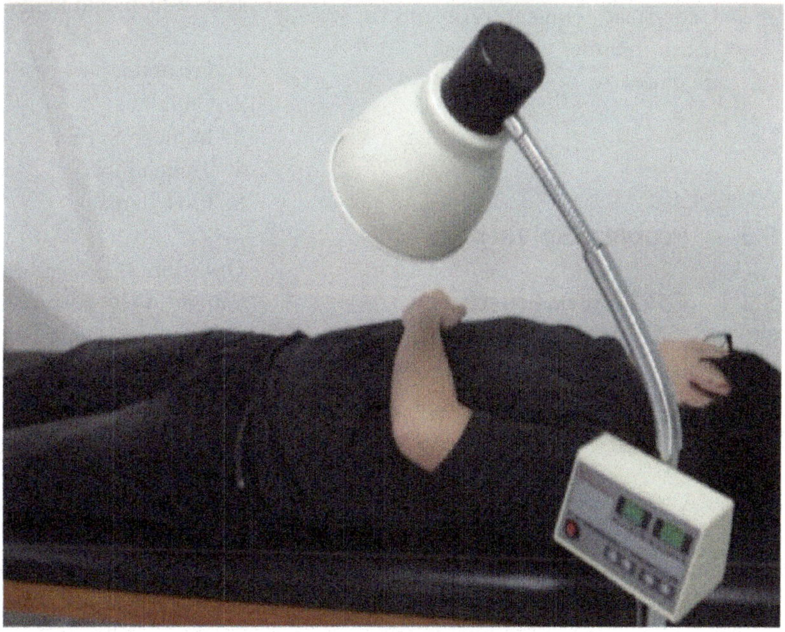

Fig. 5.17 Infrared therapy for hands

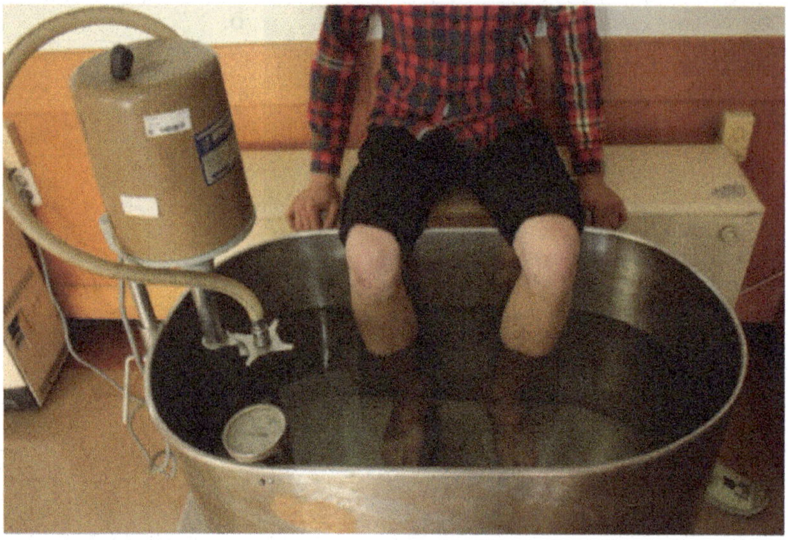

Fig. 5.18 Whirlpool bath therapy for legs

Advices for Physical Therapists

1. Keep medical evaluation and therapeutic documents on tissue damage organized.
2. Never massage before local tissue gets healed.
3. Understand joint working range, motor disturbance, functional disorder, muscular function, sense of balance, and ambulation in regard to limb amputation
4. Understand scar and dermatological disorders after the treatment.
5. Understand clinical problems of the fascia, muscle, or bones related to the treatment.

5.3 Problem Solving

5.3.1 Cold Injury, Frostbite

Choose the most suitable physical therapy intervention method for each question.

Question 1
Soldier A was working in the outdoor perimeter trenches in January–February. Later, he came to the clinic, hoping to get physiotherapy for he found pain, color change, temperature drop, and itch in his feet. What is the name of cold injury the soldier like him gets the most during winter?

1. Frostbite
2. Chilblain
3. Immersion foot
4. Trench foot
5. Frost damage

Question 2
Mrs. A sells vegetable at an outside market. During winter, after cold days passed by, she came to the clinic for rashes around her earlobes and burning skin. Which cold injury does she likely have?

1. Frostbite
2. Chilblain
3. Immersion foot
4. Trench foot
5. Frost damage

Question 3
Patient A is hospitalized for redness, edema, flushing, and aching on fingertips caused by skiing. What would be the most proper physical therapy method for patient A?

1. Escharectomy
2. Deep massage on fingertips
3. Self-dressing
4. Amputation for preventing Buerger's disease
5. Warm immersion bath or infrared irradiation

Question 4

Choose a degree of frostbite that is proper for the following symptoms:

- Damage on thin layer of skin
- Partial hyperemia
- Partial edema
- Burn
  1. First-degree frostbite
  2. Second-degree frostbite
  3. Third-degree frostbite
  4. Fourth-degree frostbite
  5. Fifth-degree frostbite

Question 5

Choose a proper treatment method for frostbite.

1. Massage the area with frostbite as quickly as possible.
2. Relieve the edema by eliminating vesicles on the frostbite site.
3. Perform warm immersion bath with water temperature higher than 43.8 °C (109.48 F).
4. Use soft tissue mobilization techniques for first aid.
5. After the surgical treatment, perform joint mobilization.

Answers

Question 1-④, Question 2-②, Question 3-⑤, Question 4-①, Question 5-⑤

References

Barker JR, Haws MJ, Brown RE, Kucan JO, Moore WD. Magnetic resonance imaging of severe frostbite injuries. Ann Plast Surg. 1997;38:275–9.

Britt LD, Dascombe WH, Rodriguez A. New horizons in management of hypothermia and frostbite injury. Surg Clin North Am. 1991;71:345–70.

Choi JK, et al. Clinical analysis of frostbite. J Trauma Inj. 2015;28(3):158–69.

Imray C, Grieve A, Dhillon S. Cold damage to the extremities: frostbite and non-freezing cold injuries. Postgrad Med J. 2009;85:481–8.

Kim SH, et al. Integumentary physical therapy. Seoul: Sky Yard Publishing Inc; 2012.

Korean Dermatological Association Textbook Compilation Committee. Dermatology. 5th ed. Seoul: Rho Moon Gak. P. Co; 2008.

Shin HK, et al. Clinical analysis of frostbite. J Korean Burn Soc. 2011;14:128–42.

Tintinalli JE, Stephan Stapczynski J, Cline DM, John Ma O, Cydulka RK, Meckler GD. Tintinalli's emergency medicine. 7th ed. New York: Mc Graw Hill Medical; 2012. p. 1331–5.

Zafren K. Frostbite: prevention and initial management. High Alt Med Biol. 2013;14:9–12.

Reference Site

http://health.mw.go.kr.

6 Photosensitivity Disorders

Wonan Kwon

ICD-10 Code
E80 Disorders of porphyrin and bilirubin metabolism
L56 Other acute skin changes due to ultraviolet radiation
L56.0 Drug phototoxic response
L56.1 Drug photoallergic response
L56.2 Photocontact dermatitis
L56.3 Solar urticaria
L56.4 Polymorphous light eruption
L56.8 Other specified acute skin changes due to ultraviolet radiation
L57.0 Actinic keratosis
L59 Other disorders of skin and subcutaneous tissue related to radiation
L93 Lupus erythematosus
Q82.1 Xeroderma pigmentosum

Learning Outcomes
After completing this chapter, you should be able to describe the following:

- The concept and categorization of photosensitivity disorders
- The symptoms and complications of photosensitivity disorders
- Test and evaluation of photosensitivity disorders
- Intervention methods concerning photosensitivity disorders
- Prevention and management of photosensitivity disorders

Key Terms
Photo test
Photopatch test
Photosensitivity disorder
Ultraviolet therapy
Erythema

6.1 Photosensitivity Disorders

6.1.1 Overview

The sunlight provides positive effects to most of the living creatures to survive by photosynthesis of the plants. However, acute or chronic exposure to the sun may cause abnormal effects to certain people. Exposure to the sun can also cause skin cancer. In general, the phenomenon of skin reacting abnormally and showing side effects to the sun in normal circumstance is called photosensitivity. The symptoms occurred or aggravated due to the sun exposure are referred to as a photosen-

W. Kwon
Department of Physical Therapy, Daegu Health College, Daegu, South Korea
e-mail: kwon1967@nate.com

J.-W. Park, D.-I. Jung (eds.), *Integumentary Physical Therapy*, DOI 10.1007/978-3-662-47380-1_6

sitivity disorder. Photosensitivity disorder includes photo-exacerbation, idiopathic diseases, genetic diseases, drug-induced photosensitivity, metabolic diseases, and neoplastic diseases (Lee et al. 2010; Kwon et al. 2013).

6.1.2 Causes

Photosensitivity disorder is caused by the exposure to the sun and at times by exposure to the sun after taking certain drugs or by interaction between the drug and sunlight. In certain cases, genetic or metabolic diseases may also cause or aggravate the disorder (http://dermnetnz.org/reactions/photosensitivity.html; http://www.akd.or.kr/akd_new2/disease/disease23.php).

6.1.3 Classification

Photosensitivity disorder can be classified by various methods. Table 6.1 shows how to classify photosensitivity disorder by the method mainly adopted by Korean Dermatological Association (DERMA) (http://www.derma.or.kr/guest/index.php).

Table 6.1 Classifications of photosensitivity disorder

Types	Photosensitivity disorders
Photo aggravative	Lupus erythematosus Erythema multiforme Actinic lichen planus Dermatomyositis Herpes simplex Atopic dermatitis Seborrheic dermatitis Darier's disease Acne
Idiopathic	Polymorphous light eruption Chronic actinic dermatitis Solar urticaria Actinic prurigo Persistent light reaction Photosensitive eczema Hydroa vacciniforme Hydroa estivale Actinic reticuloid
Genetic	Xeroderma pigmentosum Rothmund-Thomson's syndrome Cockayne's syndrome Bloom's syndrome
Metabolic	Pellagra Porphyria Hartnup disease
Exogenous drug-induced	Phototoxic reaction Photoallergic reaction Photocontact dermatitis
Neoplastic	Basal cell carcinoma Squamous cell carcinoma Malignant melanoma Actinic keratosis Bowen's disease

6.1.4 Symptoms and Complications

6.1.4.1 Photo-exacerbation

Lupus Erythematosus (LE)

Systemic lupus erythematosus is the chronic autoimmune disease mainly suffered by people at young age including women at a childbearing age (http://en.wikipedia.org/wiki/Lupus_erythematosus).

Lupus erythematosus is classified into discoid lupus erythematosus that only affects the skin, subacute cutaneous lupus erythematosus that causes wide range of symptoms, and systemic lupus erythematosus that causes lesion on the entire body. Skin trouble is one common symptom of lupus erythematosus and is found from 80 to 90 % of the patients. The symptoms include malar rash, retinitis rash, photosensitivity, and canker sore. Malar rash is an erythema (red rash) that comes out on the cheek in a flat or protruded form. It usually comes out in a symmetric butterfly-like shape covering upper part of the nose (Fig. 6.1). Arthralgia is another symptom typically found – more than 75 % – from lupus erythematosus patients. Some patients show simply arthralgia, not other symptoms of arthritis such as ardor, rash, and joint motion disorder. And kidney ailments which are found from 25 to 75 % of the patients are not recognized by patients until they progress to renal insufficiency or nephrotic syndrome. Two out of three patients show neuropsychiatric symptoms from minor to fatal symptoms. And it invades organs to cause symptoms (Kim et al. 2012; Kwon et al. 2013).

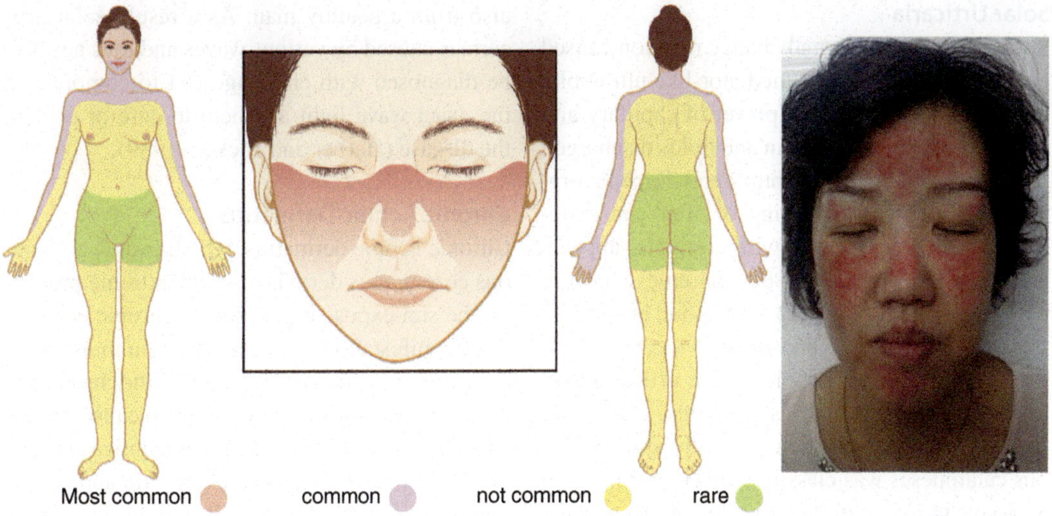

Fig. 6.1 Lupus erythematosus/most common, common, not common, rare

6.1.4.2 Idiopathic Diseases

Polymorphous Light Eruption (PMLE)

Polymorphous light eruption (PMLE), which is one of the most commonly found photosensitivity diseases, causes various forms of rashes such as papule, blister, and plaque lesion at the skin temporarily exposed to the sun (http://en.wikipedia.org/wiki/Polymorphous_light_eruption). Clinical symptoms or various forms of rashes start to appear from 30 min to 72 h after the exposure but most commonly from 18 to 48 h. Lesions normally last from 24 to 48 h but can last more than 1 week. Lesions typically appear at skin parts that are easily exposed to the sun such as the cheek, varea, arm, and dorsum of the hand. Clinical symptoms include papular, eczematous, erythema multiforme, vesiculobullous, and hemorrhage type. Small papular type which assembles to form plaque lesion, together with eczematous type, is the most typical form of PMLE. There is a tendency that this type of rash is caused more frequently by the sunlight in spring and is less likely to appear in summer. Pathological characteristics of PMLE are edema under epidermis, spongiosis under epidermis, liquefaction degeneration of second or third layer of basal cell, and perivascular infiltration of derma lymphocyte (Fig. 6.2). PMLE is usually found in women and people of young age and hardly found in the elderlies (Hölzle et al. 1987; Kwon et al. 2013).

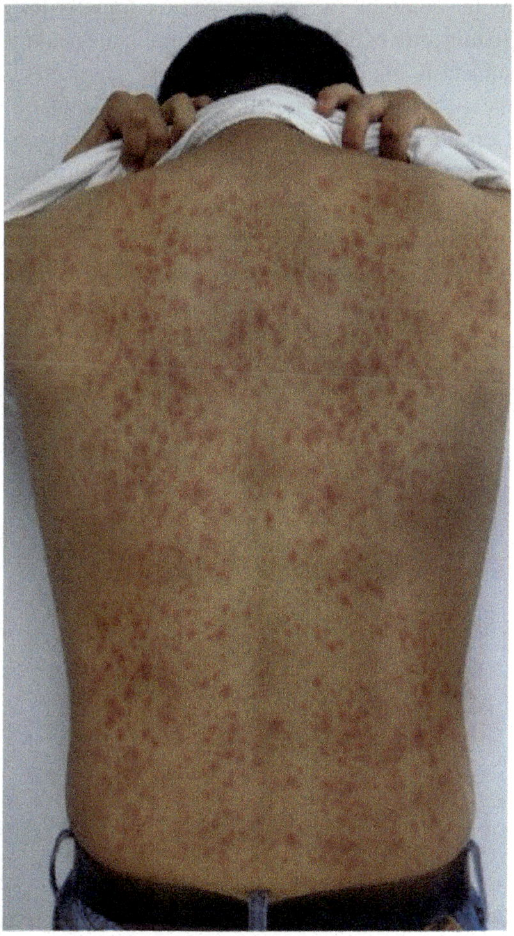

Fig. 6.2 Polymorphous light eruption (PMLE)

Solar Urticaria

Solar urticaria is a dermal change reaction caused by sun exposure because mediator-like ultraviolet ray increases transmitting power of capillary and ovarian vein to make protein and fluids discharged outside blood vessels (http://en.wikipedia.org/wiki/Solar_urticaria). During or after sun exposure, pruritus or urticaria with erythema appears at the exposed skin part but extreme exposure may cause shock (Fig. 6.3). Therefore, body parts frequently exposed to the sun such as the face or dorsum of the hand show less solar urticaria than non-exposed parts such as the arms, chest, and legs. Solar urticaria which clinically shows various catamneses was classified by Harber through a passive transfer test and reverse passive transfer test. In a passive transfer test, 0.1–0.2 mL of serum of the patient is injected to a healthy subject who is tested after 24 h if urticaria is caused by the sunlight. In a reverse passive transfer test, 30 min after being exposed to sunlight, the healthy subject is injected with 0.1–0.2 mL of serum of the patient and is tested if there is urticaria. Depending on the origin of photoreaction antigen, Leenutaphong can be classified into two different types. The first type has molecular weight of 25–45 kd and reacts to endogenous antigen and active wave within visible ray range. The second type has various active waves but reacts to photoreaction antigen of 25–1000 kd which can be found from not only solar urticaria patients but also from a healthy man. As a result, solar urticaria is caused by various waves and thus needs to be diagnosed with challenge test to comprehend the exact wave light and help to cure or prevent the disease (Harber and Bickers 1989).

Chronic Actinic Dermatitis

Chronic actinic dermatitis, which causes continuous eczematous dermatosis with extreme pruritus on the sun-exposed spot, shows chronic eczematous manifestation and decreases minimum effective dose to the ultraviolet ray and is the chronically lasting photosensitivity of unknown cause. In rare cases, it can be developed into lichenification, and in extreme cases, it can cause papule and plaque that make the whole body flush. Chronic actinic dermatitis, whose symptom is exacerbated or ameliorated, shows spongiosis due to a change in epidermis, hyperplasia from acanthosis, and perivascular infiltration of derma lymphocyte. Even a slight exposure to visible ray, ultraviolet A and ultraviolet B can cause chronic actinic dermatitis. The disease is easily provoked at outdoor-working men of middle age or above and can be exacerbated in summer or can last for a year (Won and Yoon, 2007; Uetsu et al. 2002) (Fig. 6.4).

6.1.4.3 Genetic Diseases

Xeroderma Pigmentosum

Xeroderma pigmentosum is the rare cutaneous disorder inherited by recessive chromosome. It is

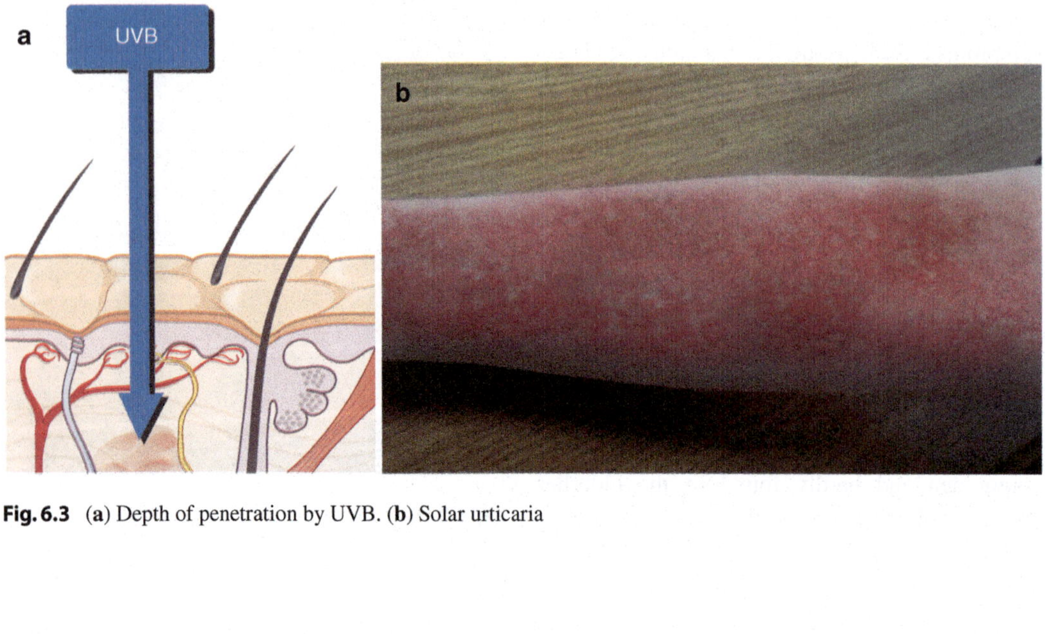

Fig. 6.3 (**a**) Depth of penetration by UVB. (**b**) Solar urticaria

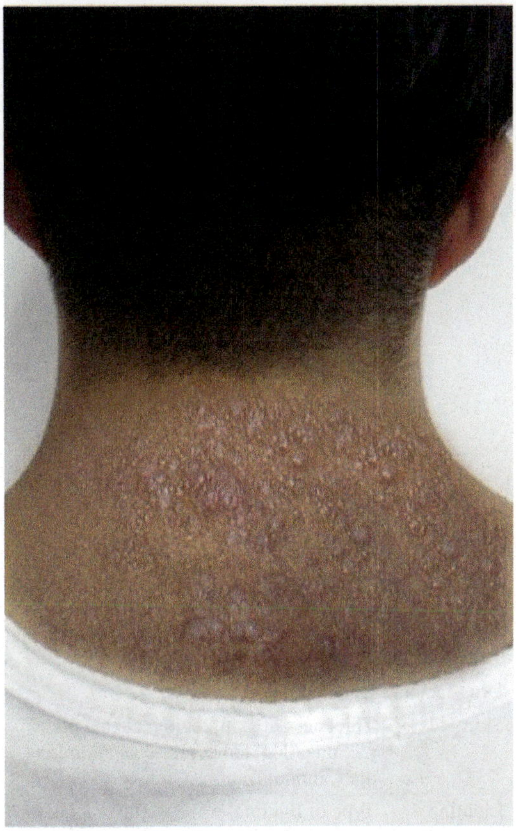

Fig. 6.4 Chronic actinic dermatitis

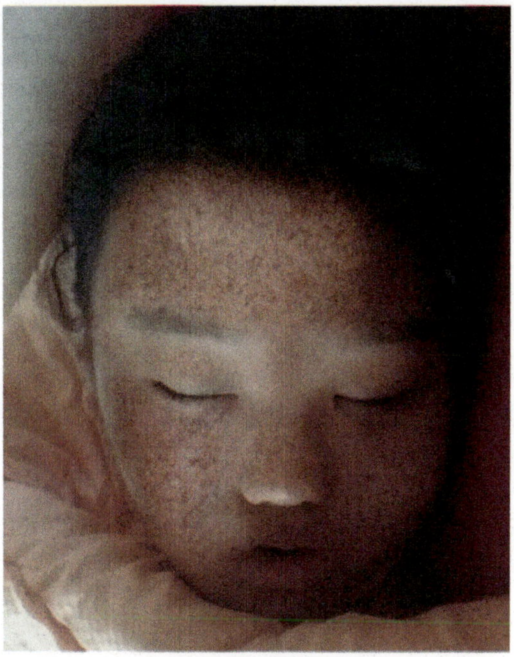

Fig. 6.5 Xeroderma pigmentosum

known to be caused by nonexistence of DNA endonuclease which is an enzyme necessary for regeneration of DNA damaged by ultraviolet ray. When exposed to sunlight, ultraviolet ray damages DNA of the skin, and if the DNA endonuclease is absent, the DNA is irrecoverable, and conclusively the sun-exposed area shows symptoms such as freckle, lentigines, and telangiectasia. Symptoms of xeroderma pigmentosum such as erythema, scaling, and hyperchromatic spots appear from the face and can further develop to the neck, legs, and corpus. If early, symptoms can appear from 6 months after the birth and normally from 1 to 2 years. When consistently exposed to the sun, the skin gets dried and atrophied and capillary hemotelangiosis may be caused. There can be not only hyperchromatic but also hypochromic parts and actinic keratosis (Fig. 6.5). And those who suffer from xeroderma pigmentosum in their young age may get skin cancer such as basal-cell carcinoma, squamous carcinoma, and malignant melanoma. A patient who has xeroderma pigmentosum not only suffers from cutaneous disorders but may also suffers from visionary disorders such as dazzling, conjunctival injection, keratitis, corneal clouding, and amblyopia. He or she may also suffer from neurological disorders which cause mal-intellectual development, microcephaly, kinesioneurosis, sensorineural, growth retardation, and gonadal deficiency (http://home.megapass.co.kr/~faldo/diseases/photo.html; http://en.wikipedia.org/wiki/Xeroderma_pigmentosum).

6.1.4.4 Drug-Induced Photosensitivity

Contact dermatitis refers to cutaneous reaction exposed to an allergen (allergic contact dermatitis) and irritants (irritant contact dermatitis). It can be classified into irritant contact dermatitis, allergic contact dermatitis, and photocontact dermatitis. Photocontact dermatitis can be classified into phototoxic and photoallergic dermatitis (Fig. 6.6). Phototoxic dermatitis is evoked when an allergen or irritant is activated by sunlight. Drug-induced photosensitivity is therefore classified into phototoxic reaction and photoallergic reaction according to the mechanism. Phototoxic reaction, with abundant amount of drug and proper dosage of sunlight, can be evoked to anyone (Fig. 6.7). Photoallergic reaction, however, can only be evoked to a person who is sensitive to photoallergic materials (Fig. 6.8). Most commonly happening phototoxic symptoms include erythema reaction similar to sunburn and delayed reaction caused few hours after edema's exposure to the sun. When the drug is highly concentrated or dosage of sunlight is plenty, a patient may be hampered with walking and daily activity due to

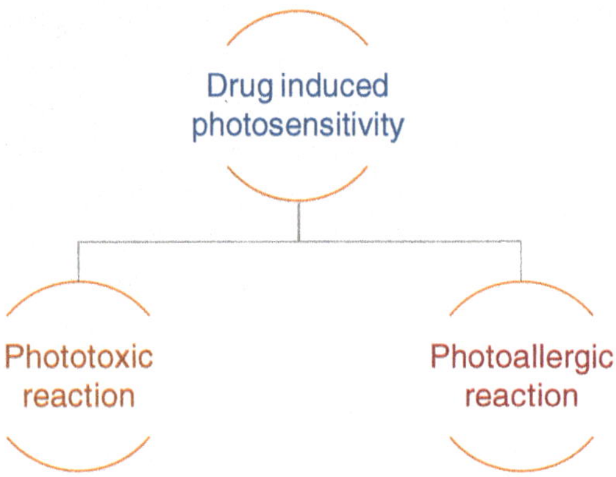

Fig. 6.6 Classification of photosensitivity by exogenous drugs

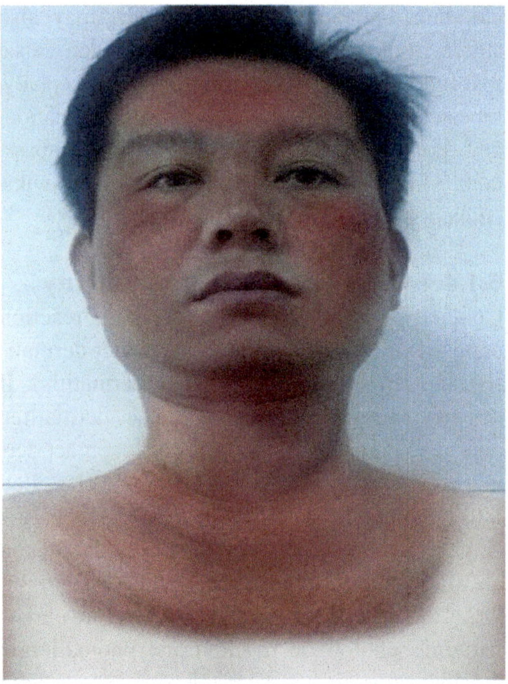

Fig. 6.7 Phototoxic reaction

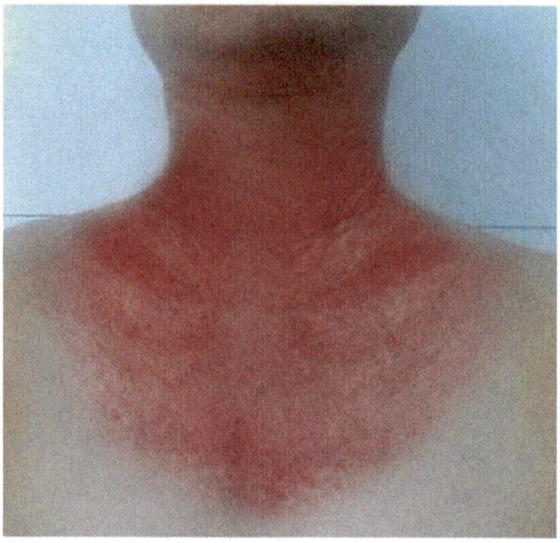

Fig. 6.8 Photoallergic reaction

Table 6.2 Various factors affecting in photosensitivity disorders

Drug factors	Detailed factors
Skin	Thickness of skin, region, degree of melanization, temperature and humidity, ages, immunization status
Lighting	Type of lighting, wavelengths, radiation time, dosage, frequency, skin vascular permeability
Medication	Medication absorption, the capacity of skin penetration, human body metabolism, excretion of drugs, radiation absorption and dispersion of drugs, period of injections

over-vesiculation. On the other hand, photocontact dermatitis causes pigmentation and in photoallergic reaction, it is normally detected by eczema. In acute phase, erythema and blister are formed, and in subacute or chronic phase, erythema and blister are abated to form scale or the skin surface as thick as leather. Lichenification or visible skinfold appears due to decreased glossiness and flexibility and occasionally papule also appears. Causal factors of photosensitivity can be classified into drug, photogenic, and cutaneous factors (Table 6.2). The typical drugs that cause photosensitivity are some sorts of antibiotics, antirheumatic, and anti-inflammatory analgesic drugs. Except for these, many other drugs may cause photosensitive reaction (Eunso 2004; Hwang 2004; Kwon et al. 2013) (Table 6.3).

Table 6.3 Drugs caused a photosensitivity disorder

Classification	Relevant ingredients
Hypertension	Captopril, diltiazem, nifedipine, felodipine
Antidiabetic	Glipizide, glimepiride
Antibiotic	Doxycycline, norfloxacin, ofloxacin, ciprofloxacin, tetracycline
Antirheumatic	Dapsone, auranofin, hydroxychloroquine, methotrexate, sulfasalazine
NSAIDS	Piroxicam, naproxen, meloxicam, nabumetone, ketoprofen, zaltoprofen
Antihistaminic	Fexofenadine
Antidepressant	Amitriptyline, doxepin, imipramine, nortriptyline, trazodone, hyperici
Diuretic	Furosemide, hydrochlorothiazide, torsemide
Depilatory	Thioglycolic acid

6.1.4.5 Metabolic Diseases

Porphyria

Porphyria is an innate metabolic abnormality of mass production of porphyrin or its precursor and is classified into hepatic and erythropoietic porphyria. Sufferers receive extreme damages such as sunburn when exposed to the sun (http://en.wikipedia.org/wiki/Porphyria). Hepatic is characterized as porphyria cutanea tarda and is often found in adult males. Intake of drugs such as alcohol and estrogen accelerates provocation of porphyria cutanea tarda which is more of acquired than congenital. Symptoms include vesicles and ulcers around the sun-exposed area, hyperpigmentation, cutaneous lesions on the cheek similar to hirsutism, and scleroderma. Vesicles easily break and form erosion and ulcer. It developed scar, pigmentation, and at times bleach until it dissipated. Local parts are easily affected, slowly recover, and may be accompanied with calcium deposition (Fig. 6.9). Typical symptoms of erythropoietic porphyria are phlyctenules and vesicles around the sun-exposed area and gradually recover yet remain a scar. Repetition of the symptom makes the tip of an ear, nose, or finger look partly broken. Red urine and erythrodontia are other symptoms, and red fluorescence appears when lighted with wood lamp. Sufferer's eyes may get keratoconjunctivitis, dazzling, ectropion, and symblepharon (Kwon et al. 2013).

6.1.4.6 Neoplastic Diseases

Neoplastic diseases – actinic keratosis, basal-cell carcinoma, epidermoid carcinoma, and malignant melanoma – will be explained in chapter 8: Skin Cancer (McKee 2005).

6.1.5 Testing and Assessment

6.1.5.1 Clinical Examination

Medical History

It is important to understand the cause of photosensitivity whose symptoms are exacerbated when exposed to the sun. A skin is the exterior layer surrounding the body and thus is most sensitive to the external environment. In recording medical history, therefore, it is necessary to comprehend the relationship between the disease and patient's age, occupation, pastime, environment, season, and climate. Whether the drug taken by the patient had any side effect should also be checked. Especially, it must be investigated under what circumstances the patient is exposed to the sun considering their occupation and activities. Also it should be investigated what kind of symptoms appeared after exposure to the sun and whether any family member has had the same symptom. This information will be the first step in diagnosing one's photosensitivity (Norris et al. 1989).

Skin Manifestation

Regarding the rash's type, shape, arrangement, distribution, color, hardness, and manifestation helps diagnosing the cutaneous disorder correctly. Cutaneous symptoms caused by photosensitivity are in various forms and thus the relation between sun-exposed part and the skin must be examined. Lesion can be primary, erythema, hypopigmentation, hyperpigmentation, papule, plaque, blister, and wheal, or secondary, scale, eschar, erosion, and scar. Squamous epithelial cell carcinoma or cutaneous appendage disorder can also be caused. These symptoms appear on sun-exposed face, neck, hands, and arms, and depending on the sufferer's occupation and pastimes, they also appear on the feet and calves. Therefore, it is important to record where exactly rashes or symptoms appeared from the sun-exposed area (Seoul University's a medical college dermatology class 2011) (Fig. 6.10).

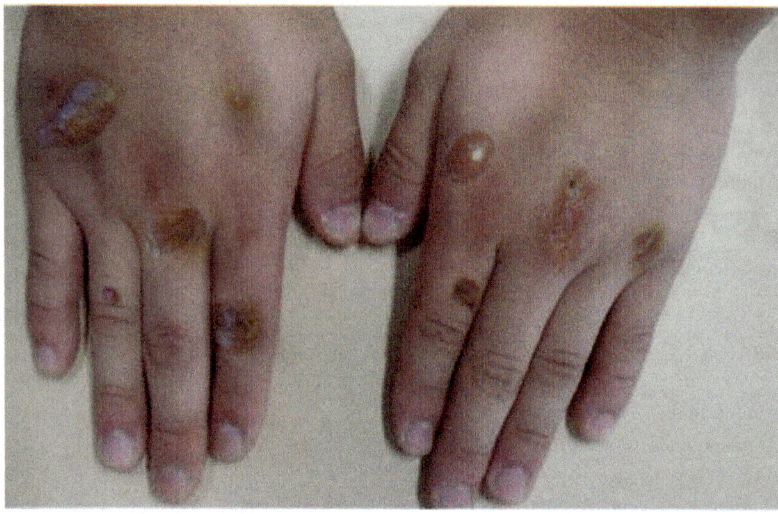

Fig. 6.9 Porphyria

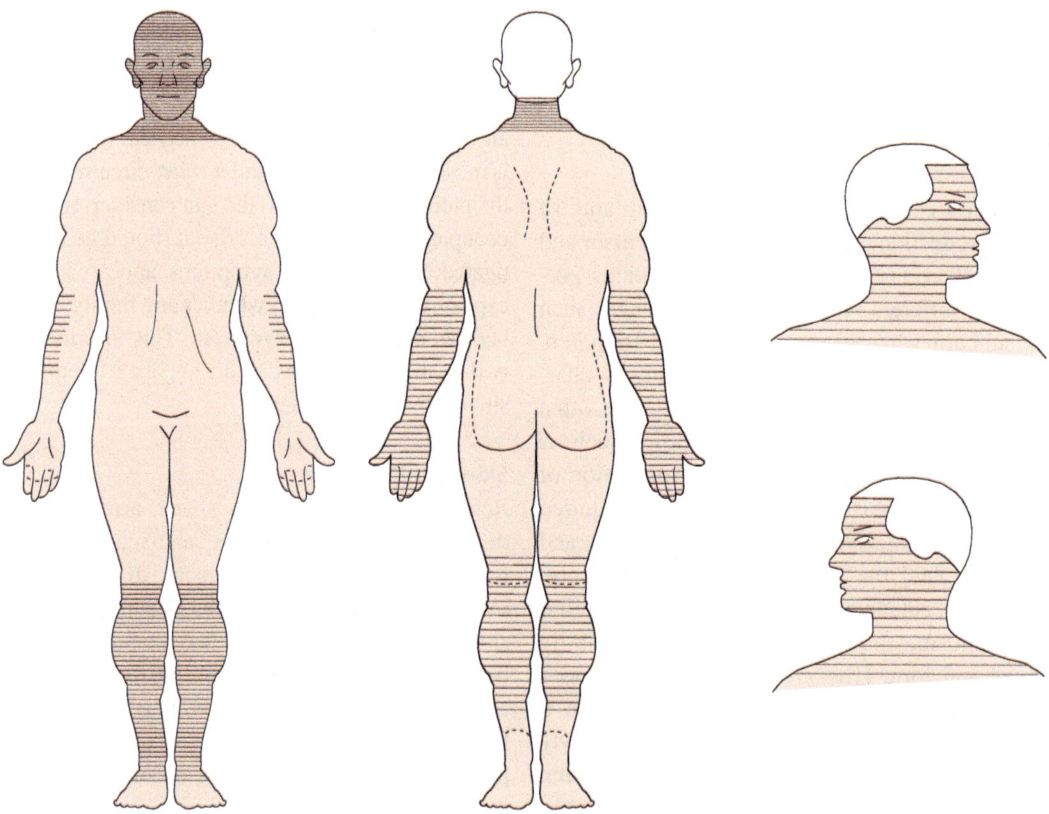

Fig. 6.10 Cutaneous sites vulnerable to photosensitivity disorders

6.1.5.2 Final Test

Photo Test

Photo test is the diagnosing methodology of exposing the skin to visible or ultraviolet ray and observing any abnormal reaction or photosensitivity. Photo test must be done to the patient who has a medical history of eczematous dermatitis or wheal as a reaction to sun exposure, or erythema, weeping eczema or hyperpigmentation appears at sun-exposed parts after taking the drug. If using a sunblock prevents symptoms from happening again, there is also a clinical reason to carry out the test. UVA, UVB, and visible ray are three typical types used in the test. There shall be no problem if the wavelength that causes the symptom is known. It is, however, unknown or more than one wavelength is involved in most cases. If the absorption of spectrum is unknown, therefore, it is recommended that all three types of ray are used to carry out photo test (Table 6.4). It is typically tested on dorsum which is distanced approximately 15 cm from the light. UVB is 20 mJ and UVA 20 J in determining minimal erythema dose (MED), while UVB is 1.5 mJ/cm^2 and UVA 0.5 J/cm^2 in examining solar urticaria. When the dosage to evoke MED is determined, so is the dosage to evoke other levels of erythema (Table 6.5). Table 6.6 shows the level of erythema. As for MED test, the result may be analyzed 48 h after the light exposure. Urticaria, papule, edema, blister, pruritus, eczematoid erythema, and folliculitis are common side effects that are followed after the photo test. MED must be checked in diagnosing photosensitivity cutaneous disorder. Polymorphous light eruption can easily be detected by photo test. When investigating the affecting wavelength as well as MED, polymorphous light eruption shows wide wavelength that causes the symptom because a wide range of lights including UVA, UVB, and visible ray all affect the skin. Therefore, it is necessary to investigate the wavelength that affects the skin for many times to diagnose the diseases correctly (Lee et al. 2013; Kim et al. 2012; Kwon et al. 2013).

Table 6.4 Type of photons for photo testing

VR (visible ray)	UVA	UVB
Monochrometer Xenon lamp	Monochrometer Fluorescent blacklight lamp Solar simulator Artificial sun	Fluorescent sunlamp High pressure mercury lamp

Table 6.5 Exposure time for a erythematic reaction

Grade	Calculating the capability of a erythema dose
Suberythema dose	1/2~2/3 of minimal erythema dose (MED, E1)
Second erythema dose, E2	2.5 times of MED
Third erythema dose, E3	5 times of MED
Fourth erythema dose, E4	10 times of MED
Fifth erythema dose, E5	20 times of MED

Photopatch Test

Photopatch test which is used to diagnose and research photoallergic reaction re-enacts the erythema reaction by antigen exposure and ray investigation. Photoprovocation test injects the suspected drug after MED gets normal and

Table 6.6 Criterion of a erythema

Erythema dose	Erythema	Exposure time	Reaction
Minimal perceptible erythema	Weak erythema	Appears within 6~8 h and disappears within 24~36 h (a day)	Erythema still exists but border are not demarcated
E1 (first erythema dose); minimal erythema doses (MED)	Weak erythema	Appears within 6~8 h and disappears within 24~36 h (a day)	Erythema still exist and border are demarcated After the repeated exposure, pigmentation changes and skin peeling occur
E2 (second erythema dose)	Weak sunburn reaction	Appears within 4~6 h and disappears within 48 h (2~3 days)	A weak ablation Itching Clear pigmentation
E3 (third erythema dose); counter-irritant dose	Severe sunburn reaction Prescription amount which is primarily used for local treatment	Erythema within 3~4 h and persist for 72~96 h (3~4 days)	Weak edema and noticeable pigmentation changes Tenderness and soreness
E4 (fourth erythema dose)	Application in topical region A brief time of applications from a short distance	It appears within 2 h and persists for more than a week	Forming rash, blister Necrosis effects Skin-destroying capacity

measures any change in the dose. In other words, information from the past medical history and photo test is referred before carrying out photo-patch test. After MED gets normal, the suspected drug is injected and photoprovocation test is done to measure any change in MED. The purpose of the test is to comprehend photoallergic reaction to external chemical materials such as medicines or cosmetics (Kim and Lee, 2009; Yoon 1994). Photopatch test normally uses UVA as a light source and uses fluorescent black light, halogen light, and artificial photoflood lamp. To test photopatch, antigen is attached in two rows between interscapulars or at lumbar area. After checking the cutaneous reaction, UVA of a patch on one side is observed. In photopatch test, UVA 5 J/cm^2 is used while in photoprovocation test, a large dosage of ultraviolet rays such as UVA 60–100 J/cm^2 and UVB 2–3 MED is used. If photosensitivity is suspected, non-tested parts of the skin should be covered to protect from ultraviolet. After ultraviolet exposure, cover the patched part so that it can be blocked from the light for 48 h. As for MED and photopatch test, test results can be interpreted 48 h after the experiment and as for photoprovocation test, 20–30 min after ultraviolet exposure. Remove both patches to observe cutaneous reaction (Fig. 6.11). It can be diagnosed with photoreaction antigen if only light-exposed part is tested positive and contagious antigen if both light-exposed and non-exposed parts are tested negative. It can be diagnosed both photoreaction and contagious if the light-exposed part reacts strongly to the light yet non-exposed part weakly reacted. Table 6.7 shows the criterion of cutaneous reaction by International Contact Dermatitis Research Group (ICDRG) (Hölzle et al. 2009; Kim et al. 2012; Kim 2004b; Kwon et al. 2013).

6.1.5.3 Histopathologic Finding

Actinic lichen planus, actinic keratosis, basal-cell carcinoma, squamous cell carcinoma, and malignant melanoma are the suspected diseases caused by photosensitivity. They are caused or exacerbated by light and can be diagnosed ultimately by histopathologic tests.

6.1.5.4 Clinical Examination

Clinical examinations to diagnose photosensitive diseases include blood test, antinuclear antibody test, and porphyria test by urine, stool, and blood test.

Table 6.7 Criterion of photopatch inspection

Mark	Decision	Feature
NT	Not tested	No reaction
+?	Doubtful positive reaction	Doubtful cutaneous reaction
+	Weak positive reaction	Nonvesicular
++	Strong positive reaction	Edematous or vesicular
+++	Extreme positive reaction	Bullous or erosive
IR	Irritant reaction	Discomfort

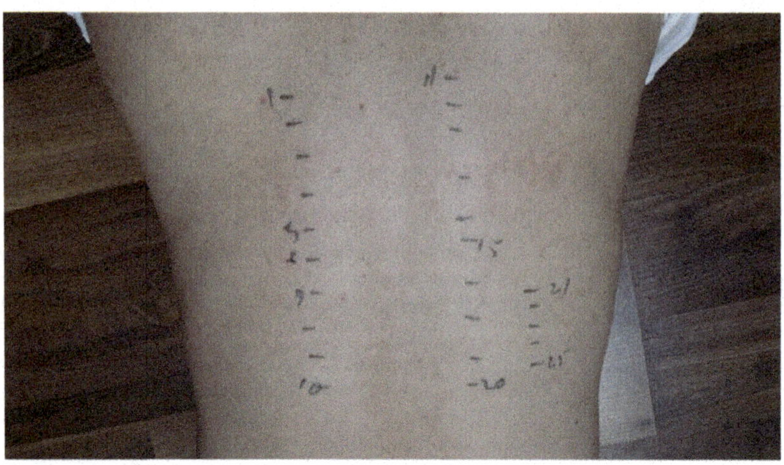

Fig. 6.11 Results of a photopatch test

6.2 Intervention

6.2.1 Intervention

6.2.1.1 Interventional Approach

Humans are exposed to various types of sunlight such as visible ray, ultraviolet ray, and infrared ray. They have positive effects on human but, at the same time, have negative effects such as photoaging and skin cancer. Outbreak of cutaneous disease is either caused by or affected by light. There is no treatment to eradicate cutaneous disease, but it can be treated by injection, light therapy, or steroid that boosts the immune system by steadily increasing the dosage of light exposure (An 2009; Kim et al. 2012).

6.2.1.2 Medical Treatment

Lupus Erythematosus

The goal of hospital treatment is also focused on how to make the disease in a stable state with no symptom. Topically, steroid injection or steroid ointment is applied and generally drugs such as nonsteroidal anti-inflammatory drug, antimalarial drug, steroid, and immunosuppressant are injected (Lee et al. 2010; Kim et al. 2012).

Solar Urticaria

Injecting antihistamine, antimalarial, and topical steroid increases minimal whealing dose (MWD) and helps in inducing tolerance. Plasmapheresis can also help the treatment (Choi 2004; Park et al. 2000).

Polymorphous Light Eruption

Topical treatment is provided to acute, subacute, or chronic dermatitis. Normally steroid ointment or emollient is applied. General injection of steroid to the acute symptom, the drug is most effective when injected 40–60 mg a day. Beware the side effects when using the drugs for a long period. Antimalarial drug or thalidomide can be used yet with small dosage for a short period (Epstein 1986; Hölzle 1987; Lee 2004).

Chronic Actinic Dermatitis

Chronic actinic dermatitis is photosensitive cutaneous disease evoked on light-exposed part and lasting chronically. It is often mistaken for other diseases such as eczema or lymphoma and thus difficult to treat. Steroid is topically applied to the suffering part depending on how serious the skin lesion is. If the lesion is serious, oral drugs such as adrenal hormone, azathioprine, and cyclosporine are used depending on whether a symptom is acute or chronic (Epstein 1986; Kim 2004a; Murphy et al. 1989).

Xeroderma Pigmentosum

Xeroderma pigmentosum is treated with wide range of surgical exeresis and skin graft. After the skin graft, 5 % of imiquimod ointment is topically applied to the surgery part. This sort of surgical treatment brings functionally and cosmetically satisfying results (Kim et al. 2012; Kwon et al. 2013; http://en.wikipedia.org/wiki/Xeroderma_pigmentosum).

Porphyria

Drug, alcohol, infection, and fast and imbalanced sexual hormones are the factors causing porphyria. In order to treat porphyria, the causing factors must be removed. Aside from this, injecting heme to vein for 3–4 days may alleviate biochemical symptoms like decreased urine levels of porphyrin and its precursor. Porphyria cutanea tarda is treated with a series of vein exeresis to decrease excessively accumulated liver iron and injection of small dosage of chloroquine, a type of antimalaria, and hydroxychloroquine. Erythropoietic protoporphyria (EPP) is treated by reducing the amount of exposed sunlight and prescribing beta-carotene, a carotenoid that reduces free radical (Kim et al. 2012; Kwon et al. 2013; http://en.wikipedia.org/wiki/Porphyria).

Photosensitivity Disorder Caused by Extrinsic Drug

A patient suspected with photosensitivity disorder caused by extrinsic drug must be examined if his or her MED level is abnormal. It must be tested if he or she shows photosensitivity if injected with specific substances of the drug because it is most important to remove the drug that causes the disease. A patient should use long-sleeved clothes, hat, glasses, and sunblock to make his or her skin unexposed to the sun. In case of acute infection, steroid, antihistamine, or nonsteroidal anti-inflammatory drug is generally used. In the chronic phase, topical steroidal ointment or emollient is applied (Hwang 2004; http://www.akd.or.kr/akd_new2/disease/disease23.php).

Actinic Keratosis

The minor lesions are treated with surgical exeresis, cryosurgery, electrodesiccation, arthroxesis, or application of topical anticancer drugs. If lesions are large, 1–5 % of 5-fluorouracil ointment or solution can be applied with topically using tretinoin cream at the same time. Decortication and CO_2 laser therapy are also applicable treatments (Won and Yoon 2007; Kim et al. 2012; Uetsu 2002; https://en.wikipedia.org/wiki/Actinic_keratosis).

6.2.2 Physical Therapy Intervention

6.2.2.1 Physical Agent Modalities

Ultraviolet Therapy

Polymorphous light eruption (PMLE) is treated with PUVA and broadband UVB. PUVA had been known to show a better result; however, narrowband UVB is being preferred recently since it is known to show the similar effect with the reduced side effects shown in PUVA. Treating solar urticaria is extremely difficult and thus it is best to minimize a patient's exposure to the sun. Therefore a patient needs to adopt skin-covering clothes, sunblock, window tinting, and shifted life pattern. Light therapies such as UVA, broadband and narrowband UVB, UVA-UVB complex therapy, and PUVA help make tolerance. UVA rush hardening is the therapy of increasing the dosage of UVA exposure little by little every 1 hour and in 3 days, making tolerance to the light. It is reported that photosensitization therapy using low dosage of PUVA or UVB with short wavelength is effective in treating chronic actinic dermatitis that shows resistance to the treatment (Kim et al. 2012; Kwon 2013) (Fig. 6.12).

PUVA Therapy

PUVA therapy has no effect by solely using psoralen or UVA; however, it is shown to be effective when psoralen, phototoxic drug, and UVA are combined. The maximum length of psoralen effect is 340–380 nm and most of the treatment

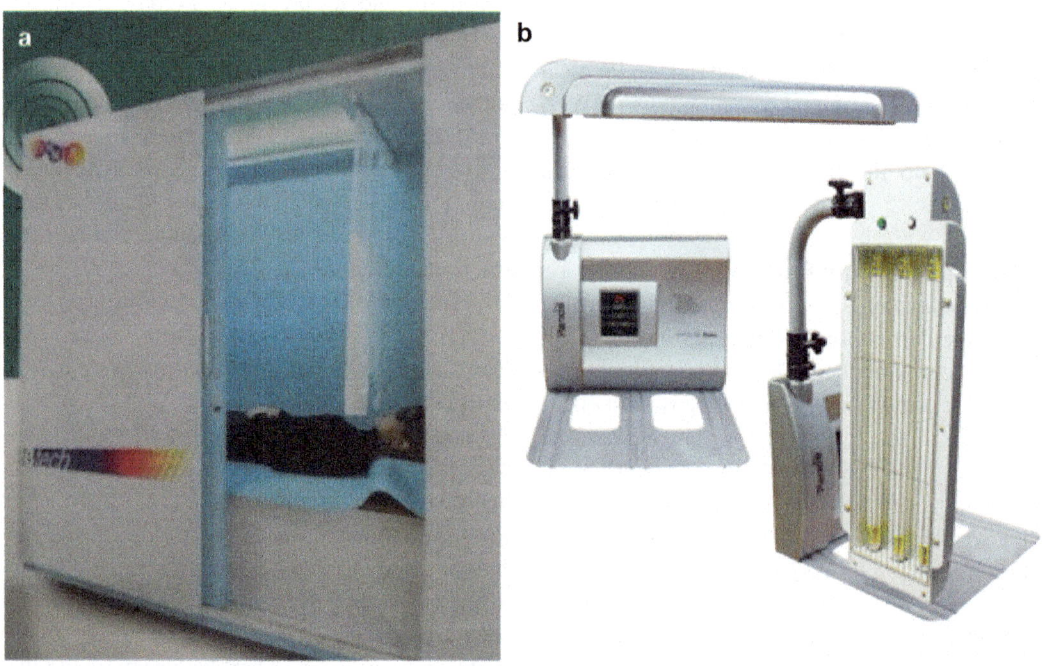

Fig. 6.12 (a) Systemic ultraviolet therapy. (b) Local ultraviolet therapy

light sources have the maximum length of 360 nm. PUVA therapy causes pigmentation and thickening of the skin and decrease in light absorption on the skin. Light exposure also causes hardening of the affected part and deters immunological mechanism due to photosensitivity. PUVA therapy includes examining UVA level 2 hours after taking psoralen and the examination is done 2–3 times a week (Lee et al. 2010; Kim et al. 2012; Kwon 2013).

Laser Therapy

Laser therapy is a method that uses a high level of photodynamic energy and transforms it into heat to destroy the specific tissues. Carbon laser, ruby laser, argon laser, dye laser, Nd:YAG laser, and copper vapor lasers are all different lasers used depending on the type of lesion, and new lasers continue to be developed. The laser is mostly used to treat vascular lesions or a retinitis lesion (Lee et al. 2010; Kim et al. 2012; Kwon 2013) (Fig. 6.13).

6.2.3 Prevention and Management

A major factor of skin photosensitivity disorder is exposure to the sun. Therefore if it is possible to avoid exposure from the sun, a photosensitivity disorder might not occur. However, it is impossible to avoid sun light, so the effective photo protection, prevention, and management is need (Kim et al. 2012; Kwon et al. 2013).

6.2.3.1 Prevention

The main cause of polymorphous light eruption is sunshine and sunscreen must be applied because the drug's ingredients absorb and react with ultraviolet radiation and causes allergic reactions. Solar urticaria patients should wear clothes that cover the skin and apply sunscreen that includes titanium dioxide or zinc oxide to protect the skin from ultraviolet rays. Patients can use sunscreen that is rated SPF 20. Removing the drug that is causing the issue is the most important thing to cure a photosensitivity disorder that has been caused by extrinsic drugs. Therapists also have to check if photosensitivity can appear from specific ingredients of the drugs and lead the patients to avoid sun exposure. Patients who have chronic actinic dermatitis must avoid the sunrays and use sunscreen before being exposed to the sun. Avoiding the sun is the only way to reduce factors for dermatitis. For cutaneous lupus erythematosus, focus on keeping them stable and asymptomatic of lupus, and educating patients can lead them to live a healthy and normal life by controlling their symptoms and activation state of the disease with medical treatments like controlling diabetes throughout their lives (Kim et al. 2012; Kwon et al. 2013).

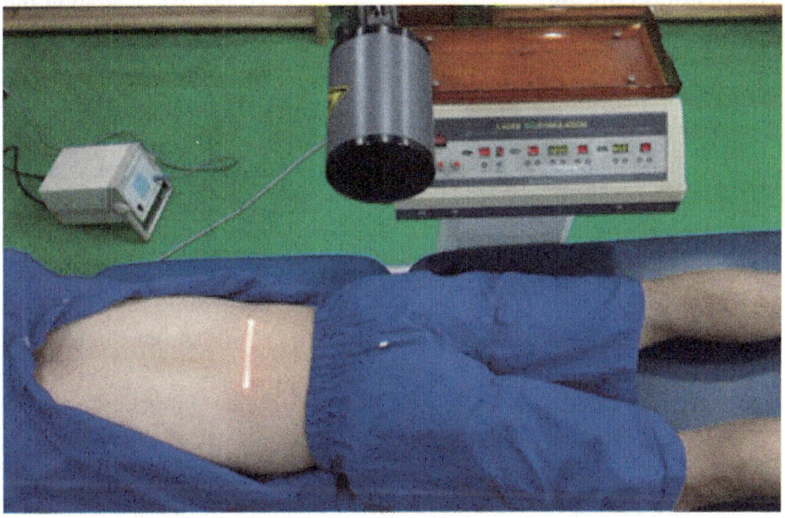

Fig. 6.13 Laser therapy

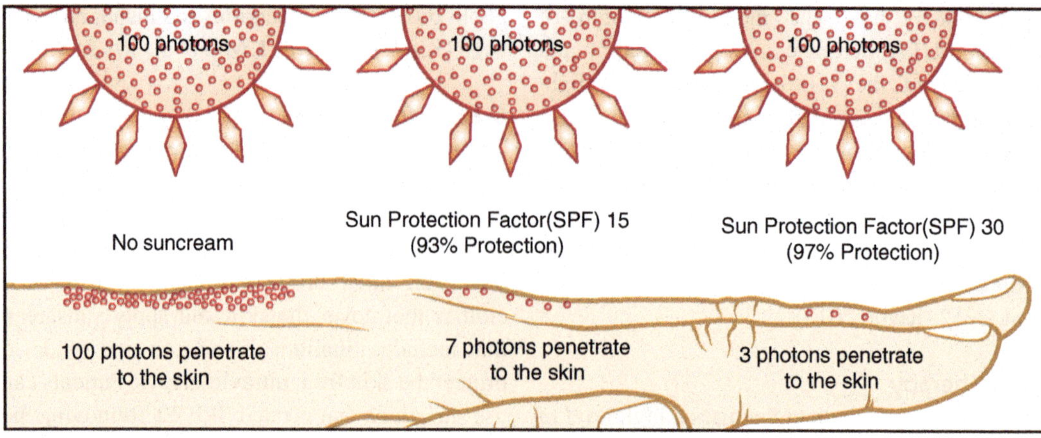

Fig. 6.14 Sun screen

6.2.3.2 Management

Use Daily Tools

It is important to protect skin from the sunlight by using clothes, sunglasses, and hats. A parasol can intercept the light but exposure can still occur through reflection. A broad-brimmed hat is better for preventing exposure from the sunlight to the face and even the neck. Black clothes are effective at blocking ultraviolet rays, but it increases the patient's heat adsorption. Patients should also wear long-sleeved shirts to reduce exposure to sunlight (Kim and Lee 2009; Yoon 1994; http://tip.daum.net/question/62014093).

The Height of the Sun

Avoiding the summer sun's strongest point in the day is more important than avoiding it in the winter. Eighty percent of the sunrays are provided from 9 am to 3 pm, and the strongest ultraviolet rays are experienced from 11 am to 2 pm. Therefore, if a patient avoids the sun during that time, it helps in managing the photosensitivity disorder (Kwon et al. 2013).

Sunscreen Preparation

In a patient's daily life, sunscreen with a sun protection factor (SPF) of 15 is recommended, and an SPF 30 sunscreen is recommended when ultraviolet rays are high. Nowadays, SPF 50 products are available. It is possible to block ultraviolet ray-A(UVA), with PA+++, but the body sweat is secreted during the summer, so using waterproof products for 15 ~ 30 min before exposure to sunlight and reapplying it every 2 ~ 4h is recommended. Also checking the sunscreen to make sure it protects from both UVA and UVB is important (https://en.wikipedia.org/wiki/Sunscreen; http://en.wikipedia.org/wiki/Xeroderma_pigmentosum) (Fig. 6.14).

PABA and PABA Ester

PABA (para-aminobenzoic acid) has a great blocking effect on UVA and 5 % of PABA concentration is widely used. PABA has the advantage of penetration through the horny layer and combining with proteins. In some extent, the sunscreen blocks the sunlight even after taking shower, swimming, or sweating. PABA ester has a better adsorption rate and persistence than PABA (Lee et al. 2010; https://en.wikipedia.org/wiki/Sunscreen).

Special Environment

Absorption of ultraviolet rays happen at a higher rate at hot sandy beaches because of the reflection of the sunrays. However, at a ski slope where the temperature is ten degrees below zero, the reflected UV rays from the snow are stronger. Trekkers who climb the snow-covered and low

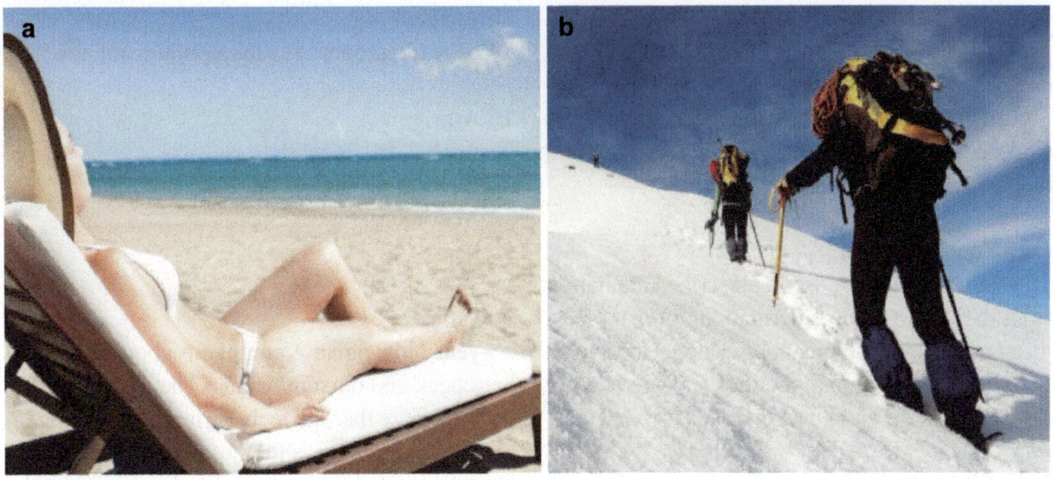

Fig. 6.15 Reflection of ultraviolet rays. (a) Beachfront. (b) High land

temperature mountains like the Himalayas and Mt. Everest have tanned skin because of the strong UV rays. So a variety of tools are needed to help them block UV rays (Fig. 6.15). Iron manufacturers and welders who treat metal with high heat need protective eye glasses because a variety of rays come from the metal and the type of ray is dependent on the type of metal (Kwon et al. 2013).

6.2.4 Patient/Caregiver Education

Due to photosensitivity disorder being caused by exposure to the sun, prevention and management is important. Therefore it is important to educate patients and caretakers on the following items (Kim and Lee 2009; Yoon 1994):

① Educate patients on preventing exposure to the sun by using long sleeves, pants, sunglasses, and broad-brimmed hats.
② Educate patients to avoid the strong UV rays that appear from 11 am to 2 pm during the summer.
③ Patients must wear sunscreen for outdoor activities. Also educate them to use a PABA ester sunscreen that has a better adsorption rate.
④ Educate patients to avoid the beach in the summer and snow-covered mountains since the dosage of UV rays in those places are high.

Advices for Physical Therapists

❶ Therapists must understand the types of photosensitivity disorders and explain them to the patients.
❷ The therapists must be able to explain the methods, the principles, and the effects of a physical therapy intervention for the photosensitivity disorder.
❸ The therapists must be able to make an exact diagnosis and apply proper intervention methods for the patients since photosensitivity disorder shows similar symptoms with a variety of skin diseases.
❹ The therapists must be able to educate the patients about proper photoprotection methods since a major factor of photosensitivity disorder is exposure to the sun.

6.3 Problem Solving

6.3.1 Photosensitivity Disorders

Choose the best physical therapy intervention method from each question.

Question 1
20-year-old woman A uses a prescribed depilatory from the department of dermatology for the aesthetic purpose as summer approached. However, a few days later, abnormal findings appeared on her skin. What is the suspected disease?

1. Dermatomyositis
2. Solar urticaria
3. Actinic prurigo
4. Chronic actinic dermatitis
5. Photoallergic reaction

Question 2
Among the photosensitivity disorders, which skin disease can be inherited to the children from their parents?

1. Pellagra
2. Porphyria
3. Malignant melanoma
4. Basal-cell carcinoma
5. Xeroderma pigmentosum

Question 3
18-year-old woman A visited the hospital because of gonalgia. After she visited the doctor, she was referred to a physiotherapy clinic for arthralgia therapy. She does not have edema, burning sensation, or lesions. However, she said that her cheeks became red. After examining her cheeks, butterfly-shaped lesion appeared on her cheeks. From what disease is she suffering?

1. Erythema multiforme
2. Lupus erythematosus
3. Actinic lichen planus
4. Atopic dermatitis
5. Atopic dermatitis

Question 4
What is the proper area for a photopatch test?

1. Arm
2. Back
3. Dorsum manus
4. Abdomen
5. Legs

Question 5
48-year-old woman A complains about itching on her cheek and dorsum manus. The symptoms she described are that she feels burning and itching on the sun-exposed areas for the past 3 years. She has been taking antidepressants for 3 years since she developed symptoms of depression 4 years ago. She has stopped taking antidepressants for photo testing a week ago and the result was normal. What is the right photosensitive reaction for her?

1. Xeroderma pigmentosum
2. Polymorphous light eruption
3. Solar urticaria
4. Chronic actinic dermatitis
5. Phototoxic reaction

Answers
Question 1-⑤, Question 2-⑤, Question 3-②, Question 4-②, Question 5-⑤

References

An SG, Jeong KH, Seo JW, Choi SH. Koreans common skin disease diagnosis and treatment. 2nd ed. Seoul: Doctorsbook; 2009.

Choi JH. 56th autumn scientific congress: symposium 5; photosensitivity disorders: solar urticaria. J Korean Dermatol. 2004;42(20):82.

Epstein JH. Polymorphous light eruption. In: Ander JE, Anderson TF, Amstrong RB, et al., editors. Dermatologic clinics. Philadelphia: W.B. Saunders Co; 1986.

Eunso L. 56th autumn scientific congress: symposium 5; photosensitivity disorders: photosensitivity disorders. Korean Dermatol Assoc J. 2004;42(20):85.

Harber LC, Bickers DR. Solar urticaria. In: Photosensitivity disease. 2nd ed. Toronto: B. C. Decker; 1989.

Hölzle E, Lehmann P, Neumann N. Phototoxic and photoallergic reactions. J Dtsch Dermatol Ges. 2009;7(7):643–9.

Hölzle E, Plewig G, von Kries R, Lehmann P. Polymorphous light eruption. J Invest Dermatol. 1987;88(3 Suppl):32s–8.

Hwang GH. 56th autumn scientific congress: symposium 5; photosensitivity disorders: prevention of photosensitivity disorders. Korean Dermatol Assoc J. 2004;42(20):87.

Kim KH. 56th autumn scientific congress: symposium 5; photosensitivity disorders: chronic actinic dermatitis. J Korean Dermatol. 2004a;42(20):84.

Kim TH. 56th autumn scientific congress: symposium 5; photosensitivity disorders: phototoxicity and photoallergy. J Korean Dermatol. 2004b;42(20):83.

Kim BJ, Lee SJ. Aesthetic dermatology. Seoul: RyoMoon Gak; 2009.

Kim SH, Koo JP, Kim GJ, Kim GY, Kim MJ, et al. Integumentary physical therapy included body shape management. Gyeonggido: Publication the Sky Yard; 2012.

Kwon WA, Kin GJ, Kin MC, Kin EY, Kin EJ, et al. Integumentary physical therapy. 2nd ed. Seoul: Beommun Education; 2013.

Lee SC. 56th autumn scientific congress: symposium 5; photosensitivity disorders: polymorphous light eruption. J Korean Dermatol. 2004;42(20):85.

Lee IH, Kim K, Park YH, Bae SS, Seo YS, Song YH, Jeong HG, Ham YU. Phototherapy. 2nd ed. Seoul: Hyunmunsa; 2010.

McKee P. Pathology of the skin with clinical correlations. 3rd ed. Philadelphia: Elsevier Mosby; 2005.

Murphy GM, Maurice PDL, Norris PG, Morris RW, Hawk JLM. Azathioprine treatment in chronic actinic dermatitis; a double-blind controlled trial with monitoring of exposure to ultraviolet radiation. Br J Dermatol. 1989;121:639–46.

Norris PG, Camp RDR, Hawk JLM. Actinic reticuloid; response to cyclosporine. J Am Acad Dermatol. 1989;21(2 Pt 1):307–9.

Park JU, Lee JH, Hwang GW, Park YR. A case of solar urticaria. J Korean Dermatol. 2000;38(11):1552–4.

Seoul University's a Medical College Dermatology Class. A dermatology class for medical college students. Seoul: Korean Med; 2011.

Uetsu N, Okamoto H, Fujii K, Doi R, Horio T. Treatment of chronic actinic dermatitis with tacrolimus ointment. J Am Acad Dermatol. 2002;47(6):881–4.

Yoon JI. Aesthetic dermatology. Seoul: Ryo Moon Gak; 1994.

Won CH, Yoon CH. Clinical study of 12 cases with chronic actinic dermatitis. J Korean Dermatol. 2007; 45(11):1144–8.

Reference Sites

Actinic keratosis.https://en.wikipedia.org/wiki/Actinic_keratosis.

Korean Dermatological Association. http://www.derma.or.kr/guest/index.php.

Lupus erythematosus. http://en.wikipedia.org/wiki/Lupus_erythematosus.

New Zealand Dermatological Society. http://dermnetnz.org/reactions/photosensitivity.html.

Photosensitive dermatitis – information of skin disease. http://home.megapass.co.kr/~faldo/diseases/photo.html.

Photosensitivity disorder – The Association of Korean Dermatologists. http://www.akd.or.kr/akd_new2/disease/disease23.php.

Polymorphous light eruption. http://en.wikipedia.org/wiki/Polymorphous_light_eruption.

Porphyria. http://en.wikipedia.org/wiki/Porphyria.

Solar urticaria. http://en.wikipedia.org/wiki/Solar_urticaria.

Summertime skin care by symptom. http://tip.daum.net/question/62014093.

Sunscreen. https://en.wikipedia.org/wiki/Sunscreen.

Xeroderma pigmentosum. http://en.wikipedia.org/wiki/Xeroderma_pigmentosum

Inflammatory Skin Disease

7

Myung-chul Kim

ICD-10 Code
B00.0 Eczema herpeticum
B08.1 Molluscum contagiosum
E02, 03.0 ~ 5, 03.8 ~ 9 Hypothyroidism
G93.3 Postviral fatigue syndrome
H18.6 Keratoconus
K13.0 Cheilitis
M32 Systemic lupus erythematosus
M33.2 Polymyositis
M35.3 Polymyalgia rheumatica
M79.7 Fibromyalgia
L20 Atopic dermatitis
L23.0 ~ 8 Allergic contact dermatitis
L23.81 Allergic contact dermatitis due to animal dander
L25.0 ~ 5, 8, 9 Contact dermatitis
L56.2 Photocontact dermatitis
L74.4 Hypohidrosis
R61.1 Generalized hyperhidrosis

Learning Outcomes
After completing this chapter, you should be able to do the following:

- Understand the concept of inflammatory skin diseases.
- Understand atopic dermatitis.
- Understand contact dermatitis.
- Understand fibromyalgia syndrome.
- Conduct diagnosis and intervention of inflammatory skin diseases.
- Solve the clinical trial problems of inflammatory skin diseases.

Key Terms
Fibromyalgia syndrome
Atopic dermatitis
Tender point
Contact dermatitis
Patch test

7.1 Inflammatory Skin Disease

7.1.1 Overview

Inflammatory skin diseases are inflammatory diseases of the epidermis and the upper layer of the dermis, which are caused by inflammatory factors. Most skin diseases are accompanied with inflammatory responses; therefore, these reactions can be developed into persistent or chronic inflammatory skin diseases. The inflammatory factors include contacts with inflammatory objects, bacteria, yeast, virus, UV, and radioactive materials as well as hereditary factors. Atopic skin disease is one of the typical inflammatory skin diseases including contact dermatitis and seborrheic dermatitis caused by bacteria or yeast

M.-c. Kim
Department of Physical Therapy, Eulji University, Seongnam-si, South Korea
e-mail: 1008kmc@hanmail.net

J.-W. Park, D.-I. Jung (eds.), *Integumentary Physical Therapy*, DOI 10.1007/978-3-662-47380-1_7

and urticaria or allergy by virus. Also, skin diseases appearing as musculoskeletal disorders include rheumatic skin disease and gout. Among the above skin diseases, atopic dermatitis and contact dermatitis will be mainly discussed in this chapter (Ahn et al. 2009).

7.1.1.1 Atopic Dermatitis

Atopy is derived from the Greek word "abnormal reaction or extraordinary." Literally, the disease is caused by various intricate reasons with repeated mitigation and recurrence. Because the causes are complicated and diverse, the disease is difficult to treat. Atopy is an allergic symptom on the skin, respiratory tract, and mucous membranes of eyes and intestine of an individual having atopic predispositions. These atopic predispositions are hereditary. Allergic dermatitis caused by atopic predispositions is allergic dermatitis, allergic rhinitis, asthma, allergic conjunctivitis, and atopic urticaria. The diseases can appear alone or with various diseases at the same time. Atopic dermatitis is a typical skin disease appearing on an individual with atopic allergy. It is chronic dermatitis often called congenital fever whose main symptoms are xeroderma and itching. Due to the immunological characteristics, it is accompanied by other allergic diseases such as hives, metal allergy, asthma, and allergic rhinitis. Also, it has a family tendency. Many people are suffering from atopic skin diseases. 0.5 ~ 1 % of total population and 5 ~ 10 % of children are suffering from atopic dermatitis. The symptoms appear within 2 ~ 6 month after birth, especially it occurs most frequently among the population less than 1 year old, and 85 % occur to those under 5 years old. It is known that the disease appears only at childhood; however, although it disappears in 50 % of the patients, 25 % prolong until the adolescent. And the remaining 25 % continue into adulthood (Fig. 7.1) (Dahl 1990).

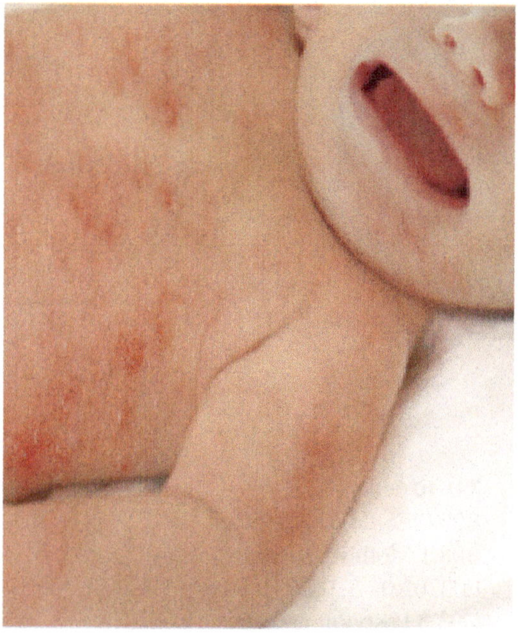

Fig. 7.1 Atopic dermatitis

7.1.1.2 Contact Dermatitis

Contact dermatitis is eczematous dermatitis caused by external substances, and it can be classified into allergic contact dermatitis and irritant contact dermatitis. Allergic contact dermatitis is a delayed hypersensitivity reaction (type IV cell-mediated immunity) caused by allergens or antigens. Dermatitis does not occur in normal people, but it can develop if an antigen susceptible person is exposed to allergens. Dermatitis is mostly acquired, and the symptoms appear about 1 week after exposure to the antigens. The primary symptom is itching. Most people tend to scratch or rub the skin, and itching appears sporadically or continuously. The degree of symptoms may vary depending on the body site of each individual. Irritant contact dermatitis is a disease caused by a nonallergic reaction, and certain concentration of stimulation can cause dermatitis to almost everyone. Although the irritants are known to damage the skin and cause inflammation, its pathogenesis is unknown. The most common symptom is rashes on the irritated areas; itching, swelling, and blisters may appear as well. More than 80 % of the occupational dermatitis is irritant contact dermatitis. However, who has the mild and transient symptoms of irritant contact dermatitis, they don't want seek hospitalization (Fig. 7.2) (Cheol 1997).

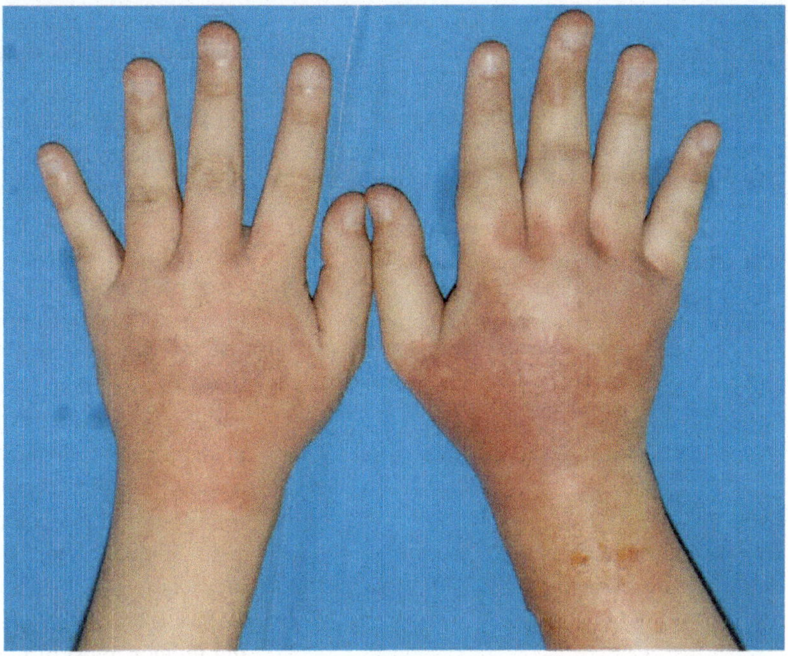

Fig. 7.2 Contact dermatitis

7.1.2 Causes

7.1.2.1 Atopic Dermatitis

Although the cause of atopic dermatitis is unknown, it is related to genetic factors and immune deficiency. In addition, the skin dryness, characteristics of feeling itchy more easily than nor normal, bacterial/viral/fungal infection, and emotional and environmental factors act together to cause atopic dermatitis. In particular, there is food relevance during early childhood. Atopic dermatitis developing within the first year of birth is usually caused by food, and after the second year, other substances are involved in atopic dermatitis. The season is related during the childhood. Mostly, it worsens in winter and summer when sweat glands are stimulated. In adults after puberty, the condition can become worse by stimulants, environmental factors, psychological factors, and endocrine factors (Dahl 1990).

7.1.2.2 Contact Dermatitis

Allergic Contact Dermatitis

The factors of allergic contact dermatitis (ACD) are related to genetic factors, antigen concentration, exposure time, and immunological tolerance. The additional factors are friction, pressure, heat, cold, and existing skin diseases. A simple chemical substance that causes allergic contact dermatitis is hapten[1]. After penetrating into the skin and binding to mediated proteins, hapten acts as a complete antigen and contacts with Langerhans cells. Langerhans cells deliver antigens to T cells, and then the antigen contacted T cells proliferate in mesenteric lymph nodes. A certain portion of activated T cells becomes memory T cells. When the same antigen penetrates into the skin, the memory T cells detect the antigen and cause inflammation by releasing chemical agents (interferon-gamma, interleukin-2) (Jung and Han 2008).

Irritant Contact Dermatitis

Chemical and biological factors are involved in irritant contact dermatitis (ICD). Among them, the light stimuli are soap, detergent, and solvents such as alcohols, and the strong stimuli are highly acidic or alkaline products. The household goods like cosmetics rarely cause dermatitis because skin irritation tests are performed before it is

[1] Hapten: An incomplete antigen that cannot elicit immune responses by itself.

Table 7.1 The causes of contact dermatitis

The causing substances	
Animals and plants	Sumac, ginkgo, mango, *Asteraceae* plants, oriental tussock moth, sea urchins, jellyfish
Metals	Nickel (accessories, watches, glasses, etc.), chromium (glass, leather, plating, etc.), mercury, etc.
Cosmetics	Base compounds, preservatives, antioxidants, etc.
Skin ointment	Base compounds and preservatives, some pharmaceutical compounds
Others	Rubber products, leather products, plastic products, clothing, shoes, paper, various substances can be contacted in the workplace

commercialized. Other common causes of contact dermatitis are shown in Table 7.1 (Cheol 1997).

7.1.3 Classification

7.1.3.1 Atopic Dermatitis

Atopic dermatitis is classified into three age groups. For the first age group, it occurs at age 2 months ~ 2 years; the second group at 2 ~ 10 years, the period when childhood eczema appears; and the third group at adolescence and adulthood (www.google.com).

Atopic Dermatitis in Infants (2 Months to 2 Years)

Infantile atopic dermatitis is often known as congenital fever appearing at 2–6 months after birth. It occurs in 1–3 % of the total infant population (www.wikipedia.org). It starts with slightly swollen spots on the cheeks, red spots, blisters, and scab on the face and head, and it may spread to the whole body. Most of the symptoms disappear, and food hypersensitivity is reduced from age 2. Usually, it occurs acutely on the face, head, and inner parts of the limbs. Eczema usually appears on the face. Especially, a number of fine blisters are formed on both cheeks, the discharge is secreted after the burst, and the scab appears as a form of pruritic erythematous (itchy and hyperemic skin condition). In some cases, the discharge flows heavily, and scratching or rubbing causes infection, so hardened pus or scab eventually causes the skin thickness (Fig. 7.3) (Dahl 1990).

Pediatric Atopic Dermatitis (2 ~ 12 Years Old)

Pediatric atopic dermatitis appears in 3 ~ 10-year-old children. The skin becomes dry and itchy, and it convulsively worsens. It usually appears on the face, neck, inside of elbows, behind the knees, hips, and eyelids. Compared with that of infancy, effusion is drier and less abundant. The skin wounds remain due to the continuous scrapping, and the skin thickens like leather. It is accompanied by rhinitis or asthma. The depression and anxiety worsen itching because this disease occurs during the emotionally immature period. Also, if the itching becomes worse at night, it may cause poor academic achievements due to lack of sleep. Although some cases progress during infancy, most of them occur in 3 ~ 7-year-old children. It appears on the elbows, knees folded inside, around the mouth, and in the wrists, eyelids, neck, and face. The crack is generated around the ears secreting discharges and forming scabs. A symptom such as athlete's foot (dermatophytosis) appears on soles like adults. Because dermatophytosis usually does not occur in children, the symptom is related to atopic dermatitis. Especially, the patients experience that body folds thicken, complain of severe itching, and often cannot sleep at night due to itching. Symptoms worsen most frequently during winter, and then summer, spring, and fall follow in sequence. It accompanies with nervous disposition because of itching, and the patients are annoyed and emotionally unstable. The symptoms become severe due to such psychological stress, and the vicious cycle goes on (Fig. 7.4) (Dahl 1990).

The Juvenile Atopic Dermatitis (12 ~ 20 Years Old) and Adult Atopic Dermatitis (After 20 Years Old)

Atopic dermatitis continues after 12 years old, and it may be accompanied by asthma and allergic rhinitis. The skin dryness and itching of the juvenile atopic dermatitis and adult atopic dermatitis are more severe than pediatric atopic dermatitis. The skin lesions are more localized,

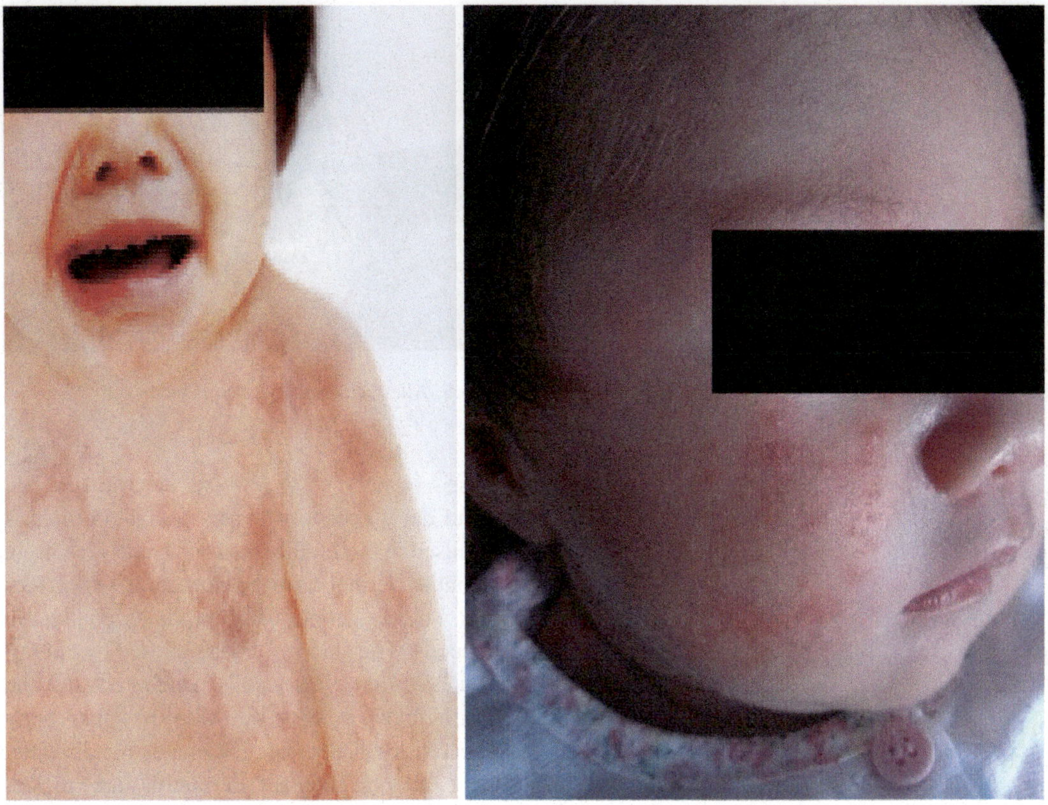

Fig. 7.3 Atopic dermatitis in infants

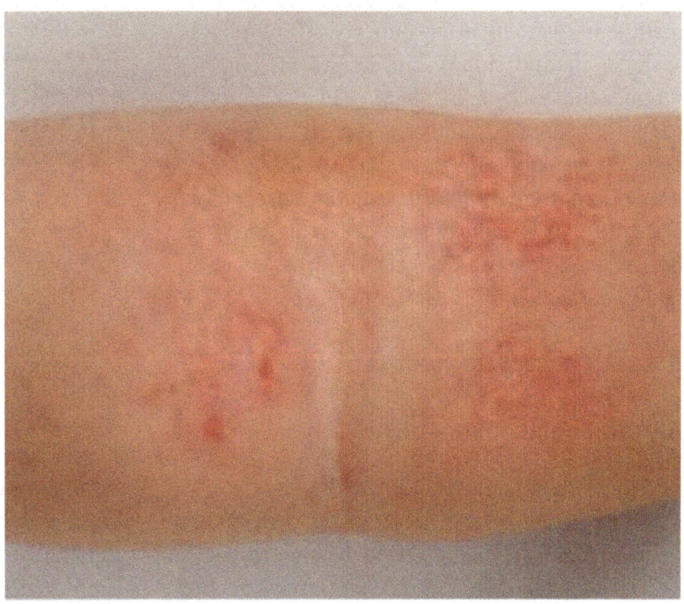

Fig. 7.4 Atopic dermatitis in children

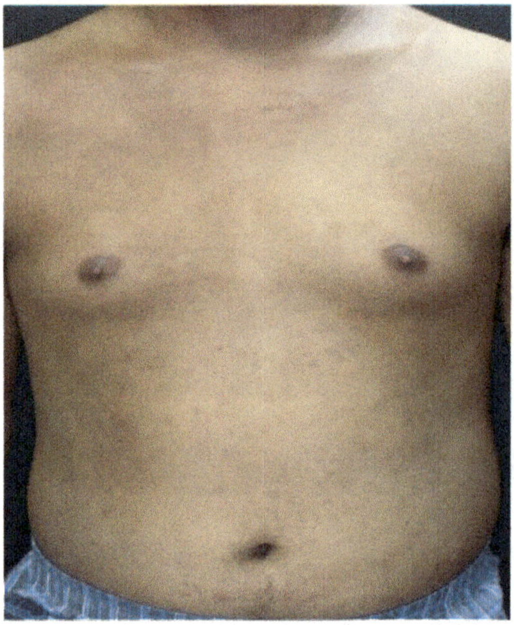

Fig. 7.5 Atopic dermatitis in adults

and thick eczema is formed around the folding parts of the arms, legs, forehead, neck, and eyes. Keratin formed in acute phase and erythematous lesions appear. If the disease becomes chronic, it leaves thick leatherlike skin. Chronic eczema and rash mainly appear on the face, neck, and scalp in adults, and nipple eczema is one of the features of atopic dermatitis in women after puberty. If itching is severe, an individual suffers from chronic fatigue due to lack of sleep, and it results in decreased learning and working efficiency and energy reduction. In particular, as a matter of aesthetic, it hinders interpersonal relationships. Therefore, it is appropriate to treat before it becomes severe (Fig. 7.5) (Der-Petrossian et al. 2000).

7.1.3.2 Contact Dermatitis

Allergic Contact Dermatitis

① Allergic contact dermatitis caused by metals

As application ranges and the usage frequencies of metals have become diverse, individuals are now more exposed to direct or indirect contact with metals or metal salts used in accessory, jewelry, electric devices, and daily necessities. This contact dermatitis caused by metallic materials may result in contact dermatitis to the workers at workplaces as well as people using products containing metals. The skin reaction is caused by chemical substances or metals penetrated into the skin in basic state by sweat or other body secretions. The most problematic metals causing allergic contact dermatitis are nickel, chromium, and mercury (Fig. 7.6).

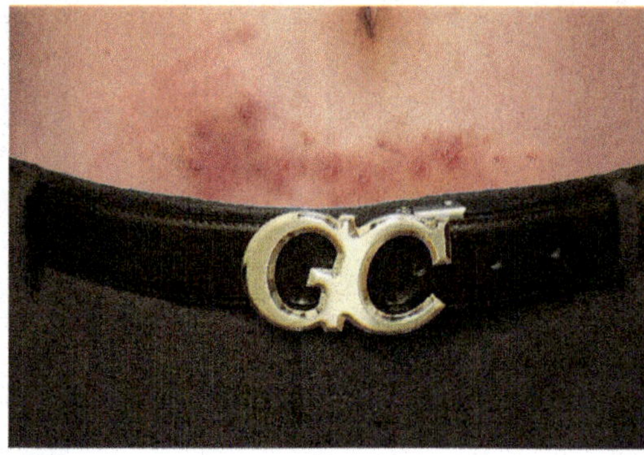

Fig. 7.6 Allergic contact dermatitis by nickel

② Allergic contact dermatitis caused by cosmetics

Due to the nature of the cosmetics usage, the skin reaction typically occurs on the face, hands, and arms, and more than half of the dermatitis cases caused by cosmetics appear on face. Generally, skin care products, shaving cream, and deodorant are the causes of dermatitis, and the products cause severe swelling and redness within a few hours. The major cause of allergic contact dermatitis due to cosmetics is fragrance contained in cosmetics and then preservatives and base components (Kim et al. 2006).

③ Allergic contact dermatitis caused by plants

Contact dermatitis caused by plants is classified into allergic, irritant, phytophotodermatitis, and pseudophytophotodermatitis. Among them, allergic contact dermatitis is the most common with the highest frequencies. The form of dermatitis caused by plants varies. The small blisters are formed first, and then considerable edema is accompanied later. Usually, the symptoms appear in few hours to few days after the contact. Sumac and ginkgo tree causes contact dermatitis in South Korea. Particularly, skin exposure to sumac causes rash, and if sumac is burned, boiled, or ingested, it can lead to systemic allergic reactions.

④ Allergic contact dermatitis caused by dyes

The problematic dyes causing allergic contact dermatitis are mostly dyes of cloth, hair, henna, or tattoo. Of the fabric dyes, disperse dyes cause skin sensitization, and the components of azo and anthraquinone dyes irritate the skin as well. In addition, the main component of hair dye PPDA (paraphenylenediamine) causes many side effects because of its strong antigenic factor (Hong et al. 1991).

Irritant Contact Dermatitis

① Irritant contact dermatitis caused by detergent

Detergent is classified into light and heavy detergents according to the intensity of the cleaning action and into household and industrial according to its application. The household detergents are classified into clothing (laundry soap, powder/liquid detergent), cosmetics (facial and bath soap, shampoo, hand cleaners), kitchen (liquid detergent for dishes and vegetable), and residential (bathroom). A typical soap or detergent does not irritate the normal skin, but it may act as an irritant if the skin is already damaged.

② Irritant contact dermatitis caused by oil

Irritant contact dermatitis caused by oil occurs in many workers who are exposed to various types of oils. It appears as folliculitis on the arms, femoral region, or closely contacted body parts with oil-contaminated clothes. Follicular occlusion and irritation by oil are assumed the causes of the disease. In severe cases, it is cured leaving a scar.

③ Irritant contact dermatitis caused by cosmetics

Irritation associated with cosmetic uses is classified into objective and subjective irritation responses. In many cases, irritant contact dermatitis occurs by weak stimulation, but patients often do not seek hospitalization due to the mild symptoms (Fig. 7.7) (Kee et al. 1995).

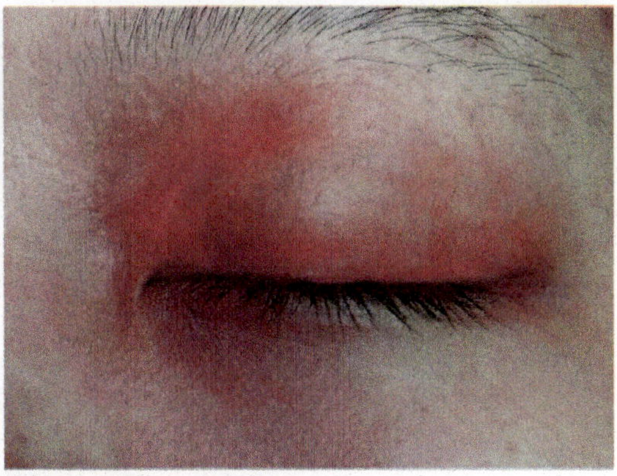

Fig. 7.7 Irritant contact dermatitis by cosmetics

7.1.4 Symptoms and Complications

7.1.4.1 Atopic Dermatitis

Symptoms

Among the symptoms including severe itching, dry skin, rash, gangrene, scab, and peeling skin (scales), severe itching is the most noticeable feature. Skin rash occurs due to scratching rather than itching due to skin rash. The degree of itching is so severe that one scratches until bleeding, and in this case, the vicious cycle of itching and scratching continues. It is problematic that blister and scab formed by external wound when scratching cause the secondary bacterial infection. Also, the unbearable itching may cause distraction and poor academic achievements. Psychological damage or emotional wound might occur because of bullying or teasing from other children. Due to the shallow sleep, it is difficult to become a physically and mentally healthy child. The mental problems worsen the skin status or the skin lesions may result in mental changes. An individual easily becomes depressed due to severe emotional changes and overly sensitive even with a little stress and may feel chronically insecure. Also, the patients seem to be nervous because they are sensitive and impatient (Ahn et al. 2009).

Complications

Atopic dermatitis may accompany with a number of complications. The external wound formed by

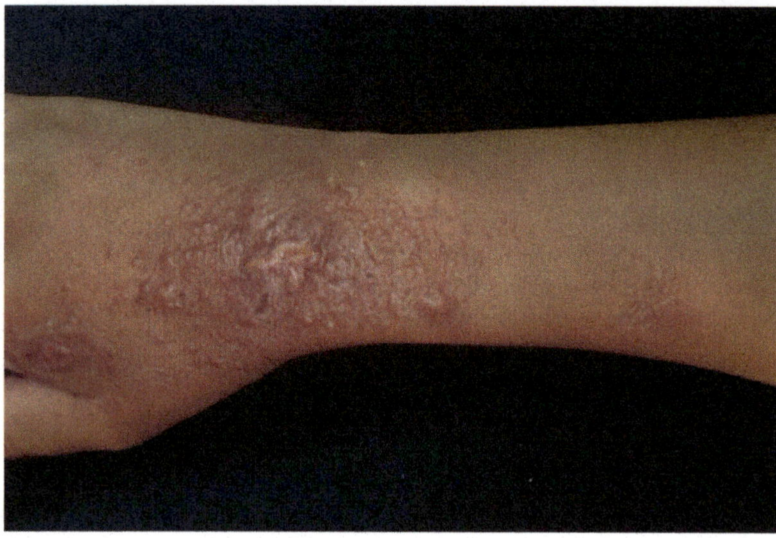

Fig. 7.8 Erythema and rash by contact dermatitis

scratching due to severe itching may cause secondary bacterial infection such as staphylococcal infection (superantigen), and water warts, a type of molluscum contagiosum, are formed due to viral infection. Also, extensive eczema herpiticum lesion occurs and generally the frequency of the pityriasis increases. Although it is rare in severe atopic dermatitis patients, a special type of cataract also occurs (Dahl 1990).

7.1.4.2 Contact Dermatitis

Symptoms

The symptoms of the primary irritant dermatitis and allergic irritant dermatitis are similar, and they are mainly erythema and swelling associated lesions in the form of eczema. In some cases, acne lesions, urticaria lesions, erythema multiforme, pigmentation, and granulomatous lesions may occur. Irritant dermatitis is limited to the allergen contacted areas of the skin, whereas allergic dermatitis is more widely spread on the skin. Erythema appears immediately in contact dermatitis as a form of common rash. Rash in allergic contact dermatitis may not appear until 24 ~ 72 h after the exposure to the allergen. Bleb, welt, or hive appears as a colony on the area of the skin exposed directly to the allergens or irritants. Also, itching and burning sensation are also common symptoms (Fig. 7.8).

Complications

One should avoid contact with allergens. If contact dermatitis has already occurred, it has to be treated according to the general principles of eczema. The symptoms of acute contact dermatitis are characterized by redness, swelling blisters, and gangrene. The bullous lesion has to be dried using cold wet dressing and then lots of creams or lotions should be applied. In chronic contact dermatitis characterized by keratin and lichenification[2], greasy ointment or creams are effective. After applying medicaments, sealing helps cure the disease faster. If the disease is spread systematically or topical agents are not effective, systemic antihistamine and steroidal adrenocortical hormone can be helpful (Bong et al. 2006; Kee et al. 1995).

7.1.5 Testing and Assessment

7.1.5.1 Atopic Dermatitis

There are no biological indicators that can accurately diagnose atopic dermatitis. Although the diagnosis is based on clinical symptoms, the most widely accepted diagnostic criteria were proposed by Hanifin and Rajka in 1980.

[2] Lichenificaton: The thickened state of the skin like leather due to scratching or rubbing.

Also, the concentration of serum IgE[3] is increased in approximately 80 ~ 90 % of the atopic dermatitis patients, and this secreted IgE causes mast cells to release histamine, a substance causing itch (Dahl 1990).

The Essential Diagnostic Criteria

The symptoms can be observed when diagnosing atopic dermatitis are as follows, and at least three of the criteria have to be met in order to diagnose atopic dermatitis (www.medcity.com):

① Atopic disease (asthma, allergic rhinitis, accompanied history of atopic dermatitis, etc.) appeared in patients or family member
② Severe systemic itching (pruritus)
③ Chronic and recurrent eczema
④ The appearance and distribution of relatively commonly appearing eczema according to the age

The Supplementary Diagnostic Criteria

The supplementary diagnostic criteria for atopic dermatitis can be conducted by observing various skin conditions. Distinctively dry skin, keratosis pilaris (goose bumps), bumpy skin around pores, immediate skin reactions (urticaria), nonspecific eczema on the hands and feet, nipple eczema, cheilitis, pityriasis rosea (psoriasis), etc. are needed to be confirmed. The eyes, neck, and excessive wrinkles of the palm are also important indicators. Besides the skin conditions, atopic dermatitis also can be diagnosed by ophthalmic findings such as recurrent conjunctivitis, keratoconus, and atopic cataracts (Ahn et al. 2009).

Food Allergy Test

If the symptoms of atopic dermatitis patients are related with food allergy, patients' medical history can be used when testing for allergy. Although there is no accurate statistics of the incidence of food allergy in atopic dermatitis patients in Korea, generally 20 out of 110 atopic patients showed atopy becomes worse by ingesting certain foods, and this incidence is lower than the United States showing 30 % in atopic patients. The most common foods causing atopy in children are milk, eggs, peanuts, fish, soy, wheat, and nuts. In adults, peanuts, nuts, fish, and shellfish are known to cause allergic reactions. In addition, food additives can cause hives according to recent studies, but their effects on atopic dermatitis are insignificant in most cases.

Allergy symptoms caused by food vary from person to person. Rubbing eyes can often be observed in infants, children often complain of itching, and hives appear on the face and body. Vomiting, diarrhea, and stomachache may occur, and eye or lip swelling may lead to difficulty in breathing. Typically, such common allergic reactions appear immediately after the food ingestion, but the atopic dermatitis patients are characterized by erythematous rash accompanied by itching on the existing site of atopic dermatitis. Continuously eating allergy causing food worsens the symptoms of atopic dermatitis (Dahl 1990).

7.1.5.2 Contact Dermatitis

History Taking

The diagnosis of contact dermatitis is conducted by multifaceted interviews asking patient's medical history, age, gender, occupation, hobbies, and all the substances expected to be in close contact.

Patch Test

It is a method used to identify skin reaction by attaching allergens to the skin. After attaching, the skin reaction is read on the second and fourth days. If the dermatitis is widely spread, the test might show false-positive because of other skin hypersensitivities, so it is recommended to repeat the test several weeks after the first try. The substances commonly causing contact dermatitis specific to body parts are hair dyes, hair lotions, shampoo, permanent drugs in the head, and cosmetics on the face. Lipstick, toothpaste, denture, chewing gum, and food may cause dermatitis in the lips and around the mouth. Also, earrings, necklace, eyeglass frames, perfume,

[3] Serum IgE: It is one of the immunoglobulin presenting in body fluids, and its concentration increases at immune disorder and parasitic infection.

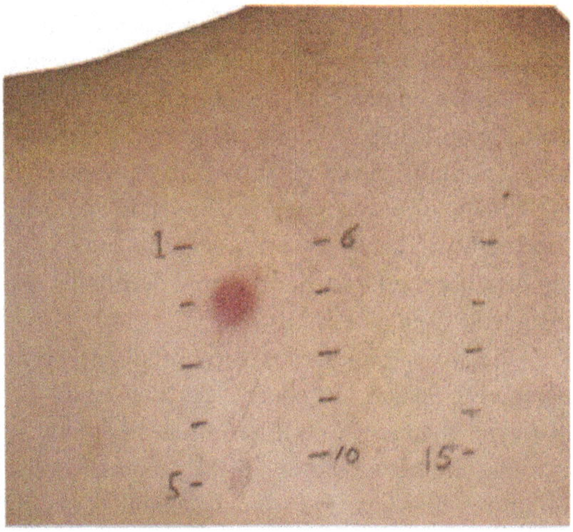

Fig. 7.9 Patch tests

and metal buttons can be potential causing agents, so the suspected elements should be detected during the history taking (Fig. 7.9) (Kim et al. 2008).

7.2 Intervention

7.2.1 Interventional Approach

Prior to the physical treatment of inflammatory skin diseases, gender, race, personal habits, occupation, lifestyle, general health status, and medical and surgical history are checked, and current status, major complaints, functional status, and the activity levels are identified. And then, the skin condition is examined, being divided into local and systemic areas. First, as a local area examination, observation, palpation, and picture evaluation are conducted. And then, itching, hives, rash, skin pigmentation such as wrinkle and rash, skin color change, and swelling are examined. As a part of the whole-body screening, temperature changes, hair changes, and wet skin like hyperhidrosis or dry skin like hypohidrosis are examined. Since inflammatory skin diseases may cause the secondary infection spread to other body parts or other people, regular assessments should be recorded daily as shown in Table 7.2 (Marilyn 2006).

Table 7.2 Daily assessment

Assessment items (check every day) yes/no changed contents
New symptoms?
Worsening symptoms?
Medication changes?
Vital signs changes?
Lab values changes?
Skin changes?
Activity changes?
Changes in sleep patterns
Changes in equipment needs?
Changes in caregiver needs?
Obstacles to performing activities?
Dietary needs/recommendation?

A score table can be used for other skin disorders

7.2.2 Medical Management

7.2.2.1 Atopic Dermatitis

Since atopic constitution fundamentally cannot be cured, it is better to avoid the causing substances and receive appropriate treatments instead of aiming for the complete cure. The treatment prospects are unpredictable and the outcomes vary; sometimes, it is curable, the treatment is either effective or not, eczema continues until puberty, and symptoms can be controlled to some extent in some cases. Typically, the skin becomes dry, and eczema appears again or becomes severe if the skin is irritated, and the symptoms can appear intermittently throughout the entire life. For the treatment of atopic dermatitis, discussion between the patient and caregivers as well as other people is needed. It is recommended that the patients do not wear tight-fitting clothes, cut nails short, and avoid wool fiber products and excessive heat. Also, minimizing skin becoming wet and exposure to irritants such as oil are necessary. It is recommended to stay away from dogs and cats which can cause acute exacerbations. Likewise, help from other people as well as patients themselves is required in treating atopic dermatitis. Commonly used atopic dermatitis treatments are introduced in Table 7.3. The fundamentals of the atopic dermatitis treatment are removing the causing substances and maintaining moisture as described previously. Also, appropriate medical treatments are required.

Table 7.3 Treatment of atopic dermatitis

Treatment	Indications
Emollient	Eczema, ichthyosis
Topical steroids	Eczema
Topical tacrolimus	Steroid-resistant dermatitis
Tar bandage	Lichenification, dermatitis accompanying old wounds
Oral antihistamine	Pruritus
Oral antibiotics	Accompanying bacterial infections
Food regulation	Food allergy/dermatitis resistant to conventional treatments
Medium-wave ultraviolet (UVB), cyclosporine, azathioprine	Severe dermatitis resistant to conventional and topical treatments

Proper steroid therapy, immunoglobulin therapy, phototherapy, or immunomodulator such as cyclosporine A is used. But the fundamental cure is impossible because the exact etiology of atopic dermatitis is unknown. Atopic dermatitis patients have to use water-based cream and emulsifying ointment such as emollient regularly in order to minimize the drying skin. Skin softeners moisturize dry skin, help to eliminate the thought of scratching, and minimize the need of topical steroid application. Bath emollient is also helpful. The principle of using topical corticosteroids is selecting steroids with high efficacy and low titer. In childhood, applying 1% of hydrocortisone twice a day is recommended. Ointments are more preferred than creams. For infection by external wound or eczema, topical fungicide or topical antibiotics can be applied for 7 days alone or in combination with steroids. Coal tar or ichthammol is applied on dermatitis accompanied by thick skin or wound, and sealed bands should be used before sleeping. In addition, wet wrap can be used on exudative dermatitis (Figs. 7.10 and 7.11) (David 2010; Lee and Noh 2010)

7.2.2.2 Contact Dermatitis

① Topical Treatment

Topical treatment minimizes the drug exposure to other organs other than the skin, it is safer compared with systemic drugs, and the side effects appear locally. For effective topical treatment, not only appropriate drug selection is needed, but affected site, the state of the affected skin, concentration of the appropriate base material, application method, and the duration maximizing the efficacy and minimizing the side effects also should be considered. The frequency of drug use does not affect the efficacy of topical drugs, but excessive application may cause unnecessary irritation or side effects by systemic drug exposure. Figure 7.11 shows the topical treatment of contact dermatitis from time to time (Kee et al. 1995).

ⓐ Acute Phase

The typical acute skin lesions are erythema, vesicles, and blisters. If the lesion is stimulated by severe itching, gangrenes follow. Therefore, wet dressing is widely used for acute phase when gangrene exists, and it softens infected sites and reduces symptoms by cleaning dirty exudates and crust. Generally, if the itching is severe, cold wet dressing is effective, and if there is no itching, warm solution is effective. Usually, it is important to control acute inflammation by using gauze moistened with cold saline, potassium permanganate (disinfecting agent), or burrow's solution to cover the affected areas for 10~15 min 3~4 times a day. Since thin-skinned areas are likely to generate more side effects, weak steroids should be applied on the face, underarms, or folding areas of the skin if possible.

ⓑ Subacute Phase

During the subacute phase, exudates are generally reduced, the surface of the lesion becomes dry, and erythema without clear boundaries and keratins are formed. If acute inflammation disappears and develops into the subacute phase, wet wrap therapy should not be practiced. Excessive wet wrapping does not only make lesion dry and hypersensitive with other stimuli, but it makes cracks on the lesions which increase the chances of the secondary bacterial infection.

ⓒ Chronic Phase

During the chronic phase, the purpose of medical treatments is addressing dry skin. At chronic phase of contact dermatitis, lesions become drier, keratinized, and thickened. During this period, it is important to use various humectants often and topical steroid ointments. Applying lotions is good only for a moment. Since it evaporates easily, it makes skin dry. Ointment is more easily spread on the skin, so it protects and hydrates the skin by sealing and lubricating action compared with cream or lotion. In some cases of severe chronic lesions, the sealing treatment with topical steroids is used. The sealing treatment can display early side effects of the drug use, so extra care is required. There are a few patients in severe cases which require oral or injectable steroid application; in this case, it should be used in a short period of time, and the doses should be reduced as the symptom improves (Jang 2011).

② Systemic Treatment

In many cases, the symptoms of most contact dermatitis improve with topical treatment, but in some cases, if the lesions are extensive, the systemic treatment of steroid is followed. In addition, to relieve itching, antihistamines or stabilizers are used.

ⓐ Steroid

Steroids are a powerful immunosuppressive and anti-inflammatory agent by inhibiting gene expression, so it can be used in systemic treatment. Contact dermatitis responds well on systemic steroid

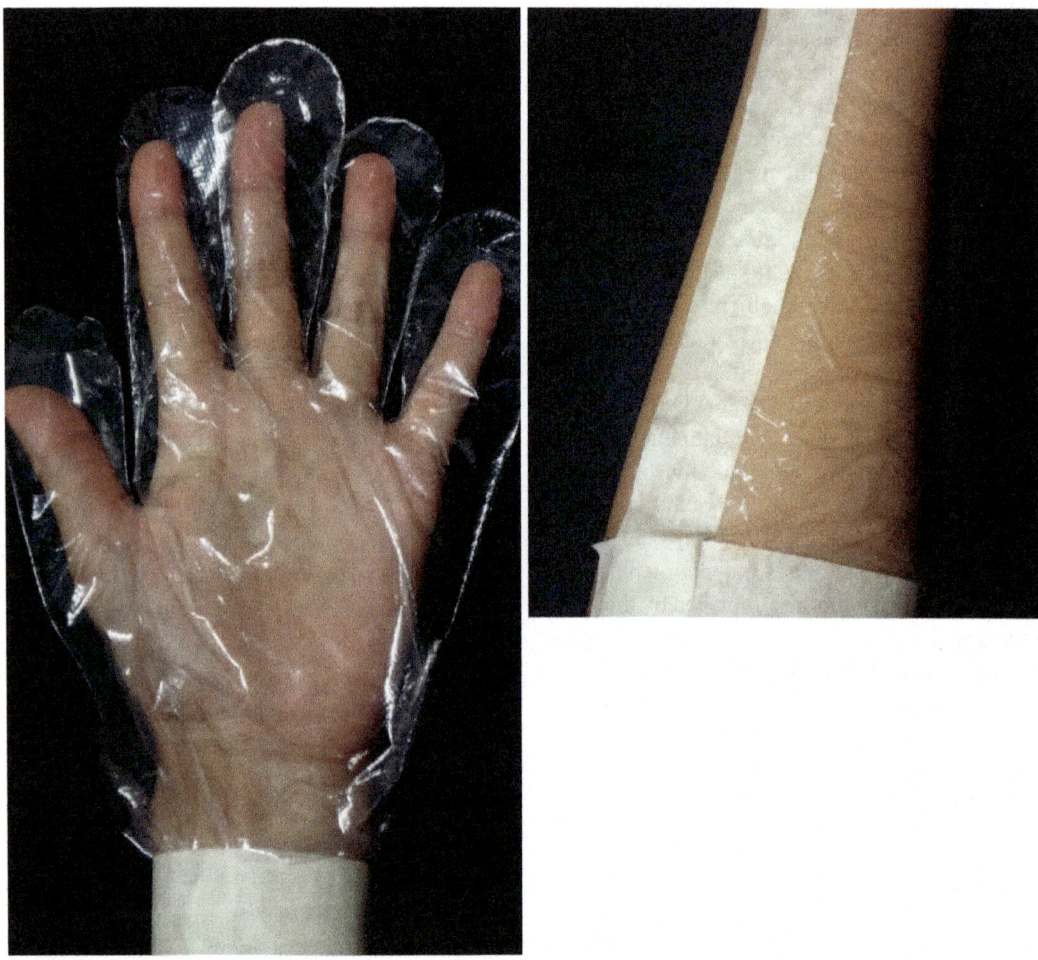

Fig. 7.10 Wet wrap

administration in short period of time, and the lesion and symptoms improve within 48 h of the treatment. It is appropriate to use short-term systemic steroid therapy once daily usually in the morning when the lesion occupies more than 25 % of the body surface area. During the systemic steroid treatment, blood glucose level, electrolytes, and lipid conditions should be checked. Polyuria, thirst, abdominal pain, sleep disorders, neurosis, weight gain, and increased blood pressure may appear, and cataract and glaucoma also should be checked regularly.

ⓑ Antihistamine

Often, the administration of antihistamine is required to relieve itching of contact dermatitis. The drug efficacy varies depending on the individual response, and selecting the appropriate drugs is needed depending on the state of eczematous lesion or reaction conditions (Hong et al. 1991).

7.2.3 Physical Therapy Intervention

7.2.3.1 Exercise Therapy

Atopic Dermatitis

One of the exercise methods emphasized for atopic dermatitis patients is low-intensity aerobic exercise. Avoiding severe exercise, it moderately contracts or relaxes the muscles in order to reap the maximum benefit. It is recommended to work

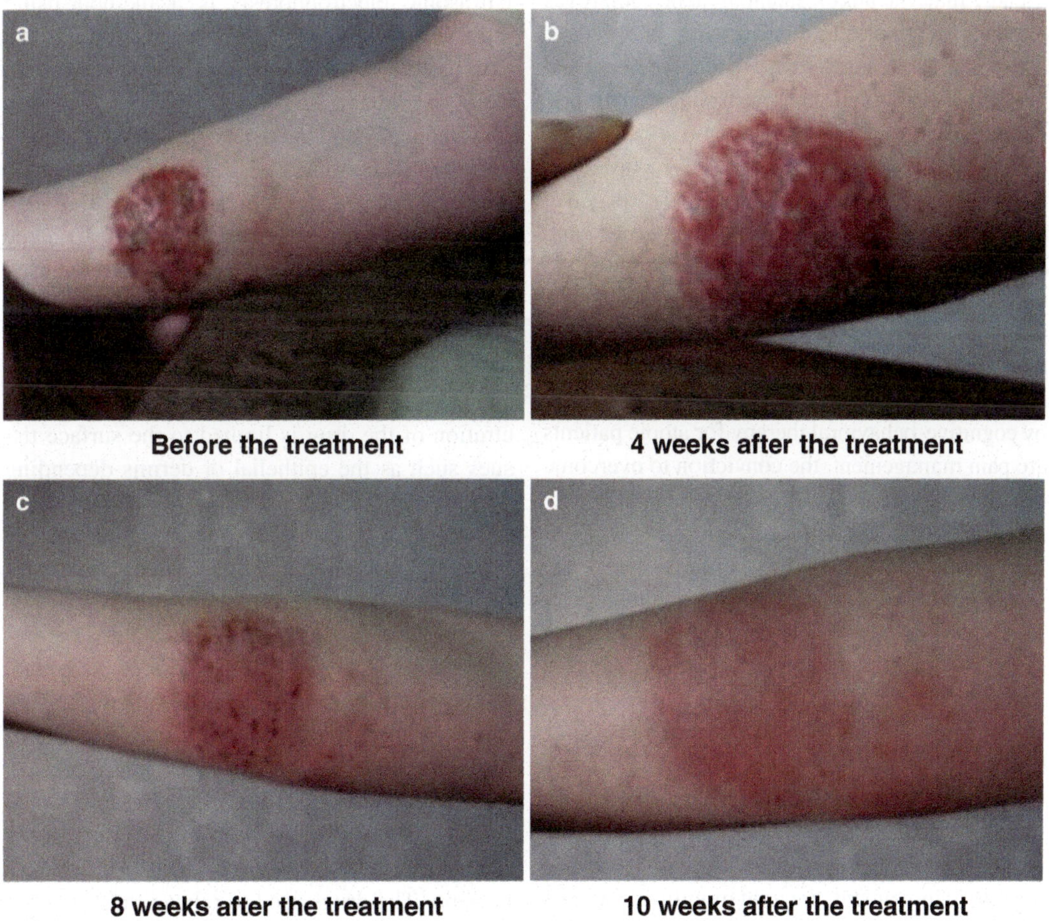

Fig. 7.11 The treatment process of contact dermatitis. (**a**) Before the treatment. (**b**) 4 weeks after the treatment. (**c**) 8 weeks after the treatment. (**d**) 10 weeks after the treatment

Table 7.4 Cognitive-behavioral model

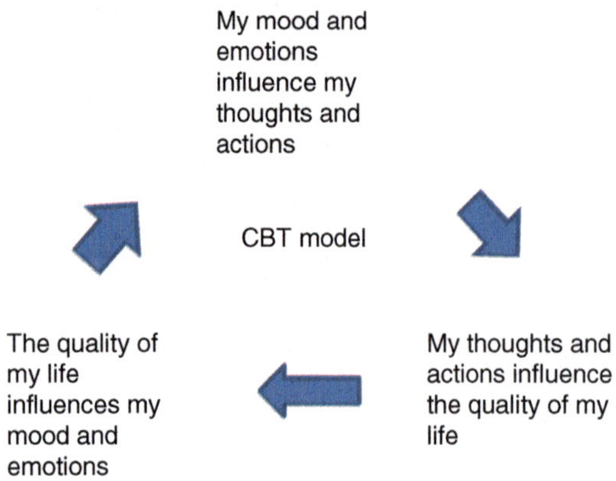

out 40~85% range of the maximum exercise capacity for starters. Especially, walking in clean air improves body functions and reduces stress. Also, low-intensity aerobic exercise in an eco-friendly material built residential facility improves physical functions and reduces symptoms (www.apta.org). In recent years, psychological and behavioral treatment approaches are emerging. Particularly, research on cognitive-behavioral therapy, CBT, is active (Table 7.4). According to the cognitive-behavioral treatment, negative thoughts reduce expectations of the success and the efficiency of the performance and suppress the motivation. Theoretically, patients can solve the problems and promote the changes in real life if they can switch the negative thoughts into the positive thoughts. The positive effects of the changes by cognitive-behavioral therapy for atopic patients are pain management, the conviction to overcome disability, less dependency on others, and improvement of physical activities. Therefore, cognitive-behavioral therapy and aerobic exercise inspire the patients to have a desire of life and maintain positive psychological states leading positive results in skin inflammation, pain, fatigue, and physical functions (Marilyn 2006).

Contact Dermatitis

Contact dermatitis is the lesions that occur locally. If the lesion is systematic or appears around the joint, playing an important role in long-term movement, the joint mobility decreases due to dryness and decreased elasticity. In this case, mild self-stretching helps minimizing the hypomobility of the skin tissues and soft tissues and improves blood circulation. But the caution is needed because the extensive stretching may cause skin injury. In addition, cardiovascular conditioning exercises including walking, bicycling, running, etc. promote blood circulation and stimulate the lymphatic flow. This type of exercise enhances the body immunity; therefore, it is effective in improving dermatitis. However, since the acute phase accompanying blister and rash interferes the process of skin repair, it is appropriate to start exercise after the wound has healed accounting the skin condition. If scarring occurs, joint movement is also necessary for skin or muscle repair (Jung and Han 2008).

7.2.3.2 Physical Agent Modalities

Ultrasonic Electrophoresis

Ultrasonic electrophoresis is a method using ultrasonic waves for the drug penetration into the skin tissues. If 3 W/cm^2 of ultrasound is applied, the permeability into the cell increases by 200%. The frequency and intensity of ultrasound used in ultrasound electrophoresis vary depending on the drugs used, but conventionally 1~3 MHZ frequency has been widely used. Even if the same drugs are used, the strength of the treatment used in ultrasound electrophoresis is slightly different depending on the degrees of the diseases. But, the typical intensity and frequency of the ultrasound can be used. However, 3 MHZ is used if the penetration of the drug is limited to the surface tissues such as the epithelial or dermis depending on the depth of the treating tissues. If deep penetration of the drug is necessary, applying 1 MHZ is better. Generally, to get thermal and iontophoresis effects at the same time from ultrasound electrophoresis, continuous ultrasound is recommended. If only iontophoresis effect is wanted, then pulsed ultrasound is recommended. The intensity of the ultrasound depends on the drug, minimum 1 W/cm^3 or higher intensity is applied, and the drug concentration has to be about 10%. And the drugs used in ultrasonic electrophoresis are dissolved into water, glycerol, or aqueous paraffin. The drugs used to relieve inflammation are nonsteroidal anti-inflammatory drugs, hydrocortisone, dexamethasone, cortisone, and cortisol. Salicylate and phenylbutazone are used for

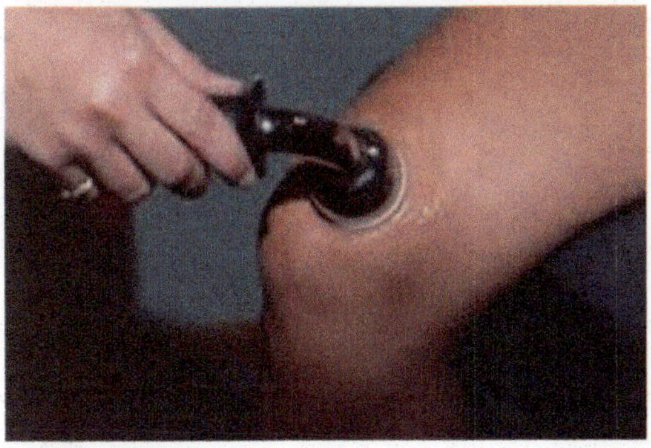

Fig. 7.12 Phonophoresis

antipyretic-analgesics. And steroid-based drugs including lidocaine or Decadron are often used in combination with local anesthetics to alleviate the pain (Fig. 7.12) (Jang 2011).

Anodal Galvanism

If the continuous direct current is applied to the body, local blood circulation increases by skin blood vessel stimulation. The increased circulation promotes redissolution of the inflammatory products. Due to the effects of the direct current, the continuous direct current is widely used in chronic and persistent inflammatory diseases. Therefore, if noninfectious inflammation of the skin, contusion, or edema exists, anodal galvanism using direct current is widely used. To get the maximum benefits from the anodal galvanism, the low-intensity current is applied for long period of time. The current strength 0.15 ~ 0.25 mA/cm^2 is used starting from 15 min and gradually increasing 5 min at a time to reach 30 min. However, it is recommended that the current strength and treatment time be adjusted to the condition of the patients, and it is recommended that patients receive treatment everyday if possible until the condition improves. The same size of the electrode as a surface area of the body is used in the treatment. To reduce the skin resistance, the electrode is moistened in warm solution. If the patients complain of unpleasant hot flushes during the treatment, the electrodes with insufficient moisture should be considered first rather than excess current might have been applied. Insulation should be considered when using galvanic bath, and 91.9 ~ 100.04 (8 F) (33.3 ~ 37.88 C) of water bath temperature is appropriate; especially the patients should be aware of electrolyte burn (Fig. 7.13) (Min et al. 2009).

Iontophoresis

Iontophoresis is effective in reducing inflammation of soft tissues and topical areas of the skin. Hydrocortisone, a typical drug used for iontophoresis, reduces or stops the inflammatory responses in soft tissues by stabilizing cell membranes. Also, trolamine salicylate inhibits prostaglandins and the chemical substances that are essential in processing inflammation. All hydrocortisone or trolamine salicylate can be applied in a form of ointment. Before the treatment, patients take comfortable position and wash the skin areas rubbing gently with brine or alcohol. When hydrocortisone is used for iontophoresis, the active electrode should be connected to the positive electrode, and when trolamine salicylate is used, it should be connected to the negative electrode. And the inert electrode moistened with water or brine should be placed in more distal parts of the skin than the active electrode. The current strength is initially started from 0 mA and gradually increased until the patients feel slight burning sensation. The overall treatment time is 15–20 min (Fig. 7.14) (Korean Dermatological Association 2008).

Phototherapy and Other Therapies

Phototherapy used in atopic dermatitis is applied to the patients with reluctant to use oral and topical applications of corticosteroids. The extended effects can be expected as an advantage. Typically used phototherapy in atopic dermatitis is high capacity UV (UVA1). In particular, it is effective in acutely worsened lesions. Usually, the efficiency of broadband ultraviolet B [(BBUVB); 270 ~ 350 nm] can be expected, but some burning sensation or deterioration of dermatitis is known to occur frequently. In addition, phototherapy using the narrowband ultraviolet B, NBUVB, also has been reported that it is effective in atopic dermatitis in some degrees. UV irradiation is known to be effective in contact dermatitis or allergic dermatitis. In addition, oxygen spray treatment, spraying oxygen to the skin, is a method that cleanses the skin by applying oxygen and then massaging the skin. A more classical and popular

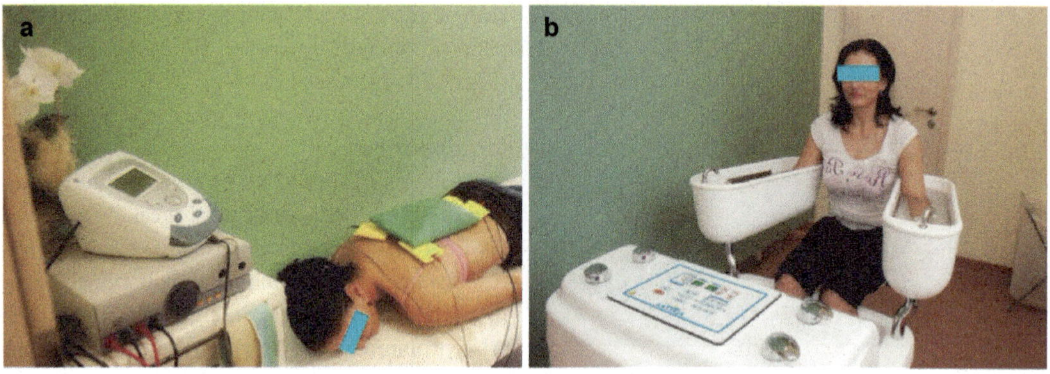

Fig. 7.13 Galvanic current therapy (**a**). Anodal galvanic current therapy (**b**). Galvanic bath

Fig. 7.14 Iontophoresis

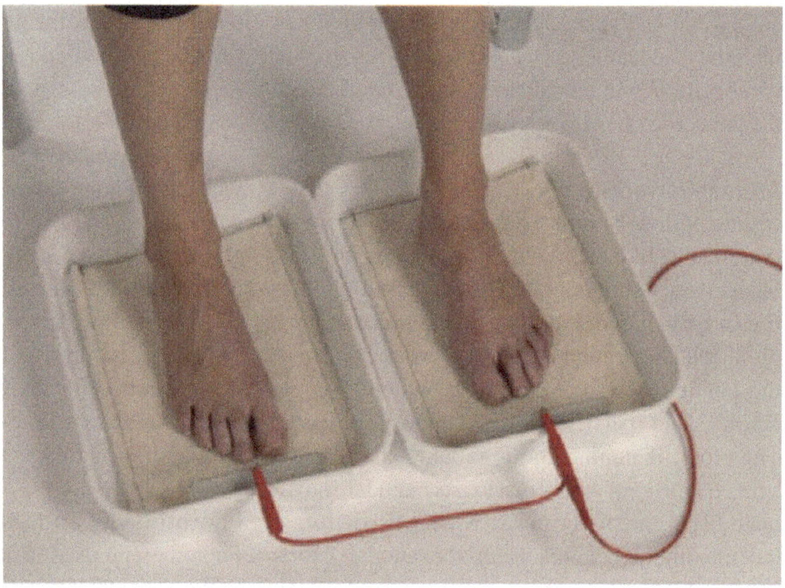

therapeutic method is adding drugs into a whirlpool bath (Jacuzzi) which sterilizes fungus or bacteria causing dermatitis (Der-Petrossian et al. 2000; Hudson-Peacock et al. 1996).

7.2.4 Prevention and Management

7.2.4.1 Atopic Dermatitis

There is no ideal treatment that completely cures dermatitis. The therapeutic methods for each patient should be selected considering their age, sex, economic status, and the site and degree of the inflammation. In addition, avoiding exposure to harmful elements including unhealthy lifestyle and dietary habits, considering that everyday life is a process of the treatment, and continuing to practice the therapeutic methods allow the patients to escape from atopic dermatitis. The incidence of food allergy in pediatrics is very high. If the period of the treatment lasts for months even the patients respond to the treatment, and if the symptoms worsen and the disease relapses immediately after stopping drugs, the food allergy is suspected. In this case, patients should eat according to the prescriptions of doctors. After the food intake, the skin, urine, and feces conditions should be checked. The atopic dermatitis patients should wash their face or bath with warm water and use neutral or slightly acidic soap without color and scent if soap has to be used. Also, after the bath, wiping gently with a towel rather than rubbing the skin and applying moisturizer before the body becomes dry within 3 min are appropriate. Moisturizer increases the moisturization of the horny layer of keratin and makes the skin soft and flexible compensating insufficient protective effects of skin lipids (Moon 2009). Therefore, it is possible to reduce the external use of steroids. Applying moisturizer protects not only the skin weakened by atopic dermatitis, but it also prevents the skin becoming dry which prevents further deterioration of atopy as a long-term prevention. A rough surfaced garment makes skin sensitive even the skin of normal people. If the symptoms appear, the cotton products, which do not irritate the skin but absorb sweat and ventilate the skin, should be used. In particular, the clothes with tight armpit, neck, or waist cannot release sweat and cause inflammation and itching, so wearing loose-fit clothes is recommended. Also, wearing pajamas and long-sleeved clothes when sleeping is recommended because itching becomes severe at night. Residual detergents left when washing clothes should be avoided, and clothes stored in a closet for a long time and new clothes should be washed before wearing. Removing house dust mites does not always improve symptoms of all atopic dermatitis patients, but it showed remarkable effects in some patients. Therefore, it is necessary to have a habit of managing beddings and carpets thoroughly which are the major habitats. Washing blankets, pillows, carpets, etc. with boiling water once every 2 weeks and drying at least for 4 h are recommended. Also, the bedroom with sunlight and well-ventilated rooms should be chosen. During the clear day, opening the windows and ventilating the room to prevent dust accumulation and lowering the humidity are needed. Particularly, many studies showed that using eco-friendly materials when building or remodeling a house is effective in reducing atopy symptoms. Plants are the only organisms that can make nutrition by themselves on earth. Everyone can feel refreshing feeling and sense of vitality when walking in the mountain with dense trees. It is due to the effect of "phytoncide," a mysterious substance released by trees of the forest. Phytoncide was first named by Waksman, a Russian-born American bacteriologist in 1943. According to Dr. Waksman, the fresh forest scent is caused by phytoncide released by trees when people walk into the forest, and it is a volatile substance that kills microorganisms including *Staphylococcus aureus*, *Streptococcus*, etc. "Phyton" from the word phytoncide is "plant" in Greek and "cide" means "kill" in Latin. It means released from the plants and kills other organisms. Phytoncide gives psychological stability, strengthens the cardiopulmonary function, and suppresses the growth of bacteria, so it has a wide range of effects in preventing diseases such as atopic dermatitis, asthma, or allergic rhinitis (Fig. 7.15) (Ahn et al. 2009).

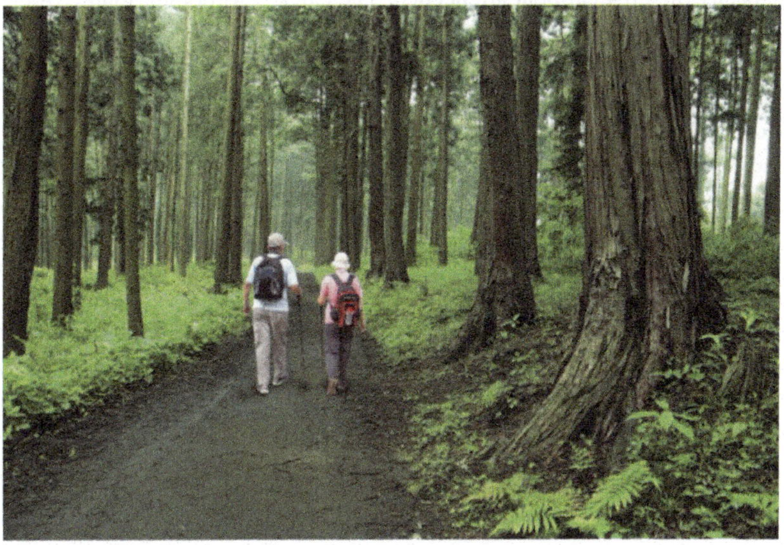

Fig. 7.15 Phytoncide

7.2.4.2 Contact Dermatitis

Since contact dermatitis is caused by allergens causing irritation or allergic reaction, it is important to reveal the exact cause and avoid allergens. The patients should know where the allergens are discovered and avoid them. In addition, the patients should be aware that the same chemical substances have different names. The most important self-management at home is washing. After the exposure to known allergens or irritants, it is recommended to remove and inactivate allergens by washing with soap and cold water. If blisters are formed, cold wet dressing 3 times a day for 30 min alleviates the symptoms. The most important management method is never scratching which might lead to the secondary infection. Also, in terms of administering drugs, corticosteroid is used to treat topical regions as a form of cream or ointment, but if the allergic reaction of the skin is relatively large or the symptoms are severe, oral administration or injection should be used (Jung and Han 2008).

7.2.4.3 Patient/Caregiver Education

The awareness of infectious skin diseases and strong action for health are necessary. Patients with bad habits or behavior which worsens the disease should be modified with the help of experts through behavioral modification. Also, finding and practicing the actions that can ensure the stability of daily life movement and functional movement and strengthening the capacity of self-treatment are needed. The caregivers should assist the patients to avoid harsh soap, inflammatory stimuli factors, the aggravating factors, and inducing agents such as extreme temperature. The patients can reduce the energy consumption generated through daily life by careful thoughts, judgment, and plans. For example, taking a shower can make atopic patients easily become tired because the action of taking a shower itself creates a hot and humid environment. However, sitting on a shower seat and taking a shower using an atopic soap with handheld foam towel can reduce energy consumption (Marilyn 2006).

7.3 Fibromyalgia Syndrome

7.3.1 Overview

The concept of fibromyalgia was first introduced by Hench in 1976, and the term fibrosis was first used by Gowers in 1904 which is generally recognized as pain generated by fibrous tissues. The cause of the disease is unknown yet, so until 1976, the disease was regarded as nonarticular rheumatism, which is neurological rheumatism different from rheumatoid arthritis (RA) and osteoarthritis (OA) due to the lack of objective diagnostic methods (Bennett 1993). Fibromyalgia syndrome (FMS) is a chronic pain disorder accompanying aches, pain, stiffness, and general fatigue all over the musculoskeletal system, and the cause of the disease is unknown. Therefore, fibromyalgia is sometimes misdiagnosed as myofascial pain syndrome, polymyalgia rheumatica, polymyositis, hypothyroidism, metastatic carcinoma, rheumatoid arthritis, chronic fatigue syndrome, or systemic lupus erythematosus. Through the Copenhagen Declaration in 1992, fibromyalgia syndrome with muscular pain, instead of joints, was defined as a chronic disease appearing throughout the musculoskeletal system accompanied by chronic fatigue, nonrestorative sleep, and general stiffness (Buchwald 1996).

7.3.2 Causes

Although many researchers try to reveal the causes of fibromyalgia syndrome through various approaches, the exact cause is unknown. It only suggests four characteristic aspects.

7.3.2.1 Lack of Sufficient Sleep

Looking at the sleep EEG of fibromyalgia syndrome patients, alpha-wave appears throughout the sleep stages which acts as a factor preventing deep sleep (sleep stage 3~4). Through EEG, the low wave change was detected in fibromyalgia syndrome patients on their frontal lobe. This frequency change causes reduced concentration, short-term memory, and multitasking ability doing a number of works at the same time causing so-called fibro fog (Boissevain and McCain 1991)[4].

7.3.2.2 Abnormal Neurobiochemical Reaction

Due to the reduced serotonin precursor tryptophan, it is hypothesized that metabolic disorder of the serotonin disturbs deep sleep (sleep stage 3~4) and causes the inconvenience of the whole body, depression, and pain. Serotonin is synthesized from tryptophan, stored in synaptic vesicles in nerve terminals, and released regulating sleep, pain transmission, feeling, and aggressiveness. Particularly, in the spinal cord, it is known to inhibit nociceptive afferent neurons and activate motor neurons at the same time (Burckhardt et al. 1994).

7.3.2.3 Sympathetic Nervous System Disorders

The hypothesis is that the activity of the sympathetic nervous system influences the microcirculatory changes in muscle tissues. Particularly for the fibromyalgia syndrome patients, hypoxia in the muscle is caused by the sympathetic nervous system disorder after exercise. As an experiment supporting this hypothesis, the muscle tender points and increased fatigue and pain appeared when fibromyalgia syndrome patients attempted to exercise for 25~48 h repeatedly. This phenomenon is similar to the symptoms appearing during the hypoxic state of muscles (Kim et al. 2008).

7.3.2.4 Local Tissue Factor

Muscle disorders (inflammation or myopathy) were not found on the cadaveric dissection of quadriceps muscle of the thigh in fibromyalgia syndrome patients. Many other scholars have made a conclusion that it is not a muscle-related disorder. Instead, the abnormal changes of local tissue cells are revealed by many researches. The abnormal pattern of mitochondria and the formation of lipofuscin inclusion cause nonspecific changes in local tissues such as angular fiber atrophy and abnormal alignment of filaments. Many scholars explain that muscle hypoxia is the cause of nonspecific changes. The other change in local tissues is 30~40% reduction of cross-sectional area of the muscle fiber during the muscle contraction of fibromyalgia syndrome patients causing low physical activities due to fibromyalgia syndrome. Following the low physical activity of the patients for 4 years, it was related to the number of tender points, and the pain played a role as an obstacle of muscle contraction (Kim et al. 2008).

7.3.3 Symptoms

In 1990, the American College of Rheumatology, ACR, defined fibromyalgia syndrome as 11~18 tender points in muscle tissues appearing on both sides of the body resulting in pain persisting for more than 3 months. Figure 7.16 depicted 18 sites of tender points. In addition, tender points or pain described here is defined by complaints of pain when given less than 4 kg/cm^2 using algometer (Buckelew et al. 1996). Generally, fibromyalgia syndrome has tender points, tePs, and trigger points, TrP. TrP forms taut band on the muscle and triggers radiating pain, soreness, or tingling feeling when compressed. TePs, located in muscles, ligaments, tendon, and periosteum tissue, are more limited to local pain by pressure than reflective pain sending stimulation to proximal sites. Palpation of tender points can be promoted by constant pressure (4 kg/cm^2) using the thumb, index finder, or ring finger until the nails become white. The threshold of the tender points differs by regions, but it is about 2 kg/cm^2, and the tester discovers spasm when palpating redness or tenderness area of the skin. The tender points can be found compressing with thumb or index finger by following each step until the patients say "stop," avoid, or grimace due to the pain. Tender point index can be classified as shown in Table 7.5 (Buchwald 1996).

7.3.4 Test and Assessment

The simple diagnostic methods for fibromyalgia syndrome are X-ray, neurological examination,

[4] Fibro-fog: Cognitive impairment caused by fibrositis.

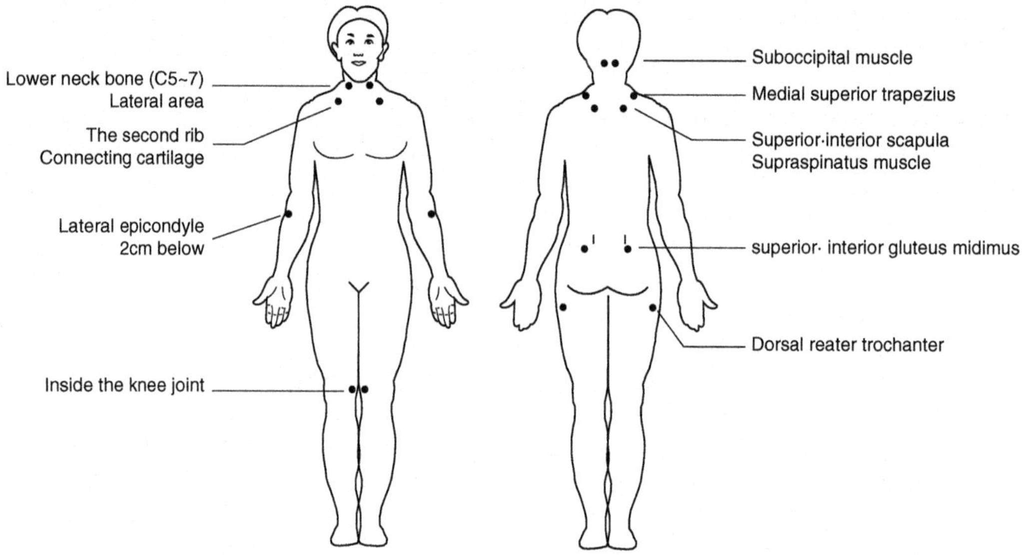

Fig. 7.16 Tender point position

Table 7.5 Tender point index

0	No tenderness
1	Tenderness with no withdrawal
2	Tenderness and withdrawal
3	Tenderness and exaggerated withdrawal
4	Untouchable

and the range of motion test of joints. Also, since fibromyalgia syndrome may sometimes appear along with other problems, the close examination is required. Therefore, Carrie and Lori suggested the classification of fibromyalgia syndrome into genuine and pseudo as shown in Table 7.6 (Bennett 1993).

7.4 Intervention

7.4.1 Interventional Approach

Fibromyalgia syndrome is mostly caused by habitual behavior or repetitive stimulus in daily life. The honest conversation about the life patterns of the patients with their family and experts is needed. Also, as it is reported that it most commonly occurs in ages from 30 to 55, work environment where the patients are exposed during their most economically active age is important. Prior to the treatment, the patients should actively cooperate in training about pharmacotherapy and exercise therapy considering the above record. The therapists must conduct differential diagnosis on easily confused diseases such as chronic fatigue syndrome (Burckhardt et al. 1994).

7.4.2 Medical Treatment

The drugs fibromyalgia syndrome patients are taking are mainly used to control pain and improve sleep disorder. Nonsteroidal analgesic, antidepressants, and benzodiazepine are the main drugs, and sometimes narcotic analgesic is taken together. Also, tricyclic antidepressants (amitriptyline) or cyclobenzaprine reduces morning stiffness, pain, and fatigue and induces deep sleep resulting in increased body energy (Boissevain and McCain 1991).

7.4.3 Physical Therapy Intervention

7.4.3.1 Exercise Therapy

Exercise is the most effective way of long-term managing the intervention in fibromyalgia patients. Since the abnormal muscles use low energy, it increases fatigue and causes pain by microtrauma. Women with fibromyalgia syndrome typically have a low functional body

Table 7.6 Classification of fibromyalgia syndrome into classic and pseudo

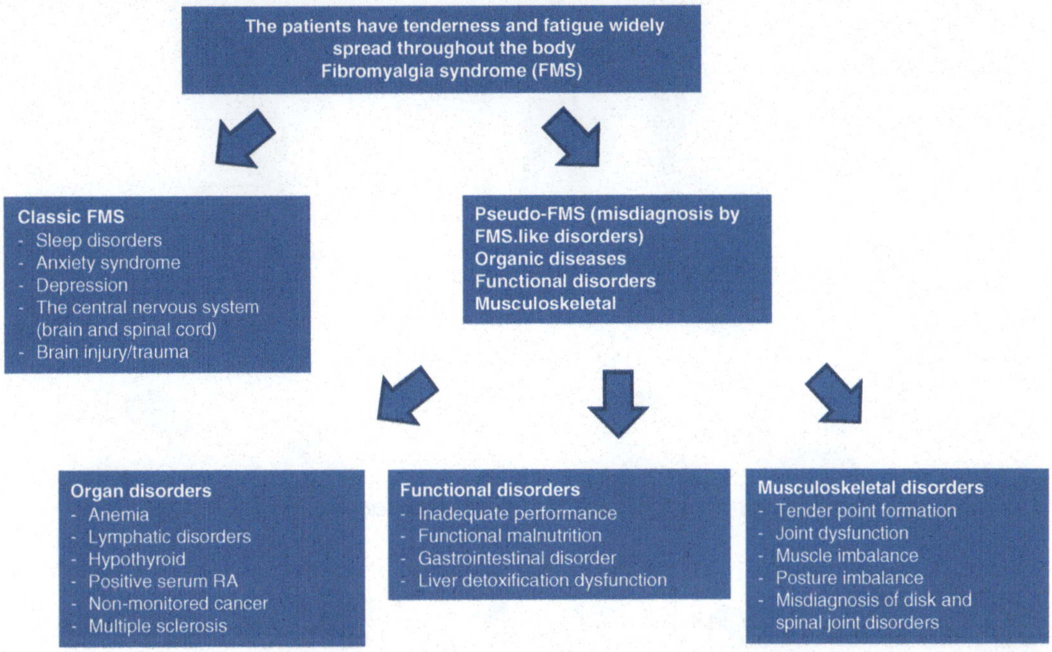

score compared with normal women. For example, the isometric endurance test for the shoulder muscle in female fibromyalgia syndrome patients showed 35 % of the normal women. Fibromyalgia syndrome in women presumably gives difficulties in transporting, pushing, or pulling loads which result in preventing the movement of the arms. Before practicing exercise programs, partial restriction on the patient's eating habits through diet is recommended. The program consisted of posture exercise, self-stretching (Fig. 7.17), low-load/repetition strength training, and low-load aerobic exercise (cycle, swimming, walking). Especially, because the maximum stretching appears as a result of the limited range of motion rather than the discomfort with the increase of the exercise range, the fundamental principle of self-stretching should not exceed the limited range of the pain. The proper aerobic exercise method for fibromyalgia syndrome patients is starting exercise 5 min a day from low intensity to 30~40 min gradually increasing 1 min at intervals of 3~4 days. 3~4 times a week are appropriate and 85 % of the maximum heart rate of each age group is ideal. For fibromyalgia syndrome patients showing low activity index, typical exercise is more effective than pharmacotherapy or special physical therapy. The exercise therapy for fibromyalgia syndrome is suggested as an interventional plan for four disabilities. They are stress, posture mobility disorders, and muscular and cardiovascular endurance disorders (Table 7.7) (Burckhardt et al. 1994).

7.4.3.2 Manual Therapy

The main purpose of manual therapy is relaxation of the strained belt on tender points. It is applied to improve pain control and functional movements. Ischemic compression is giving continuous pressure until the tender points are inactivated after finding the tender points. If the patient is trying to protect tender points by muscle contraction due to pain, the therapeutic effects cannot be expected. Therefore, to apply ischemic compression, the tender points are continuously compressed with the thumbs until the patients can endure after the muscles are relaxed by maximum stretching (Fig. 7.18) (Kim et al. 2008).

7.4.3.3 Physical Agent Modalities

Physical therapy should focus mainly on increasing the strained band in the muscle

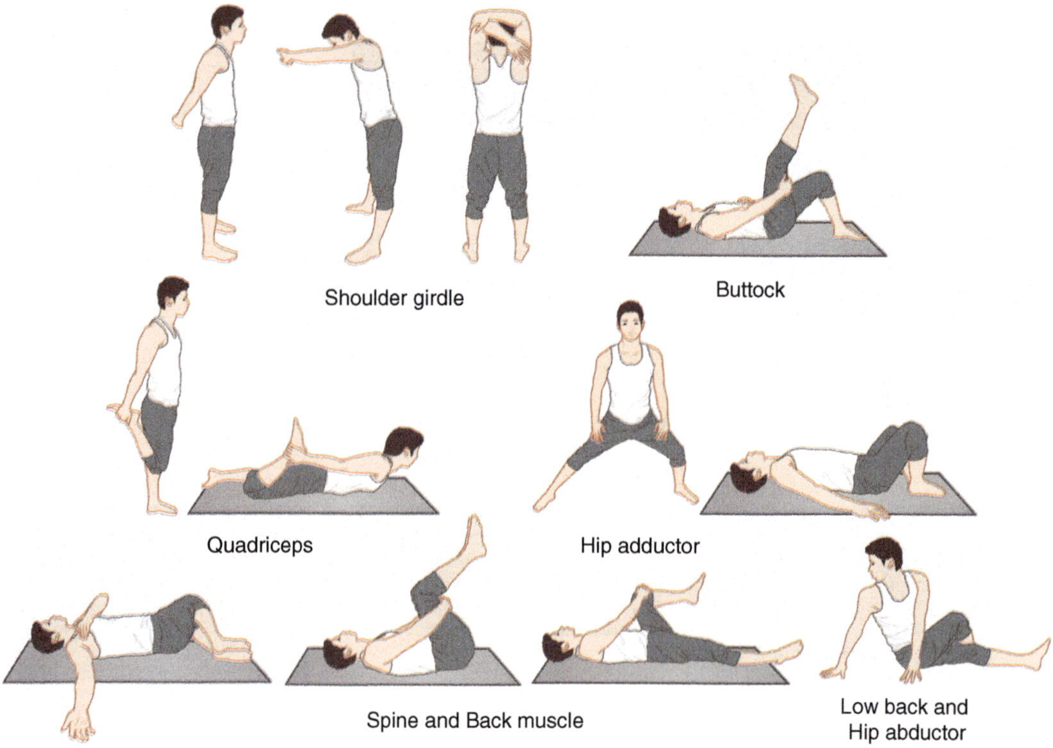

Fig. 7.17 Self-stretching

where tender points are and removing the tender points which cause other pains and worsen the symptoms.

Therefore, physical therapists should instruct clinically applied physical agent modalities to the patients so that they can use thermotherapy appliances (moist heat packs, heating pad, and warm whirlpools) at home to improve local blood circulation and reduce muscle stiffness and tension (Fig. 7.19). Also, teaching patients to use cryotherapy appliances (ice pack, ice massage, and cold shower) helps in preventing pain by local anesthetic effects and pain transmission. Besides, transcutaneous electrical nerve stimulation (TENS), interferential current therapy (ICT), or massage techniques using appliances are used to relieve the pain. Hyperstimulation analgesia is used to enhance blood circulation, strained band stretching, and local anesthetic effects. Hyperstimulation analgesia is a very old pain control method and the application ranges vary from home remedy to scientific therapeutic methods. The typical hyperstimulation analgesia methods are mustard plasters, hot wax, spray, and needling. A simple brief intense cold is used recently. Particularly, because it can break pain-spasm-pain cycle through intramuscular stimulation in a short time, using electrical stimulation during needling is one of the effective therapies treating tender points (Buckelew et al. 1996).

7.4.4 Prevention and Management

7.4.4.1 Prevention and Management

Because there is no exact cause of fibromyalgia syndrome, the prevention and management in daily life are important. The self-management for happiness is important by finding how to relieve stress and recovering from fatigue through enough sleep. Also, changing working environment prevents local muscle diseases caused by fixed position for a long time, and the brain stimulation by new environment actively releases hormone like serotonins. Besides, the comprehensive treatments such as exercise therapy and regular sleep

Table 7.7 Exercise therapy for patients with fibromyalgia syndrome

Beginning stage (week 1) middle stage (week 2) terminal stage (week 3)
Objectives: stress and pain management
Relaxation
Progressive relaxation
Spontaneous breathing
Breathing
Stretching
Objective: musculoskeletal balance
The skin surface anesthesia (fluoromethane spray) and stretching joint motion exercise
Neuromuscular facilitation stretching: stop and relaxation-contraction and relaxation
Strain-counterstrain
Closed chain kinetic exercise
The initial aerobic exercise
Stationary bicycle, non-load equipment exercise, easy aquatic exercise: walking underwater, underwater gymnastics
Objectives: maintenance
Continuation of stretching
Overall strength training
Resistant tubing and other equipment exercise and closed chain kinetic exercise
Aerobic exercise
Non-loading to loading exercise
Jarring activities: ski training machine
Stationary bicycle, treadmill
Aquatic exercise: aerobic exercise, flotation belt

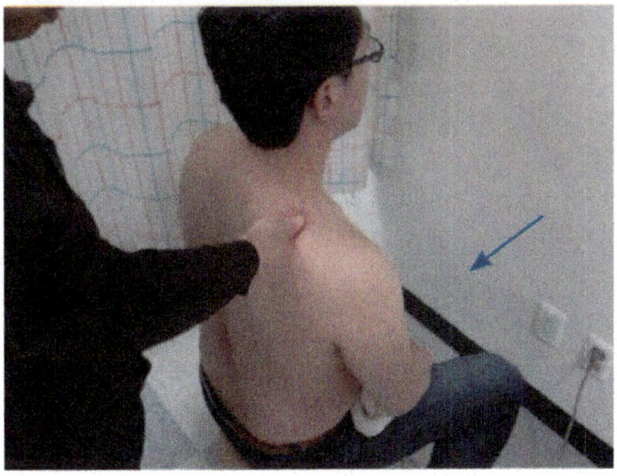

Fig. 7.18 Ischemic compression therapy for tender points

habits for pain reduction and muscle strength, pharmacotherapy for sleep disorder and other symptoms, deep breathing, muscle relaxation or

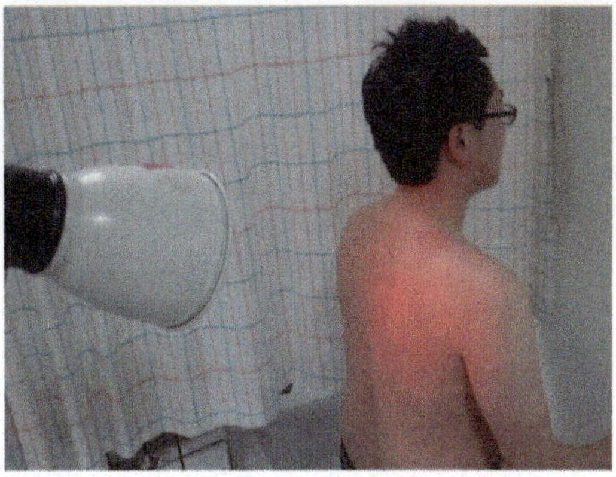

Fig. 7.19 Infrared therapy for tender points

psychotherapy for stress relief, and less fat and fiber-rich food intake are helpful. Therefore, it is most important self-managing that the treatments are made by daily life instead of regular treatment by life patterns (Burckhardt et al. 1994).

7.4.4.2 Patient/Caregiver Education

Researchers, long-term observing fibromyalgia syndrome patients who participated in an educational intervention program, emphasize that inspiring the confidence of patients is the most important factor in treatment. Fibromyalgia syndrome patients can change their problems, and it is more important that they recognize these treatments are essential before thinking they can do something. In addition, continuous education should be received including the disease process, coping strategies of fibromyalgia syndrome, stress awareness and management, sleeping pattern, nutrition, pain management, cognitive-behavioral intervention program, medication, body conditioning, etc. For the training related with food intake, caffeine, alcohol, or nicotine intake should be avoided or reduced because they disturb sleep patterns or energy recovery. Because carbohydrates increase serotonin production during low-protein intake and sugar increases serotonin, their consumption is recommended. Also, supplements such as calcium, magnesium, or multivitamin intake are recommended. In addition, the training on the energy-conservation method after food intake is needed. The education on technically required time to increase productivity and maintaining harmony and balance during the process of energy consumption and reproduction is needed. The assistive device are trained to decrease tension and minimize the strength consumption due to the hypermobility that fibromyalgia syndrome patients are often experienced. The patients can master the methods about consuming the minimum energy required in maintaining body functions (Kim et al. 2008).

Advices for Physical Therapists

❶ Do not fear about the skin diseases and engage in treatment with positive attitude.
❷ Atopic dermatitis is a skin disorder sensitive to the environment, so the overall check of the treatment environment is needed.
❸ For contact dermatitis, diagnosis is needed whether the disease is infectious through patch tests prior to the treatment for the therapists themselves.
❹ Prevent the deterioration of the skin disease by checking the fatigue test from time to time when aerobic exercise was applied for inflammatory skin diseases.
❺ Know the differences between fibromyalgia syndrome and myofascial pain syndrome.
❻ The most important principle in the treatment of fibromyalgia syndrome is psychological stability of the patients and education.

7.5 Problem Solving

7.5.1 Inflammatory Skin Disease

Choose one highly possible method for physical therapy intervention or test from each questions.

Question 1
After 27-year-old woman "A" moved into the big city, atopic dermatitis progressed rapidly and showed drug resistant. What is the appropriate physical therapy for this patient?

1. TENS
2. Frequent bathing
3. UV phototherapy
4. Steroid ointment
5. Codman's exercise education

Question 2
A 40-year-old man working in a workshop making metal crafts had rash and an itching symptom on his fingers for 2 weeks. Blisters appeared on his fingers accompanied with pain for few days, so contact dermatitis was diagnosed. Choose the correct answer.

1. Perform infrared therapy.
2. Conduct pressure and strong stretching exercise on the fingers.
3. Perform patch test on various metallic materials.
4. Wind compression bandage to reduce swelling of the fingers.
5. Use hot wet dressing to reduce blisters on the hands.

Question 3
A 40-year-old woman complained about fatigue without any reasons for 5 years; especially, she suffered from musculoskeletal pain and stiffness. The symptoms are similar to rheumatoid arthritis, but rheumatoid factors are not detected and tender points gradually increased. What is the correct physical treatment method for this woman?

1. Relaxation-resistance exercise
2. Plyometric exercise
3. Relaxation and aerobic exercise
4. Strength exercise through diet
5. Low-load/high-repetition aerobic exercise

Question 4
What is the correct electrical therapy attenuating and spreading unusually concentrated positively charged hydrogen or potassium ions on inflammatory lesions to reduce inflammation?

1. Anodal galvanism
2. Interferential current therapy
3. Medical galvanism
4. High-voltage pulsed galvanic current therapy
5. Chloride iontophoresis

Question 5

What is the correct ray typically used in atopic dermatitis?

1. UVA1
2. UVA2
3. BBUVB
4. NBUVB
5. Infrared

Answer

Question 1-③, Question 2-③, Question 3-③, Question 4-①, Question 5-①

References

Ahn SG, et al. Common skin disease of Koreans. Seoul: Doctor's Book 13. 2009.

Bennett RM. Fibromyalgia and the facts: sense or nonsense. Controversies Clin Rheumatol. 1993;19(1):45–59.

Boissevain MD, McCain GA. Toward an integrated understanding of fibromyalgia syndrome I: medical and pathophysiological aspects. Pain. 1991;44:227–38.

Bong KJ, Myoung OK, Seok DP. Three case reports: irritant contact dermatitis due to buttercup (Ranunculus sceleratus). Korean J Dermatol. 2006;30(6):886–91.

Buchwald D. Fibromyalgia and chronic fatigue syndrome. Similarities and differences. Rheum Dis Clin North Am. 1996;22:219–43.

Buckelew SP, Huyser B, Hewett JE, et al. Self-efficacy predicting outcome among fibromyalgia subjects. Arthritis Care Res. 1996;9(2):97.

Burckhardt CS, O'Reilly CA, Wiens AN, et al. Assessing depression in fibromyalgia patients. Arthritis Care Res. 1994;7(1):35–9.

Cheol HL. Review: skin tests for irritant contact dermatitis. Korean J Dermatol. 1997;35(1):1–10.

Dahl MV. Flare factors and atopic dermatitis; the role of allergy. J Dermatol Sci. 1990;1(5):311–8.

David J. Dermatology: an illustrated colour text. 4th ed. Seoul: Koonja Publishing Inc.; 2010.

Der-Petrossian M, Seeber A, Honigsmann H, Tanew A. Half-side comparison study on the efficacy of 8-methoxypsoralen bath-PUVA versus narrow-band ultraviolet B phototherapy in patients with severe chronic atopic dermatitis. Br J Dermatol. 2000;142:39–43.

Hong JK, Kyeong JH, et al. Allergic contact dermatitis due to topical medicaments in Korea. Korean J Dermatol. 1991;29(1):32–40.

Hudson-Peacock MJ, Diffey BL, Farr PM. Narrow-band UVB phototherapy for severe atopic dermatitis. Br J Dermatol. 1996;135:332.

Jang SH. Symposium2: contact dermatitis and skin allergy; therapeutic approaches. Korean J Dermatol. 2011;49(1):95.

Jekler J. Phototherapy of atopic dermatitis with ultraviolet radiation. Acta Derm Venereol Suppl. 1992;171:1–37.

Jung JY, Han KH. Allergic contact dermatitis in Korea. Seoul: MD World Publisher; 2008.

Kee CM, Hee CE, et al. An epidemiological study of contact dermatitis in Korea (1986–1993). Korean J Dermatol. 1995;33(3):445–52.

Kim HM, et al. Dermatology. 1st ed. Seoul: Koonja Publishing Inc.; 2006.

Kim MC, et al. The review of fibromyalgia syndrome. Korean J Neurol Phys Ther. 2008;4(1):83–98.

Korean Dermatological Association. Dermatology. Seoul: Ryo Moon Gak; 2008.

Lee M, Noh H. Dermatology: an illustrated color text. Seoul: Koonja Publishing Inc.; 2010.

Marilyn M, Katherine BH. Integumentary Essentials: Applying the Preferred Physical Therapist Practice Patterns. SLACK Incorporated; 2006;1–17.

Min Chul K, Sung Ae K, Sang Lip C, Kyu Suk L. Case report: a case of allergic contact dermatitis from silmazine® cream. Korean J Dermatol. 2009;47(6):710–3.

Moon BK. Moisturizer and skin barrier. J Skin Barrier Res. 2009;11(1):64–80.

Reference Sites

APTA. www.apta.org.

Google. www.google.com.

Medcity. http://www.medcity.com.

Wikipedia. www.wikipedia.org.

Skin Cancer

8

DongYeop Lee

ICD-10 Code

C44 Other and unspecified malignant neoplasms of the skin

C44.9 Other and unspecified malignant neoplasms of the skin, unspecified

C44.90 Unspecified malignant neoplasm of the skin, unspecified

C44.91 Basal cell carcinoma of the skin, unspecified

C44.92 Squamous cell carcinoma of the skin, unspecified

C44.99 Other specified malignant neoplasms of the skin, unspecified

I89.0

Lymphoedema, not elsewhere classified

C43

Malignant melanoma of the skin

Including morphology codes M872-M879 with behavior code/3

Excluding malignant melanoma of the skin of the genital organs (C51-C52, C60.-, C63.-)

C43.0

Malignant melanoma of the lip

Excluding vermilion border of the lip (C00.0-C00.2)

Learning Outcomes

After completing this chapter, you should be able to describe the following:

- Types of skin cancer
- Causes and risk factors of skin cancer
- Classification of skin cancer
- Complications and clinical signs of skin cancer
- Physical therapy diagnosis and intervention of skin cancer
- Problem solution of skin cancer
- Clinical problems of lymphedema therapy

Key Terms

Basal cell carcinoma
Lymphedema
Lymph
Massage
Malignant melanoma
Squamous cell carcinoma
Skin cancer

D. Lee
Department of Physical Therapy,
Sun Moon University, Asan, South Korea
e-mail: kan717@hanmail.net

J.-W. Park, D.-I. Jung (eds.), *Integumentary Physical Therapy*, DOI 10.1007/978-3-662-47380-1_8

8.1 Skin Cancer

8.1.1 Overview

Skin cancer occurs when one is exposed to ultraviolet ray, one of the sunlight, in general. Skin cancer is divided into melanoma and nonmelanoma, and nonmelanoma skin cancer occurs in 90 % of skin cancers (Lee et al. 2013; http://www.cancer. gov). A 5-year survival rate of nonmelanoma cases is very high – more than 99 % – while melanoma cases have very high fatality rate, 22nd highest fatality in all cancers, provided that its survival rate depends on therapy methods. The recent epidemiologic researches in Europe and the USA have reported that the incidence rate of melanoma cases continuously increases over the world including the USA (Catherine and Kenda 2010; www.medcity.com). Skin cancer, one of the skin tumors, is the most common and fastest-growing cancer described by the American Cancer Society, affecting almost all Caucasians (http://www.cancer.gov; www.u.arizona.edu/~witte/ISL.htm). Also, skin cancer, mostly occurring due to sunlight irradiation, is found to be significantly decreased by sunlight exposure prevention for 20 years after the birth. Among the skin cancers, melanomas are found to occur in high-income countries, where Caucasians live. The incidence rate is ten times higher than that of low- and middle-income countries. For example, thirty people per one hundred thousand are reported to suffer from skin cancer in Australia and New Zealand while one person per one hundred thousand in Africa or Asia, which seems relatively small (Table 8.1) (Hildebrandt et al. 2002; Park et al. 2010).

Table 8.1 Major features of skin cancer

Incidence rate	Basal cell carcinoma or squamous cell carcinoma, most of which have high complete recovery rate, occurs more than one million times annually. The most fatal cancer (skin cancer) is rare, and total 62,000 cases have been reported annually
Fatality rate	Total death recorded was 11,200 in 2008; of that, 8420 died from skin cancer and 2780 died from other skin cancers
Risk factor	An excessive ultraviolet exposure by sunlight, clean skin, coal tar, resin, creosote, arsenical, radium, chronic immunosuppression, and heavy skin pigment (for the melanoderm) skin cancer in dark-skinned people are ignored due to their dark skin pigments
Warning signal	Abnormal skin state, especially proliferation of the nevus or other dark pigments and change of mole size and color
Prevention and initial check	Avoid the sun (10:00 am to 04:00 pm) when ultraviolet ray is high; use sunscreen; skin basal cell carcinoma and squamous cell carcinoma often make macule with red prominent boundaries, or pale waxlike pearly knot is formed. Melanoma generally seems dark-brown or dark, which multiplies like small nevus, changes its size and color, and then becomes ulcerating and bleeds when experiencing slight attractive. They begin to proliferate from the size of a small nevus, become bigger, change their color, become ulcer, and cause hemorrhage even with the mild damage
Medical handling	There are four ways in medical handling [operation, electricity cauterization (tissue damage caused by heat), radiation therapy, and cryotherapy (tissue damage caused by cooling)]. Malignant melanoma requires wide and deep excision and removal of surrounding lymph nodes
Survival rate	Basal cell carcinoma or squamous cell carcinoma is almost completely cured through initial checking or treatment. However, skin cancer causes metastasis quickly. Because of this, Caucasian shows low 5-year survival rate due to this disease

Source: refer to pathology for therapists (Catherine and Kenda E-Public, 2010)

8.1.2 Causes

Skin cancer, of which the risk factors are family history, race, scar, and burns, can occur when one is exposed to sunlight. Malignant skin cancers are divided into squamous cell carcinoma, skin cancer, and basal cell carcinoma (http://www.icd10data.com; http://apps.who.int/classifications/icd10/browse/2015/en). The most important factor of squamous cell carcinoma (squamous cell carcinoma) among them is long-term exposure to ultraviolet ray. The risk of skin cancer may increase if DNA is damaged by ultraviolet ray without DNA repair after the damages. Another occurrence case is that one's immunity is depressed chronically after an organ transplant. Also, for precancer-period lesions (such as accumulated ultraviolet ray exposure, burn, keratoma senile, and Bowen's disease), skin cancer can result from radiation therapy, inhalation of herbicide including arsenic, chronic skin irritation and inflammation, exposure to local carcinogen (tar and oil), and hereditary problems (such as xeroderma pigmentosum and albinism).

Accumulated sunlight exposure and intermittent sunlight exposure are the most common causes of basal cell carcinoma; besides, immunosuppression, hereditary vulnerability, and immunization sites are rare causes. Basal cell carcinoma is likely to occur more frequently in adults infected by HIV. Especially, it occurs on the neck or face of workers, who work outside, because they are exposed more.

Skin cancer (malignant melanoma) can occur in the race that has blonde hair, red hair, fair skin color, and blue eyes. Those people who are exposed to burn and belong to Celtic and Scandinavia act as risk factors. Gene is related to gene mutation that produces melanin pigment to protect the skin from ultraviolet ray (Lee et al. 2013; http://www.kostro.or.kr/). In addition, the disease occurs more in Caucasians, especially, more often to those who has a risk of being exposed to long-term sunlight. Skin tanning business can be regarded as a risk factor of generating skin cancer. For the pilot and flight attendants, the exposure to ionizing radiation from the space is a factor that increases the incidence of malignant melanoma (http://www.icd10data.com).

In other words, most of the malignant melanoma is associated with its intensity rather than the time of exposure to sunlight, which is because most of the people suffering from melanoma work inside but are exposed to intense, however limited, sunlight in weekends or during the vacation (Table 8.2) (Jung Dam 2010; http://apps.who.int/classifications/ icd10/browse/2015/en).

Table 8.2 Inducing risk factor of malignant melanoma

Family history
Race: the Celts and Scandinavian
Hair (blond hair or red)
Striking freckles over the back
Past history
More than three times of bullous burn medical history (before the age of twenty) In the case that exposure to sunlight while working outdoors during adolescent summer for 3 years Existence of keratoma senile (horn-shaped growth)

8.1.3 Classification

Based on the tumor tissue initiating sites, skin cancers can be classified as primary skin cancer and metastatic skin cancer. Primary skin cancer means the tumor (glot) that begins in the skin; metastatic skin cancer means the cases where cancer tissues, resulted from other organs, are metastasized into various parts of the body or recurred on the skin. Specifically, metastatic skin cancer, which occurs in other organs but develops into skin cancer, is rare. Skin cancer frequently means the primary skin cancer resulting from the skin. The most common malignant tumors are squamous cell carcinoma, basal cell carcinoma, and malignant melanoma. Among them, squamous cell carcinoma occurs in the epithelium, and it can be detected in the skin with hair.

8.1.3.1 Squamous Cell Carcinoma

Occurred by long-term exposure to sunlight and chemical substances, squamous cell carcinoma has higher incidence rate than other skin cancers, especially, in elders. It is one of the malignant tumors, originated from the keratinocyte of the epidermis, and appears in the scalp, lower lips, external ear, and hands. Its biological characteristics (e.g., causes, size and depth of cancer, anatomical position, and metastasis by histological properties) are more complicated than those of basal cell carcinoma. Among the skin cancers in Korea, squamous cell carcinoma and basal cell carcinoma account for the highest percentage. It is a skin cancer often found in elders and middle-aged population, showing the incidence rate in male twice higher than that of in women

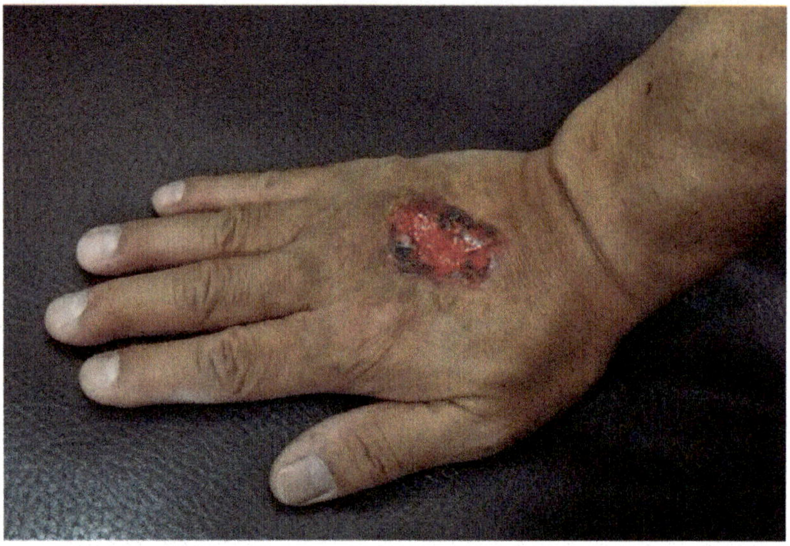

Fig. 8.1 Skin squamous cell carcinoma placed "centeralization" (ex) Skin squamous cell carcinoma

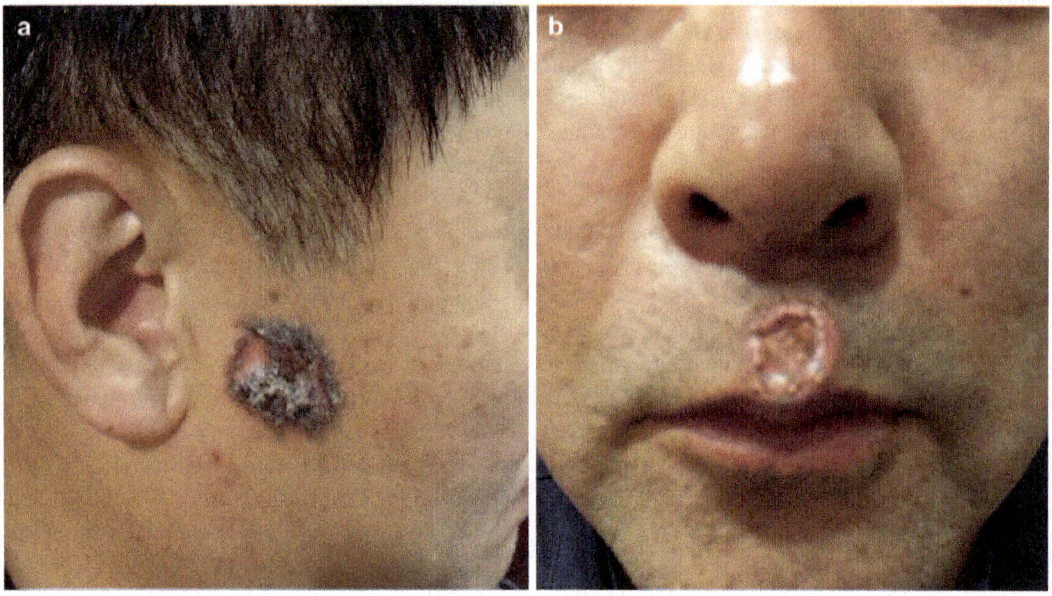

Fig. 8.2 Skin basal cell carcinoma. (**a**) Basal cell carcinoma on side of the ear (**b**) upper lip basal cell carcinoma

(Wust et al. 2002). Ninety percent of it occurs in the lips and particularly the regions that were exposed to chronic ulcer, scar, and tar. So, when detected earlier, it may have positive prognosis. Squamous cell carcinoma is characterized by locally invasive and higher metastatic rate (Fig. 8.1).

8.1.3.2 Basal Cell Carcinoma

Basal cell carcinoma accounts for 65 % of the entire skin cancers, which is a malignant tumor disease of the cell mass formed by the follicle, bottom of the epidermis – i.e., basal layer (basal cell). It is called rodent ulcer and basal cell. Also, it results from skin cancer of Caucasian, showing relatively low malignancy. Basal cell carcinoma and squamous cell carcinoma are the most common nonmelanoma skin cancers with low metastatic rate. It originated from scar and burn scar and particularly developed in damaged parts with chronic exposure to sunlight. As is relatively rare, its metastasis is infiltrated locally; if not properly treated, it is metastasized into the bone, lung, and brain leading to death (Fig. 8.2a, b).

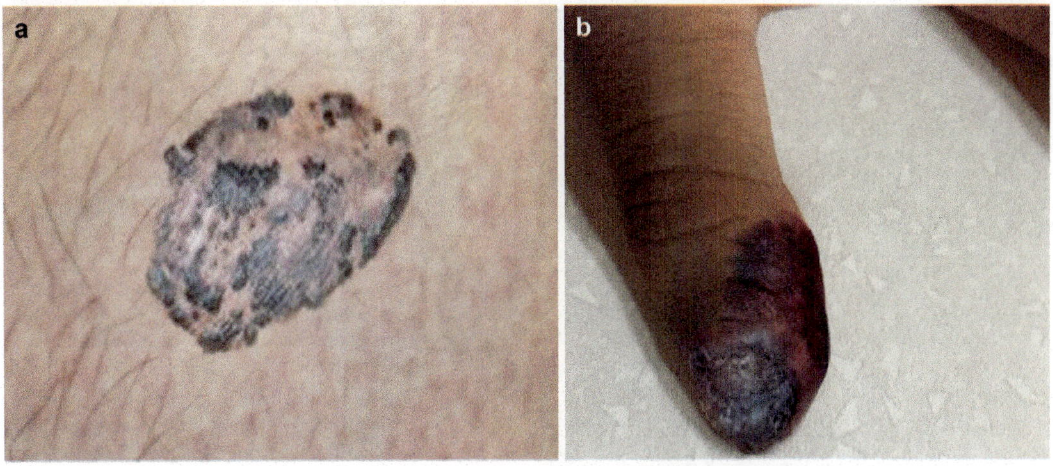

Fig. 8.3 (a) Skin cancer occurring in trunk and (b) skin cancer occurring in the finger

8.1.3.3 Malignant Melanoma

Malignant melanoma is a skin disease with the highest mortality rate. It is a malignant tumor of melanocytes that a melanin cell or nevus cell (spot) becomes malignant. It occurs in any part of the body where melanin cell exists especially in the skin (Wust et al. 2002). Malignant melanoma is a malignant tumor which spreads very rapidly and deeply through blood and may be exacerbated by sunlight irritation or stimulation of the nevus (Fig. 8.3a, b).

8.1.3.4 Keratoma Senile

Keratoma senile (actinic keratosis) is the precancer stage of skin cancer which appears in damaged part of the skin exposed to long-term sunlight. Those who are over 50–60 years of age – particularly Caucasians who become red ripe and have freckle when exposed to sunlight – have high incidence rate (Choi 2010; www.u.arizona.edu/~witte/ISL.htm; www.medcity.com).

The forms of keratoma senile lesion are small but rough and keratinized skin. Also, especially it is red in color with unclear boundary or brown keratinized lesions. Lesion is usually multicentric, and its form comes a little uplifted or flat. Also, the diameter of its keratinous papule or red to gray verrucous shape is 1–10 mm (Fig. 8.4). As highly fixed in the surface, the scale is difficult to remove and its lesion surrounds an erythema. Cutaneous horn occurs if hyperkeratosis is severe. It often appears after subsiding for weeks or months, and even it can quite occur even if keratin is removed.

It often occurs in the lower lips, and it is called actinic cheilitis. It is reported that less than 1–20 % of keratoma senile develops into flat epithelium cell cancer; however, it can grow into nonmelanoma skin cancer.

8.1.4 Symptoms and Complications

8.1.4.1 Squamous Cell Carcinoma

It can occur in a form of an ulcer, flat red part, epidermis keratin, protuberance valve, and module, and its sarcode seems red and is surrounded by scale tissue. More than 80 % of the squamous cell carcinoma occurs in the head, neck, lower lips, and ears. Systemic symptoms are accompanied by pain, fatigue, malaise, weakness, and anorexia.

8.1.4.2 Basal Cell Carcinoma

Its form is classic pearl or ivory shape. It, whose boundaries are round and slightly elevated than other skins, has small blood vessels on its surfaces. Generally, its nodules cause no pain and gradually grow to become ulcer in the center. More than 65 % of the basal cell carcinoma occurs in the head, face, and neck, followed by the body, especially the upper back and chest (Wust et al. 2002).

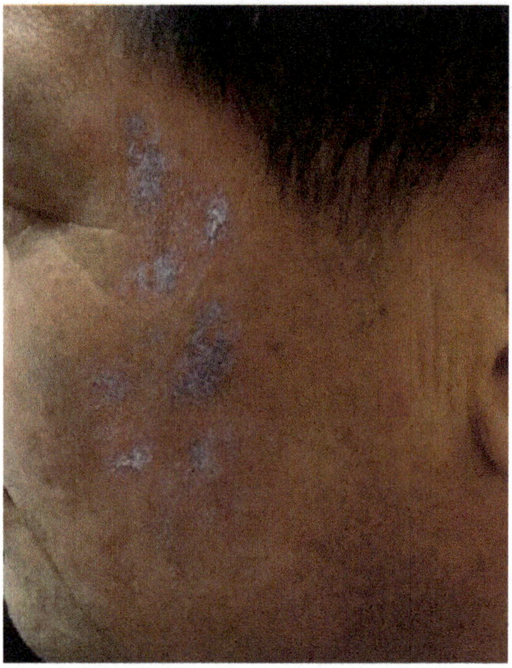

Fig. 8.4 Actinic keratosis

8.1.4.3 Malignant Melanoma

Male can suffer from skin cancer in the head and neck, while female can contact it in the leg or back during the exposure to excessive ultraviolet ray. It results from previous nevus more than 70 %. The factors affecting the therapeutic prognosis of skin cancer change by the depth of the tumor, shifting term, race, age, sex, and histological form.

8.1.5 Test and Assessment

8.1.5.1 Diagnosis of Skin Cancer

Melanoma is a skin cancer which requires a rapid recognition and monthly self-examination (http://www.icd10data.com; www.mw.go.kr). By histological examination, it is necessary to test and determine the depth of tumor as well as to assign the stage in order to distinguish skin cancer from other lesions (Fig. 8.4). The diagnosis stage of skin cancer is systemized for the progress of skin cancer by skin-layer infiltration. In the first stage, it infiltrates only into the epidermis; in the second stage, into the dermis; in the third stage, into most of the upper dermis; in the fourth stage, into the lower dermis; in the fifth stage, into the hypoderm. The higher the stage becomes, the higher the metastasis occurs. Also, biopsy or histological test is taken.

The assessment and diagnosis of cancer depend on the types of cancers, using hematological test, X-ray test, ultrasonic diagnosis, CT (computed tomography), MRI (magnetic resonance imaging), etc.

Table 8.3 The stage of skin cancer

Period	Proceeding aspects
Stage 0	Although exists cancer cells, it is surrounded by the epidermis. It is right before the cancer stage and called '*intraepithelial carcinoma*'.
Stage 1	The size of cancer exists in the dermis below 2 cm or is surrounded by the hypoderm in the dermis.
Stage 2	The size of cancer exists only in the dermis over 2 cm or is surrounded by the hypoderm (loose connective tissue, blood vessel, fat cell) in the dermis.
Stage 3	The depth of cancer progresses to deep inner region (muscle, cartilage, bone, and so forth) or metastasizes from the region that initial tumor occurs to the nearest lymph node.
Stage 4	Pass from the region where cancer occurred at early stages to the nearest lymph node and remotely metastasizes to internal organs.

8.1.5.2 Stages of Skin Cancer

During the diagnosis and prognosis, the depth and skin-infiltration degree of tumor are most important, divided into the depth of "infiltration degree of Clark" and "Breslow." (http://www.kslymph.or. kr/; http://www.cancer.go.kr/mbs/cancer/subview.jsp?id=cancer_030206030300; www.kams.or.kr)

The stages of skin cancer are classified below (Table 8.3). First, infiltration degree of Clark means how far the depth of the tumor infiltrates (Fig. 8.5). Second, Breslow law is the measurement method to check the depth of melanoma. The thinner the melanoma, the better the prognosis is. Third, the layers of infiltrated skin by melanoma are measured. Fourth, Computed tomography is essential to confirm basic pathological laboratory test, metastasis of bone scan, chest part, abdominal

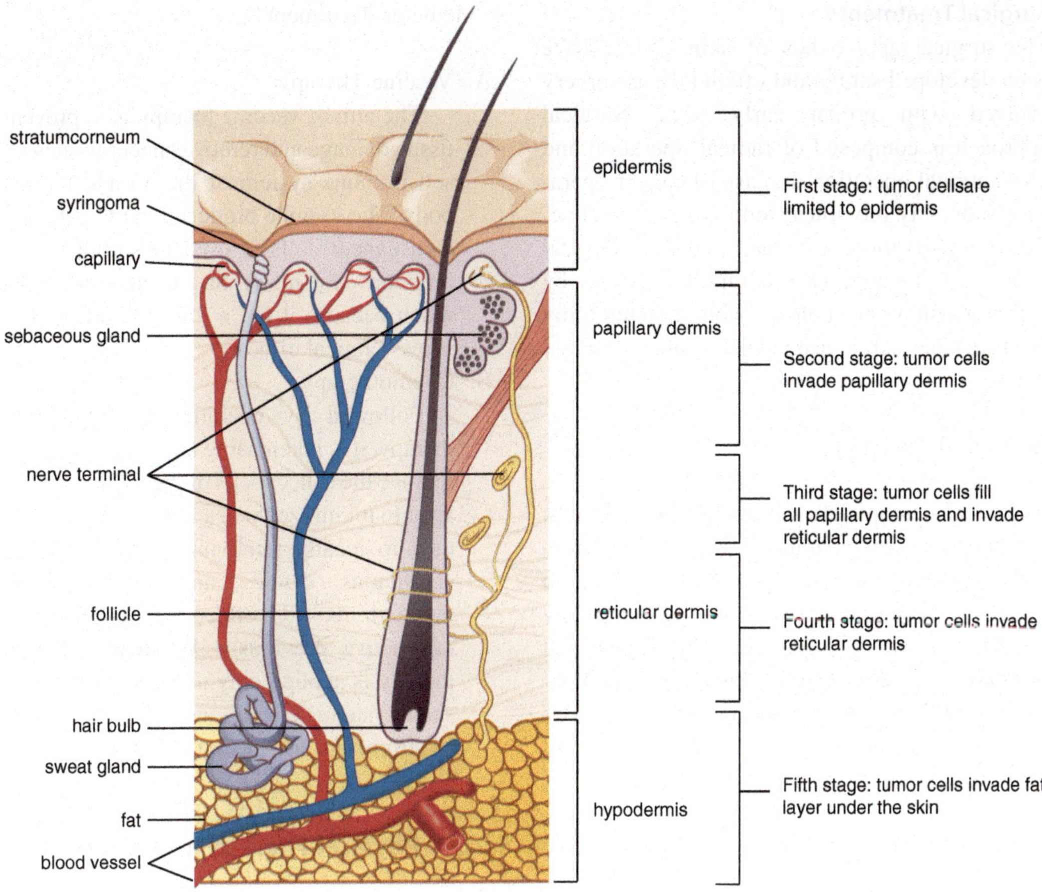

Fig. 8.5 The diagnosis of skin cancer, using Clark stage

part, central nervous system, and metastasis of cerebellar tract.

8.2 Intervention

8.2.1 Intervention

8.2.1.1 Interventional Approach

The therapeutic approach of skin cancer depends on age; thus, the small cancer of old patients can be removed by simple operation or radiation therapy while their aesthetically important parts, such as a face, have high re-occurrence possibility, which should be recovered by minimal incision. For America, physical therapists massage them, and therapeutic intervention is needed to resolve the contraction or stiffness of the face after the cancer of aesthetic face parts is operated. Therefore, it is necessary to take manual therapy by a physical therapist after the operation (Park et al. 2013a, b).

8.2.1.2 Medical Treatment

Therapeutic Goals

The medical approach of skin cancer depends on the depth, size, and location of the lesion and consists of tissue dissection (excochleation, abrasion), electrocauterization (cauterization), chemotherapy, surgical operation, and radiation therapy, which means abrasive materials or tissues by abnormal mechanical procedure. It is important to take the approach within required time because metastasis into other parts can occur if the approach for cancer is not taken sufficiently (Park et al. 2013b; Van 2002).

Surgical Treatments

The surgical approaches of skin cancer have been developed safely and efficiently as surgery evolved with proper early tests. Surgical approach is composed of radical operation and conventional operation. In case of cancer operation, radicality (complete remove), safety, functional preservation, etc., are applied. Surgical approaches show good or complete recovery by local incision or non-incision thalamotomy because the early test makes tumors found rapidly.

① Radical Operation

It means completely removing cancer tissues, which consists of operation, radiation, carcinostatic chemotherapy, etc. Among them, radiation therapy is a representative skin cancer therapy applied to those suffering from skin cancer and difficult to incision-operate. Also, it is accompanied by radiation therapy secondary to incision-operate and then remove completely the tissue of those who are suffering from skin cancer.

② Conventional Operation

It, although impossible to remove tumor tissues completely, focuses on improving the symptom of those suffering from the cancer – namely, it does not remove cancer tissues completely, but lessens the degree of symptoms.

③ Radiation Therapy

Concentrating on more radiation ray than measurement ray on the cancer, it can cure human bodies from the cancer. Radiation therapy is divided into outer radiation therapy and close radiation therapy. Mainly its period and number vary according to the type and size of cancer, and it is recommended to drink sufficient amount of water and to eat food to increase the therapeutic effects during the therapy. Radiation therapy methods depend on the type of cancer; especially, the radiation therapy of basal cell carcinoma is not allowed to those who are below 50 years old. The risk of the secondary skin cancer occurs by radiation ray, let alone its recurrence risk.

④ Medicine Treatment

A. Vaccine Therapy

The aim of vaccine therapy is to prevent tissue damage and remove cancer tissues by self-immune system of the normal human body. The vaccine produced in the patients' own cancer cells is used to stimulate the immune system. It has been considered much because it has a few side effects but shows clinical effects.

B. Chemotherapy

Followed by operation and radiation therapy, it is taken using anticancer drugs to remove the cancer cells of the tissue. It managed to minimize them and thus has contributed to locally removing cancers through continuous studies and clinical tests although its side effects are prominently destructive previously. Whereas radiation therapy is applied only to local parts, it can show systemic effects, and thus those suffering from cancers select it the most.

8.2.2 Physical Therapy Intervention

8.2.2.1 Positioning

Those suffering from skin cancer should try to maintain balanced body and to exercise stretching so as to prevent the side effect occurring in cancers. Switch off multimedia devices (such as notebook, a computer, a smart phone, etc.), and take a rest once or twice a week to reduce mental stress. Also, read a book, take meditation, or walk outside for mental rest while not using electric devices.

8.2.2.2 Exercise Therapy

Like other cancers, skin cancer results in decreasing physical abilities and causing daily lethargy by insomnia, fatigue, depression, pain, and helplessness of those suffering from other cancers. Accordingly, those suffering from these cancers can be taken by exercise therapy to improve their depressed physical functions, which involve joint exercise, strength exercise, aerobic exercise, and endurance exercise. The best benefit of exercise effects is to advance the maximum amount of oxygen intake and to improve whole body function as

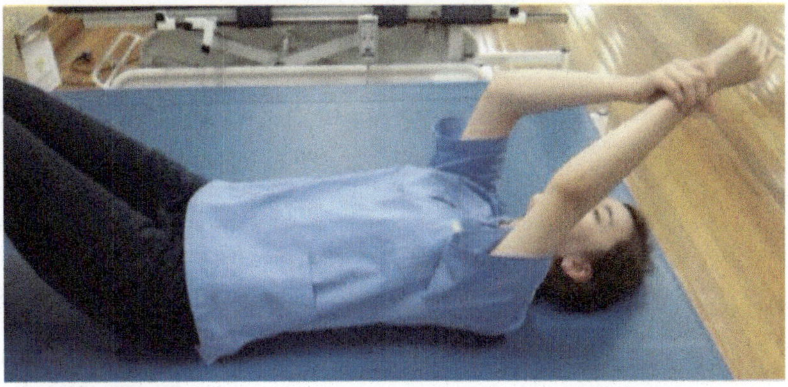

Fig. 8.6 Arm shift exercise over the other side of the head

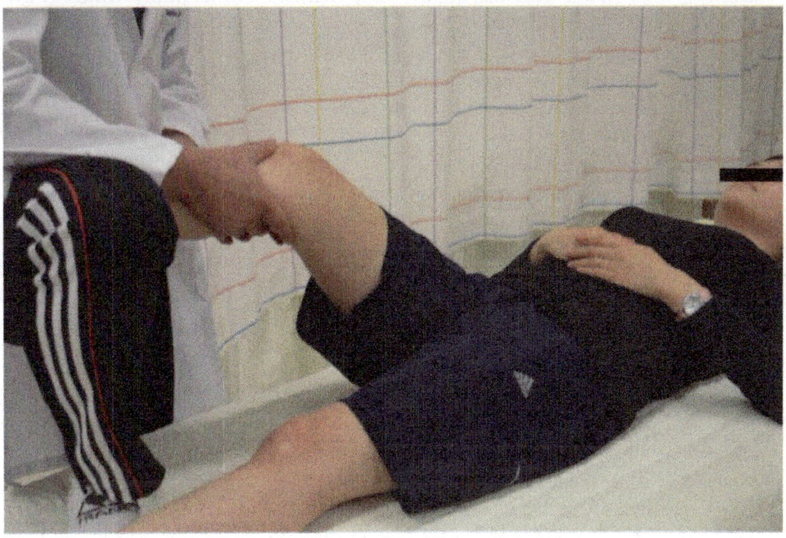

Fig. 8.7 Lower limb joint exercise of skin cancer patients

well as minimize the side effect of treatments for cancer if the aerobic exercise programs for those suffering from the cancer are offered. Benefits of exercise therapies are the following: the increase of strength by muscle contraction, the increase of blood circulation, the rise of blood return to the heart (means the whole strength of the heart), and the resistance to muscular fatigue.

Joint Mobilization Exercise

Active joint mobility exercise is taken many times a day after the patient becomes conscious or can move. Skin cancer patient must be able to take an active joint mobilization exercise on undamaged upper limbs and lower limbs as well as the body. At first, must have stage by stage, it takes soften ROM initially and, if required, active movement and passive movement are acquired at first (Fig. 8.6). The exercise of the neck, arm, and shoulder near the proximal is taken, and then the exercise to promote the mobility of the whole body is applied (Fig. 8.7). If patients cannot take an active movement efficiently, an active assistance movement and manual movement are taken at first.

Strength Exercise

If skin cancer patients are recovered rapidly, strength exercise can be taken as a part of rehabilitation program in stage. Those suffering from skin cancer show the decrease of weight and muscle mass. Especially, resistance exercise for strengthening can prevent the strength loss of non-infiltrated parts, and strength exercise is taken using isokinetic devices, isotonic devices, other resistance exercise devices and limbs of

Table 8.4 Aerobic and resistance exercise program intervention plan

Aerobic exercise program intervention	
Variable	Recommend aerobic exercise program for incipient cancer patients and healthy people who underwent cancer treatment
Type of exercise	Exercise using large muscle group (example – walking, stationary exercise bicycles, and so on)
Frequency	At least three to five times per week, low intensity, short time; those who have good physical fitness are recommended to exercise every day
Intensity	50 ~ 70 % VO2 max or 50 ~ 75 % HRR, 60 ~ 80 % HRmax
Time	Continual exercise for at least 20 to 30 min; those who have bad physical fitness are recommended to exercise in sections
Degree of progress	Progress considering physical fitness levels: consider individual conditions
Resistance exercise program intervention	
Variable	For incipient cancer patients and those who received cancer treatment is recommended
Type of exercise	Dynamic resistance exercise of concentric, eccentric exercise form, balanced exercise of the upper limbs or lower limbs
Frequency	At least one to three times per week, break at proper interval
Intensity	50 ~ 80 % of 1RM, repeat up to 6 ~ 12 times
Time	Continual exercise for at least 20 to 30 min; those who have bad physical fitness levels are recommended to exercise in sections
Degree of progress	Progress considering physical fitness levels. Consider individual conditions

patients. To prevent excessive exercise, physical therapists can block sudden accident by checking the pulse, blood pressure, and respiratory rate during, before, and after the exercise.

The types of resistance exercises applying the active exercise of concentric and eccentric shape need balanced exercise between the upper limb and lower limb. Its intensity is 50–80 % of 1RM, its repetition is 6–12 times, and its frequency is one to three times a week. After the exercise, take sufficient rest, provided that the exercise is continuously taken for 20–30 min. (Lee et al. 2013; Park et al. 2013b).

Aerobic Exercise

Light walking exercise, needed to improve systemic strength through blood circulation, should be taken by patients to stimulate cardiovascular system. The programs to take aerobic exercise effect are fixed bicycle exercise using big muscle, rowing, treadmill walking, and gradual stair climb. Its intensity is set against 50–70 % VO_2max or 50 ~ 75 % HRR (maximum heart rate reserve) and 60 ~ 80 % HRmax (heart rate maximum), and its frequency is at a minimum of three to five times a week by low intensity within a short period of time many times (Park et al. 2013b; Jung Dam 2010). It is needed to exercise continuously for 20–30 min in order to take effects (Table 8.4).

8.2.2.3 Manual Therapy

The skin can have scars resulting from the incision of skin cancer and the surgical operation. They become factors of which the adhesion to surrounding tissues makes it difficult to move the epidermis and hypodermis. Even it causes intense pain and mobility restrain. Therefore, physical therapists cannot only take skin rolling and skin relaxation technique but have the mobility of the skin and the benefit of pain solution while recognizing the recurrence risk of skin cancer. When interfering with skin cancer, the lymph massage should be applied carefully, which significantly improves the blood circulation. That is because it results in aggravating skin cancer.

8.2.2.4 Physical Agent Modalities

The therapy using physical factors includes those using cold and warmth; those suffering from tumor and skin cancer can be prescribed to pressure treatment methods (e.g., pressure stocking and pneumatic compression treatment). Also, the laser therapies for them are lower-intensity laser therapy or so. For skin cancer patients, the physical factor therapy should be applied carefully, which contributes to increase blood stream, due to the active circulation in tissues.

8.2.3 Prevention and Management

8.2.3.1 Prevention of Skin Cancer

All cancers have high recurrence rate and their metastasis can move into each part of the body, so it is important to prevent the cancer by regular medical examination. In addition, a small number of malignant tumors show poor prognosis, so the advanced management and prevention are necessary. The guidelines for the prevention of skin cancer are shown in Table 8.5.

8.2.3.2 Management of Skin Cancer

Because skin cancer, if detected early, can be almost fully recovered, the examination by a medical team is taken periodically. Also, those suffering from skin cancer show good prognosis as the therapy method for skin cancer is varied and its therapeutic effect becomes high. It's coming to the fore that self-management of in terms of therapy as well as diet. Avoid an excessive sunlight exposure, try to prevent the direct sunlight, and avoid going out from 10:00 am to 14:00 pm when ultraviolet ray becomes strong. Use the sunblock against ultraviolet ray, if owing to an unavoidable engagement. Furthermore, wear long-sleeved clothes or hats.

8.2.3.3 Patient/Caregiver Education

For those suffering from skin cancer, it is difficult for them to care for themselves, which means they need a caregiver for them. The training for a caregiver is essential in terms of prevention, so that the training of a caregiver for children should be taken exhaustively, which has been supported by the researches that severe burn by sunlight occurs mostly during the childhood and more aged group causing the higher possibility of skin cancer.

Table 8.5 Prevention guide of skin cancer

Avoid exposure when sunlight is peak (11:00 am ~ 15:00 pm)
Put on clothes made of fabric to avoid sunlight when going out
Use sunblock cream (PA++) which is higher than 15 SPF to protect sunlight
Inform children of sunlight protection
Avoid artificial tanning by sunlight
Take regular skin examination
Consult experts as soon as possible if recognizing abnormal symptom of the body and skin

8.3 Lymphedema

8.3.1 Overview

In terms of anatomical composition, the lymph system, which originally develops in the vein, consists of deep lymphatic glands and lymphatic vessels as well as shallow lymphatic glands and lymphatic vessels. Besides, it includes the thymus glands, marrow, spleen, tonsil, and Peyer's patches of the small intestine as lymphatic organs and tissues. The role of the lymph system is immunity function, body fluid balance, and infection control. In general, 18 L of the tissue fluid is removed inside the interstitium of the body, most of which is absorbed from 80 to 90%. The rest (10–20%) is removed in shallow lymphatic vessels and deep lymphatic vessels. Lymph disease is caused by the disease of blood vessel, meaning the disease which affects significantly the functional loss of the upper limbs and lower limbs due to the limb circulatory disturbances. The disturbance results from acute or chronic medical conditions of peripheral blood vessel diseases (PVD), causing a severe blood vessel disease in artery, vein, and especially lymph circulatory system. For example, it is unavoidable to take the radiation test or surgical incision of chronic lymphedema in the upper limbs, which can have physical effects on mental status in daily life. Lymphedema results from the circulatory system disorder of lymph – namely, the unbalance between the amounts of body fluid, needed to remove in interstitium, and the transportation ability. Therefore, this secondarily results from the lymphedema by side effects and complications after cancer therapy, operation, and radiation therapy. It is the disease which changes tissue and skin as well as increases edema in the upper limbs and lower limbs. In other words, it means chronic inflammation when edema is accumulated by abnormal accumulation of tissue protein. Accordingly, the physical therapists should pay attention to acquire physical therapy intervention methods by the symptom and sign, evaluation of lymphedema and to prevent the secondary infection or complications of lymphedema (www. cdc.go.kr; www.medcity.com).

8.3.2 Causes

Lymphedema resulted from various causes, meaning that lymph fluid occurs because it does not circulate through lymphatic vessels – that is, lymphatic glands are blocked or removed, the circulation of lymph fluid is not taken, it is accumulated into the body tissue, and edema occurs. In other words, it means the edema resulted from the abnormally accumulated tissues on the upper limbs and lower limbs due to the damage of the lymph system. Although lymphedema has natural causes, it generally resulted from infection, malignant tumor (cancer), venous disease, scar and wound by radiation therapy, and incision operation. Especially, those obese or old are likely to have the possibility of lymphedema.

8.3.3 Classification

By the cause of occurrence, lymphedema is divided into the first lymphedema and the second lymphedema. The International Society of Lymphology classifies incubation period into first, second, and third stage by its symptoms (Table 8.6) (Lee et al. 2013; Myers 2011).

8.3.3.1 Primary Lymphedema

It means the edema created from birth. It results from the loss of lymph circulation by the aplasia and hyperplasia of natural lymphatic vessel as well as no absorption of lymph fluid. Seventy-five percent of the first lymphedema is premature lymphedema and occurs in young women, especially after their puberty.

It has been reported that the disease is caused by abnormal genes of FOXC2 and VEGFC. Although the 3rd gene has doubt but not clearly identified (Myers 2011; An 2009).

8.3.3.2 Secondary Lymphedema

It means the second or acquired lymphedema, showing the complications after cancer operation and radiation therapy. Specifically, its 15–20 % occurs during breast cancer surgery and uterus cancer surgery with lymphatic gland removal; its 50–70 % occurs when lymphatic vessel removal operation and radiation therapy are taken.

8.3.4 Symptoms and Complications

The symptoms of edema vary in the upper limbs and lower limbs generally. The distribution of edema shows local condition and edema occurs in the other or both upper limbs and lower limbs (Figs. 8.8 and 8.9). The lymphedema of the upper limbs occurs in the incision part of armpit lymphatic gland and below the radiation therapy part. The tissue and skin with edema tend to become soft and then too hard to press during palpation. Also, patients feel heavy and tight in the part with edema and suffer from the pain in the part with lymphedema, and the restrain of mobility after edema extended into the joints. Secondarily,

Table 8.6 The stage of lymphedema

Period	Symptoms
Incubation period	Show the decrease of the ability to move lymph fluid Reveal little clinical symptoms and feel simply heavy
The first stage	It means reversible stage Edema occurs; however, skin is still flexible It takes longer to remain a little pressed than in normal state if edema part is pressed by the finger It returns to its abnormal state if an edema part is located higher than heart for long Fibrosis has not yet occurred in lymphatic vessel, and it can be cured
The second stage	Protein accumulates in tissue, and resultant fibrosclerosis makes skin not pressed if the therapy period is missed in the first stage It has low change of improving It has very high risk of infecting
The third stage	Irreversible stage Skin becomes very swollen and abnormal change occurs in the skin Functional loss takes longer with complications Known as elephantiasis; it shows that skin becomes rough and its surface turns uneven, so body fluid release outside the skin Infection incidence rate is very high, and one's life hangs in the balance without active therapy Because of its long state of fibrosis, there is rarely chance of returning to normal tissue

Source: International Society of Lymphology homepage

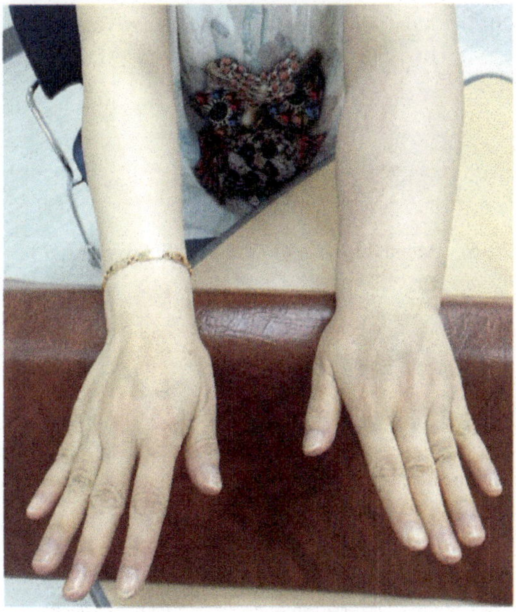

Fig. 8.8 Lymphedema of the upper limb

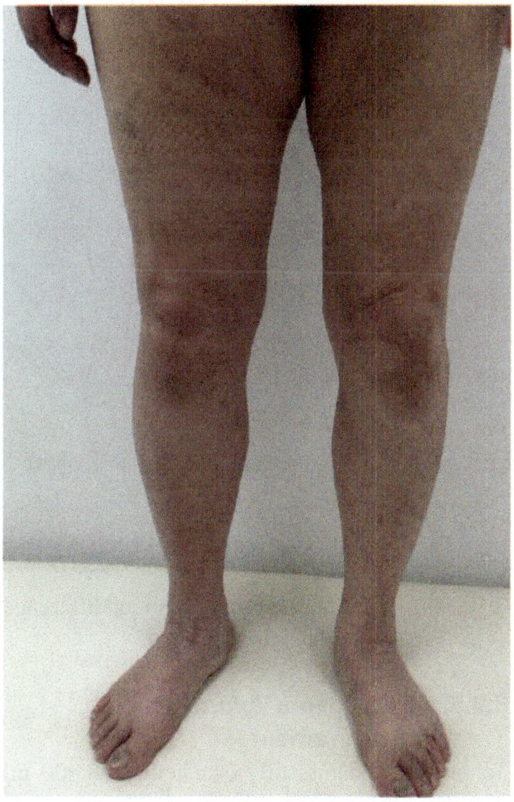

Fig. 8.9 Lymphedema of the lower limb

lymphedema has high frequency of skin infection occurrence and causes exothermic reaction, rubor, etc. The damage to the lymph system, resulting from the secondary causes, has the risk of keeping up lymphedema and generating recurrence.

8.3.5 Test and Assessment

Check those with abnormal lymph system suffering from injury, malignant tumor, lymphatic gland clearing surgery, and radiation therapy in past medical history. Confirm whether they had blood clot in their medical history, and then set and take therapeutic intervention with the prevention of lymphedema before the examination (Lee et al. 2013; Park et al. 2013c).

8.3.5.1 Radiologic Examination

For the exact diagnosis, check the increased number of leukocytes using the blood test, and check the state of lymphatic glands and lymph nodes as well as the location and aspect of lymphedema using the ultrasonic test, Doppler test, lymphography, computed tomography, magnetic resonance imaging (MRI), etc. (Fauci et al. 2010; Park et al. 2013a).

8.3.5.2 Physical Therapy Examination

Test and measure the sensibility evaluation of the skin, muscular contraction, strength, the restrain of articulation exercise, the range of movement, etc. Besides, assess differently various measurement and evaluation methods by the type of cancer and the damage extent of patients.

8.3.5.3 Self-Marking Tape Measure

Measure the other part of the upper limbs and lower limbs with lymphedema, using tapeline (Table 8.7, Fig. 8.12). Measuring the edema of the upper limbs and lower limbs is shown below (Figs. 8.10, 8.11, 8.12, and 8.13). Stand with patient feet shoulder length apart using tapeline, stand above the ground, and measure not only the bottom of the left and right metatarsal and the bottom of saber shin but also the circumference of the front of metatarsal in the largest part of the calf muscle and that of the upper end of the anklebone in calf bone.

Table 8.7 Compilation of circumference measuring table for both upper limbs and lower limbs (unit: cm)

Part	Month/day/year (12/16/2016)		Month/day/year (/ /)		Month/day/year (/ /)	
Arm	Rt.	Lt.	Rt.	Lt.	Rt.	Lt.
①	27	28				
②	24	26				
③	25	25				
④	17	19				
⑤	8	8				
Part	Month/day/year (12/16/2016)		Month/day/year (/ /)		Month/day/year (/ /)	
Leg	Rt.	Lt.	Rt.	Lt.	Rt.	Lt.
①	54	55				
②	36	38				
③	34	35				
④	28	30				
⑤	24	25				

To compare it after measuring the circumstance of both upper limb and lower limb, measure and record as it is designated

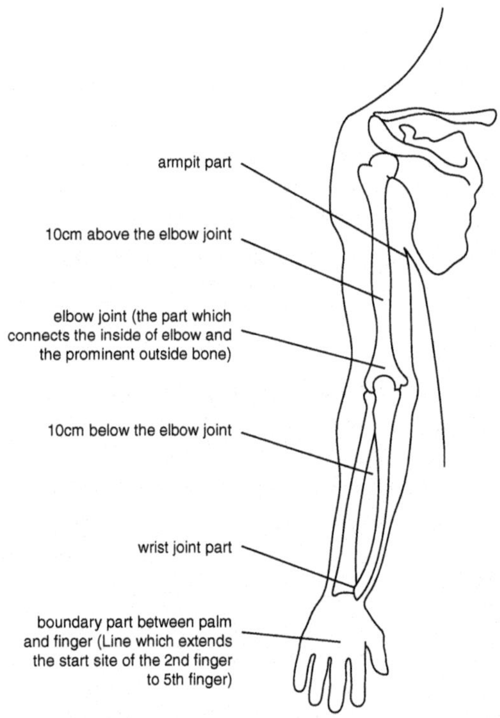

Fig. 8.10 Circumstance measuring part of the upper limb

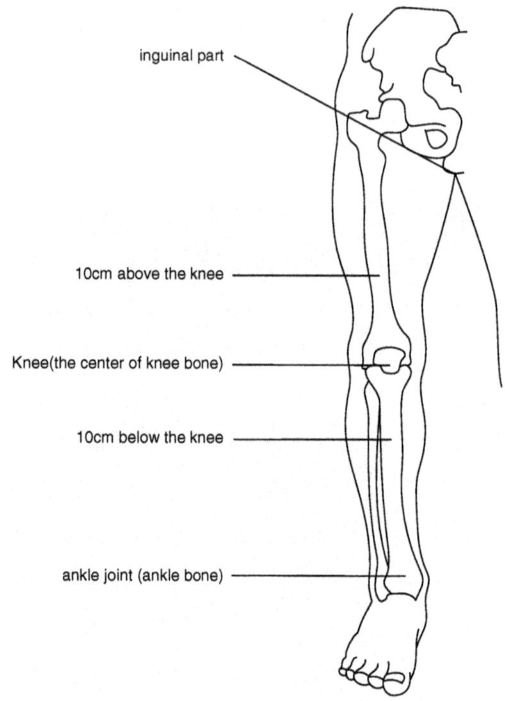

Fig. 8.11 Circumstance measuring part of the lower limb

① Measure it regularly in every week or every day.
② Measure it at the same time zone (mainly morning) with the same posture.
③ Wind tape line horizontally and measure it with appropriate pulling.
④ Compare its value when measuring those with swelling and those without swelling.
⑤ Confirm how far their measurement difference is (Fig. 8.13).

8.3.5.4 Skin Edema Volume Measurement

To measure edema, fill consistently 28,000 ml with left and right legs by their cubiti anterior, put overflowing amount of water into a beaker, and calculate the average after measuring it (Fig. 8.13) (Jung et al. 2001).

8.3.5.5 Body Composition Analysis (Inbody)

A body composition analyzer (Inbody co.) is characterized by a simple measurement using the property that residual resistance occurs in water, fat, and muscle when a little current passes, recognizing weight, body fluid, intracellular fluid, extracellular fluid, body fat, and edema degree. Placed foot at the heel part of sole shape on body composition analyzer (Inbody) (Fig. 8.15. See the body composition analyzer (Inbody, co., Ltd.)) and always reach it on the same part, spread the upper limbs by about 15° and examine with the eyes straight (Figs. 8.14 and 8.15).

8.3.5.6 Identification of Prodrome

The presymptoms include feeling height, feeling sullen, feeling one or the other of upper limbs or lower limbs, feel a stinging sensation, hot flush, rubor, hot flush, etc. (Table 8.8).

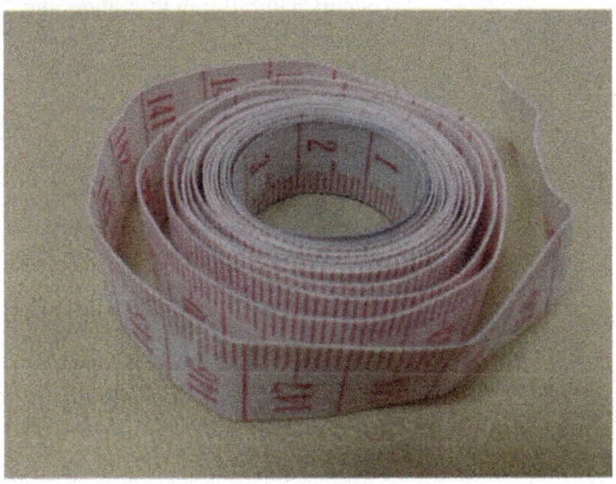

Fig. 8.12 Tapeline examination

8.3.5.7 Assessment of Symptoms and Severity

Those suffering from lymphedema can feel pricky, heavy, bulky, weak, etc., in the affected parts. For the severity of lymphedema, the International Society of Lymphology classifies into four stages, including the incubation period which shows abnormal lymphedema in the lymph system without clinical symptom (Tables 8.9 and 8.10) (Lee et al. 2013; Jung Dam 2010; Myers 2011).

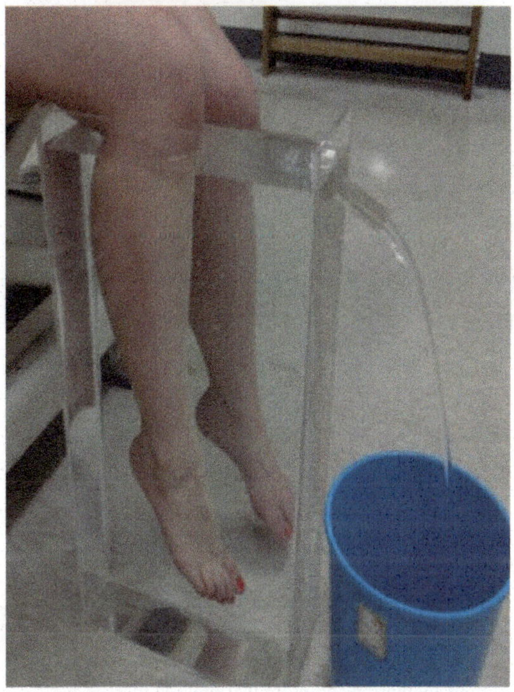

Fig. 8.14 Volume of water examination for edema measuring

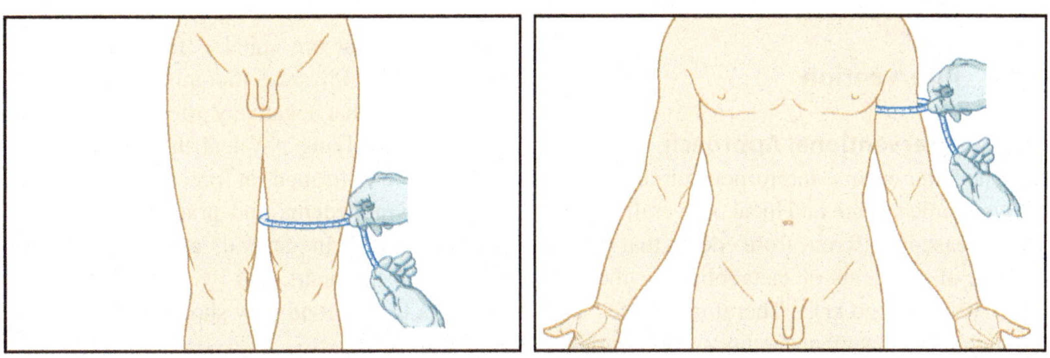

Fig. 8.13 Circumstance tapeline measuring of the lower and upper limb

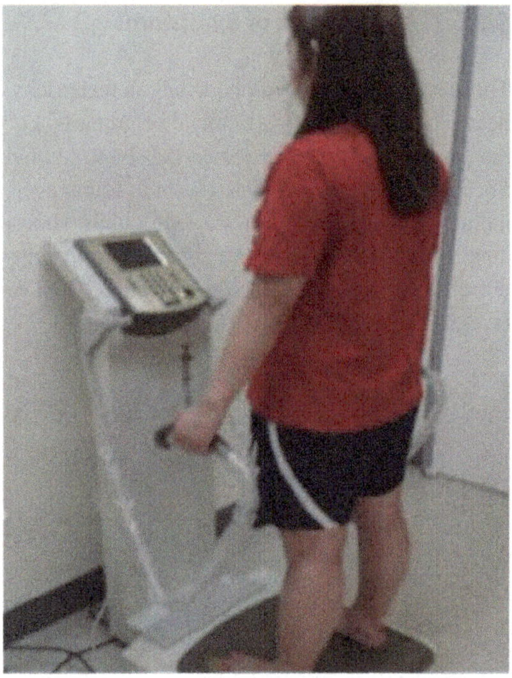

Fig. 8.15 Measure edema by body composition analyzer

Table 8.8 Self-reported diagnosis of lymphedema

Legs feel cramping
Legs feel tight when wearing shoes
Legs often feel weak
Legs often feel sore and aching or heavy
Skin of legs easily becomes red or edema occurs
There is an infection symptom such as hot flush or pain
Pitting edema(the symptom that pressed marker maintains for seconds if skin is pressed by finger end) occurs

Table 8.9 The diagnosis requirement of lymphedema

① There is edema without one or both lower limbs and upper limbs
② Earlier indentation edema is changed to non-indentation edema
③ Pigmentation, created by ulcer, varix, and stasis, does not occur; however, lymphedema is diagnosed when lymphangitis or phlegmon is detected

Table 8.10 The step classification by the International Society of Lymphology

Clinical stage	Characteristics
0 stage (Incubation period)	It is the state that the mobility of lymph fluid is damaged without edema. In reality, it can last for certain months or years before edema occurs
The first stage	It is the stage that edema naturally decreases; if pressed, pitting edema, which lasts the state, occurs, while if maintained high, edema decreases
The second stage	It is the stage that edema rarely occurs naturally; in this stage, the fibrosclerosis of tissue becomes prominent. Pitting edema occurs in the earlier second period, while pitting edema does not occur because of the fibrosclerosis of tissue, and, if edema part is maintained high, the edema of tissue decreases in the last second period
The third stage	This stage is that edema is very severe, as is known as "elephant skin disease" which changes skin. Although the skin is pressed, hypertrophic skin change occurs such as pitting edema acanthosis, fat deposition, overgrowth of verruciformis, etc.

8.4 Intervention

8.4.1 Intervention

8.4.1.1 Interventional Approach

Lymphedema occurs due to poor circulation of the lymphatic system and local or overall edema. This disease is different from edema that occurs because of problems of metabolism or the kidney (www.cdc.go.kr). Therefore, safe and affordable management methods and treatment intervention that are suitable for lymphedema are necessary. Physical therapists should prohibit methods that negatively affect lymphedema patients in applying physical therapy intervention and be informed of precautions to ease patients' lymphedema and practice to increase flow of lymph. In general, a limb should be higher than the heart, and by putting overpressure on a limb, blood flow should not be drastically increased.

8.4.1.2 Medical Management

If there is inflammation by the primary and secondary damage resulting from cancer, there is likely to be injury or acute inflammation. At this moment, care is required for excessive amount of intervention and care, and in severe cases, a quick wound dressing care and administration of antibiotics are required (www.u.arizona.edu/~witte/ISL.htm; http://www.lymphnotes.com/article.php/id/474/).

8.4.2 Physical Therapy Intervention

8.4.2.1 Postures

Physical therapists should be informed of posture which exacerbates lymphedema and preventable posture. They should have patients informed about it and manage them. Especially, patients should not be exposed to risk factors (sauna, fomentation, acupuncture, vacuum cupping therapy, injection, excessive exercise, wearing tight underwears, bruise) and should be prescribed with regular range and intensity of training (Park et al. 2010; Park et al. 2013a; Kim et al. 2008).

Supervise patients to not adopt a posture that interrupts blood circulation.

8.4.2.2 Exercise Therapy

As a way of increasing limited joint range, union, and immobilization resulting from cancer, exercise treatment should be carried out. Especially, passive and active joint motion exercises and extensional movements may affect on fluid diffusion and flow of lymph circulation. To improve weakened muscles and myatrophy, by the gradual strength exercise, lymph and blood circulation can be improved (Park et al. 2013b; Jung et al. 2001). Also, this kind of exercise treatments of cancer affects in weight loss and in lymphedema and is preventive measures. Promoting mobility exercise of the neck, your own exercise regime for improving pain, raising a shoulder blade and forearm over a head lying for stretching, and butterfly-shaped stretching methods apply to exercise treatment for cancer patients (Figs. 8.16, 8.17, 8.18, 8.19, and 8.20).

Maintaining Posture and Movement Program

Through movement of the parts where edema occurred and proper joint position, edema can be prevented. Especially, conservative methods that lift the arms and legs may induce emission of intercellular interstitial fluid by gravity and reduce hydrostatic pressure resulting from the blood vessel.

Exercise of the Whole Body

There is a good point that through exercise of the whole body, pump muscle and at part of edema move lymph fluid to a region where there is no edema, and by increasing joint working range, blood circulation can be facilitated; thereby functions of overall body improve. Generally, 30 min of exercise three or four times a week is proper, intensity of exercise slowly increases, and maximum heart rate should be increased up to 60 ~ 80 % step by step.

Breathing Exercise

Abdominal breathing using deep breath facilitates flow of lymph fluid and is used for treatment of lymphedema. Through abdominal breathing, the ventral muscle is stimulated, and by continual pumping to central lymph vessel, flow of lymph fluid is more facilitated. The order of intervention of diaphragmatic respiration is that you have patients raise their hands over the center of the stomach, slowly breathe, and feel the stomach rising and swelling. And, have them breathe out and feel the stomach down again.

Next, when patients breathe in, therapists should press the stomach, and when they breathe out, they should have them smoothly exhale by slowly relaxing.

At first, start from one to three times, and when getting used to it enough, increase to about ten times.

8.4.2.3 Manual Therapy

As a manual therapy, lymph massage (manual lymph drainage massage) and lymph effleurage increase blood circulation and lymph circulation where lymphedema occurs and act as reducing edema. That is a way of excreting exudates

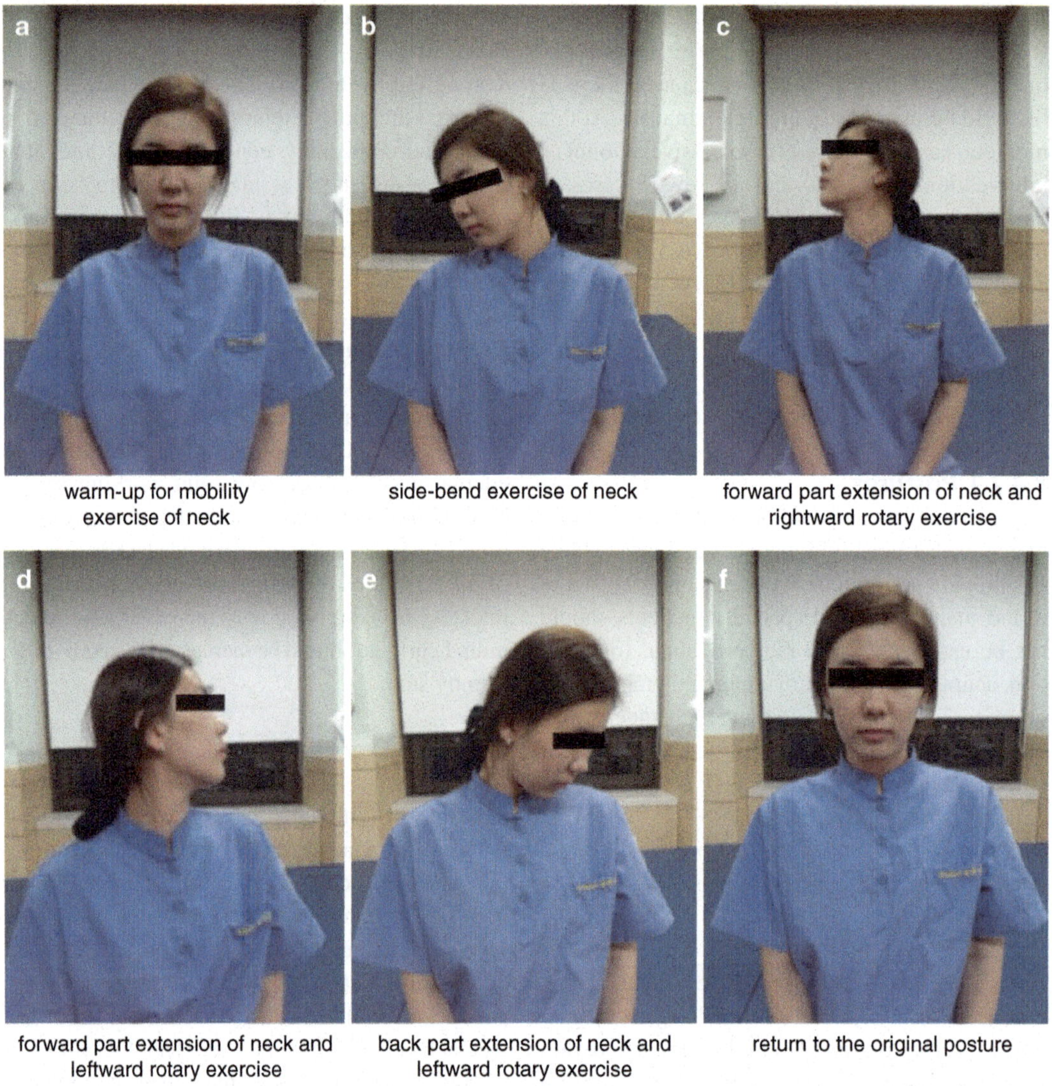

Fig. 8.16 Exercise therapy of the neck promoting mobility. (**a**) Warm-up for mobility exercise of the neck. (**b**) Side bend exercise of the neck. (**c**) Forward part extension of the neck and rightward rotary exercise. (**d**) Forward part extension of the neck and leftward rotary exercise. (**e**) Back part extension of the neck and leftward rotary exercise. (**f**) Return to original posture

occurring within the tissues far away from the tissues. To excrete accumulated body fluid, physical therapists massage with soft, slow, repetitive, and low pressure. Through effects resulting from this, blood within the vein returns to the heart without troubles, and there are sedation, reduction in pain, and relaxation effects, reduction and maintenance of edema, and so forth. Also, there is increment of lymph formation, increment of lymph blood vessel mobility, formation of collateral circulation pathways, reduction in nervous system stimulation during parasympathetic reaction stimulation, and so on. The types of lymph massage are as follows, and detailed procedures about massage order are indicated in lymph effleurage (Fig. 8.21).

Manual Lymph Drainage Massage (MLD)

During manual lymph drainage massage, with lymph vessel as center, increase to two direc-

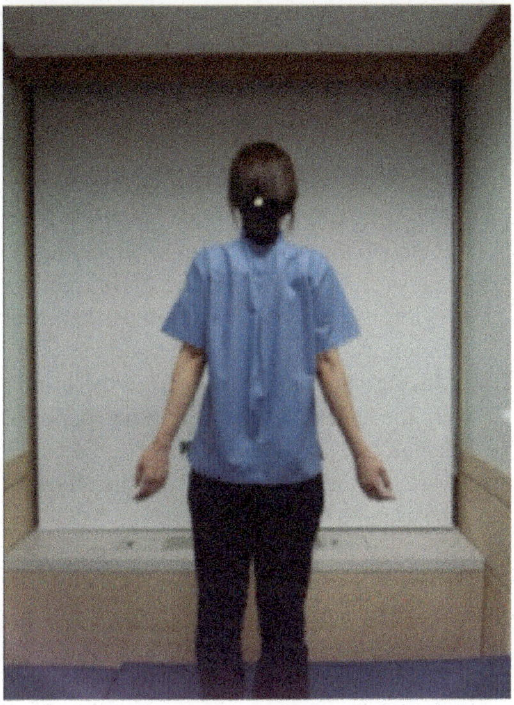

Fig. 8.17 Scapula exercise for promoting mobility

tions, and through soft pressure, prevent acute muscular contraction by a reflex, and slowly massage. In general, the order of massage application starts from the top region, neck, and chest and to a distance, and when massaging the abnormal part, start from the neck and chest or the center of the body to the arms or legs and go down to a distance. Treatment time is about 30–90 min.

Lymph Effleurage

Lymph effleurage is carried out for sedation of the skin and relaxation of tension. Massage to the direction of body of lymph vessel as if stroking and hands' pressure should be low and soft if possible, and move body fluids to forward direction. Stroking also follows lymph fluid emission order, and application order starts from the chest and moves from the near part of the body to the arms and legs and goes down (Jung et al. 2001; Kim et al. 2008). However, application direction should be carried out from the arms and legs to the near part of the chest

Fig. 8.18 Overhead exercise using one of the upper limb

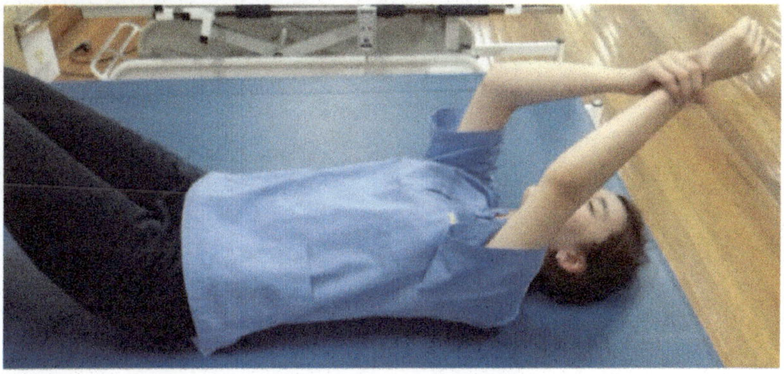

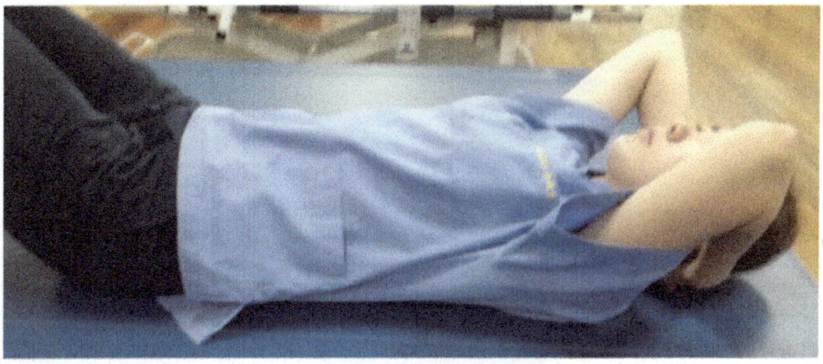

Fig. 8.19 Butterfly-shaped extensional movement of pectoralis major muscle

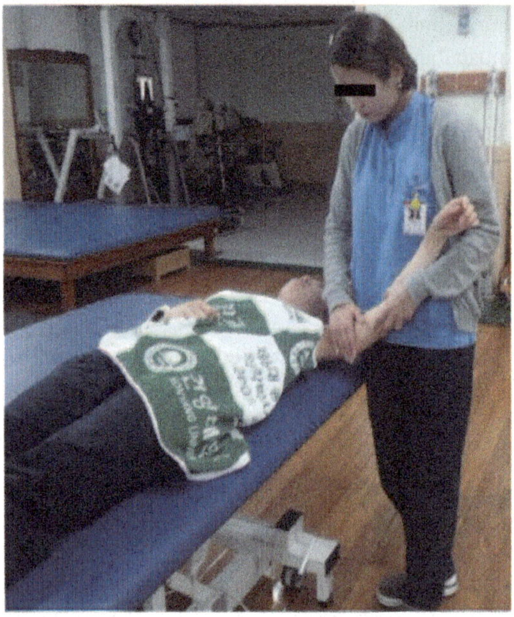

Fig. 8.20 Manual lymph massage applied to the upper limb

and body. Treatment time is about from 1 to 2 h (Fig. 8.22).

Ways to Apply Lymph Massage

① Neck and arms.

ⓐ Massage from the neck to downward.
ⓑ Massage from the armpit of the edema region to the opposite armpit direction.
ⓒ Massage from the armpit of the edema region to the same direction of the groin region.
ⓓ Massage the back region from the armpit of the edema region to the opposite armpit.
ⓔ Massage the upper arms from the elbow to the armpit.
ⓕ Massage the forearm from the wrist to the elbow.
ⓖ Massage the back of one's hand upward (Fig. 8.23).

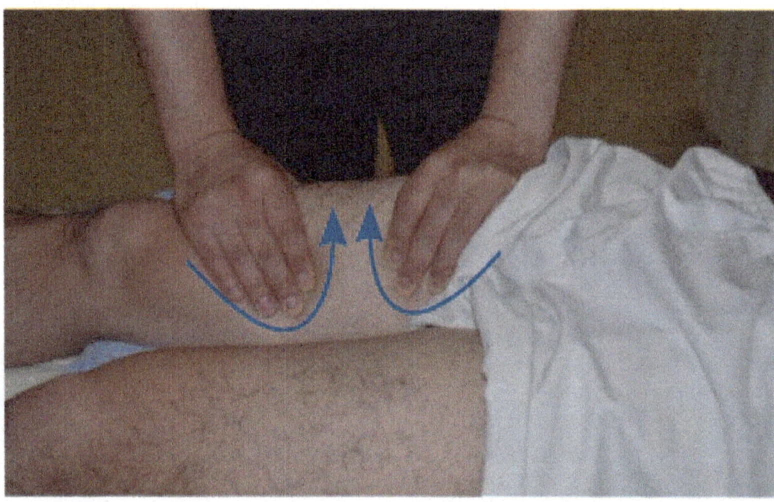

Fig. 8.21 Manual lymphatic drainage massage

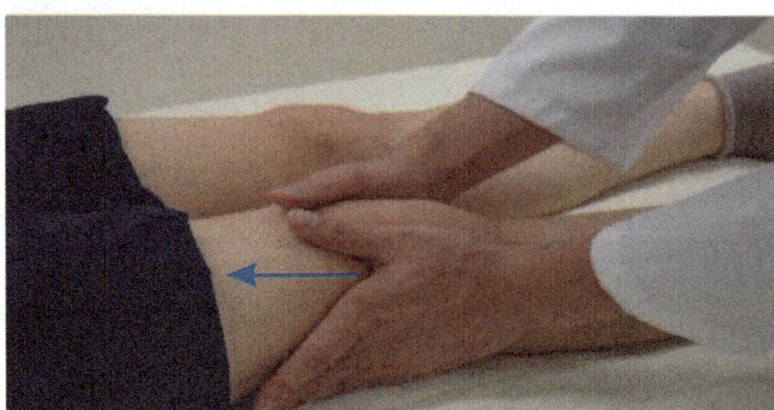

Fig. 8.22 Lymph stroke

Fig. 8.23 The order of manual lymphatic drainage massage. (**a**) Part of the upper limb, (**b**) lower limb

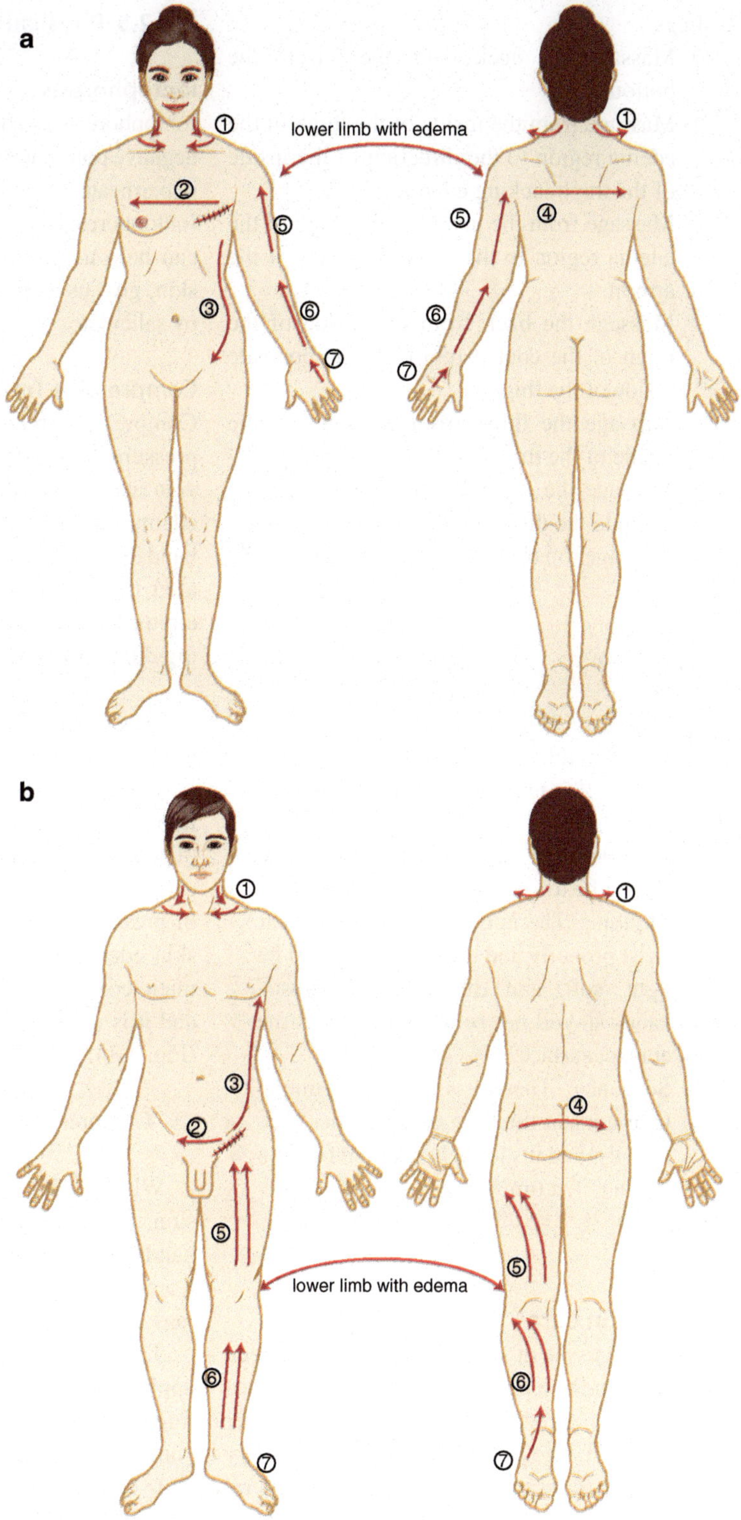

② Legs
- ⓐ Massage the neck from the top to the bottom.
- ⓑ Massage from the inside of the thigh of the edema region to the direction of the inside of the thigh lacking edema.
- ⓒ Massage from the inside of the thigh of the edema region to the same direction of the armpit.
- ⓓ Massage the back from the inside of the thigh of the edema region to the opposite inside of the thigh.
- ⓔ Massage the thigh from the knee to the inside of the thigh.
- ⓕ Massage the leg below the knee from the ankle to the direction of the knee.
- ⓖ Massage top of the foot upward (Fig. 8.23).

TIP

① Pressure: Hand pressure should be 30~40 mmHg and massage lightly and softly not to increase hemofiltration from blood vessel.
② Direction: All directions of the massage should be toward the heart.
③ Rhythm: Therapists should use their wrist properly and their hands should be light, soft, and rhythmic. Therapists' hands should not be separated from the contact surface.
④ Sequence: Therapists should maintain their contact time for about 5 s per each activity, and it should be repeated within seven to ten times.

8.4.2.4 Skin Care

Because the tissue of skin edema region has been weakened due to a cancer cell, it is a good place for germs to grow. Therefore, through proper skin care to reduce inflammation, it is necessary to prevent damage of lymph vessel. As a general method, it is important to prevent the skin from being dry and keep the skin glossy by applying body lotion or cream to the skin after a bath.

8.4.2.5 Physical Agent Modalities

Iontophoresis

Iontophoresis is a direct current of the positive and negative poles, and through skin semipermeability, it permeates free ion to the skin edema region. Iontophoresis using copper medicine at both poles can help us prevent inflammation of weakened skin, give us sterilizing action, and reduce edema by salicylate.

Compressive Treatment

Compressive treatment can maintain hydrostatic pressure of tissue and facilitate fluidity of the vein and lymph fluid. In case of severe lymphedema, using continual pressure stocking, elastic bandages, and a pneumatic compression device after the first stage, edema can be reduced, and circulation of blood and lymph increased by giving direct pressure on edema tissue.

① Pneumatic Therapy

When carrying out pneumatic treatment, it is important to know that due to hypersensitiveness of sense that tumor patients, especially skin cancer patients have, there may be pain. The intensity of pressure of pneumatic treatment for reducing skin edema is important. The pressure of pneumatic compression for this is about 0~40 mmHg and it is recommended not to exceed 30–40 min (Fig. 8.24) (Lee et al. 2012; Jung 2010).

② Compress Bandage Therapy

When applying elastic bandages for compression, the intensity of compression, direction of bandage, types of bandages should be checked. Compressive treatment is good right after lymph massage.

The method of compress bandage is easily applied with large bandages, sponge bandages, finger bandages, hands, and so on. Compress bandage using bandages should be bound softly and securely, and to prevent inhibition of blood circulation, it is desirable to use spiral or figure-of-8 bandage that binds the limbs from a distance to a body. Especially, when binding compress

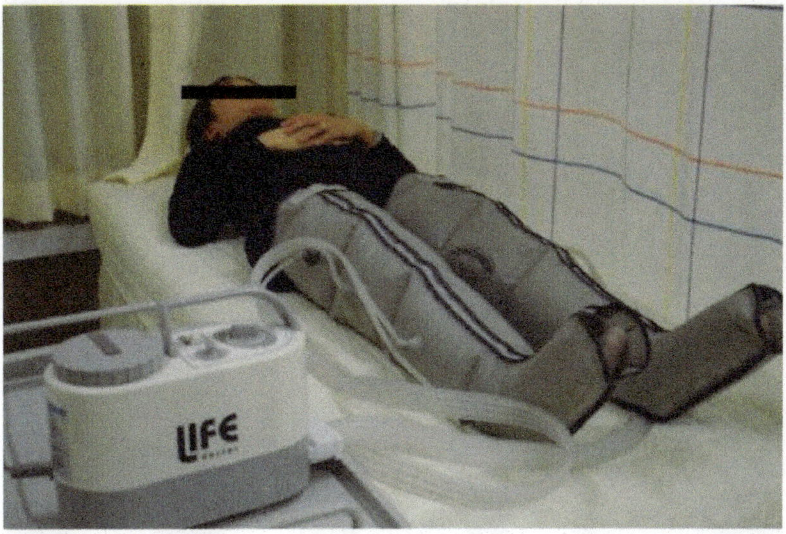

Fig. 8.24 Pneumatic therapy to reduce lymphedema

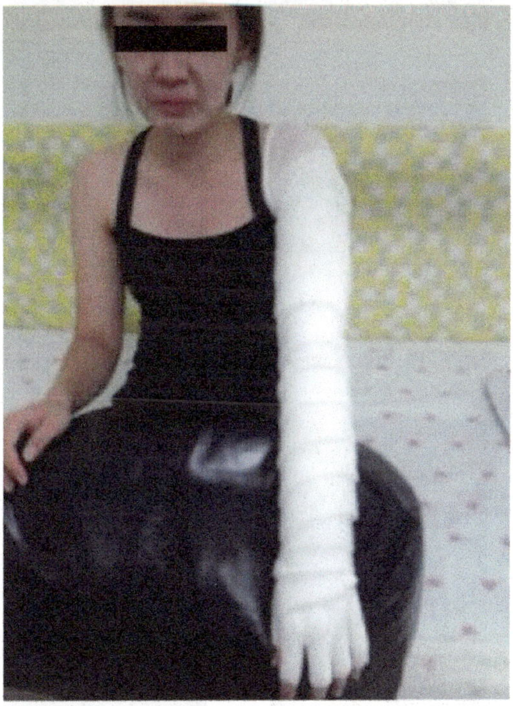

Fig. 8.25 Compress bandage therapy to reduce lymphedema

bandage, bind the end point region in layers since pressure of the region of the bottom end should be higher than the top end. At this moment, there is caution that when pressure is high and applied to not sensitive patients, there is likely to be dermolysis and stasis of blood circulation, so the amount of pressure should be adjusted. Especially, check regularly if the fingertip becomes excessively blue or white. And by bending the arms, the thumb should contact the nose. Compression order using bandages is shown in Figs. 8.25 and 8.26.

③ Pressure Stocking Method

Using stocking, by giving proper pressure during daily life, it is possible that more edema cannot be increased.

8.4.3 Prevention and Management

Lymph disease results in stasis of lymph system circulation and undercurrent of blood vessel within a body should be prevented. Physical therapists lift the arms and legs higher than heart to prevent lymphedema in cancers such as prostatic cancer, skin cancer, lung cancer, stomach cancer, and especially skin cancer occurring after the surgery. In addition, through lymph massage, compressive treatment, and exercise treatment, lymph circulation should be increased by contracting and relaxing muscles. Lymphedema can be prevented by relaxing the region of edema in the daytime with pressure

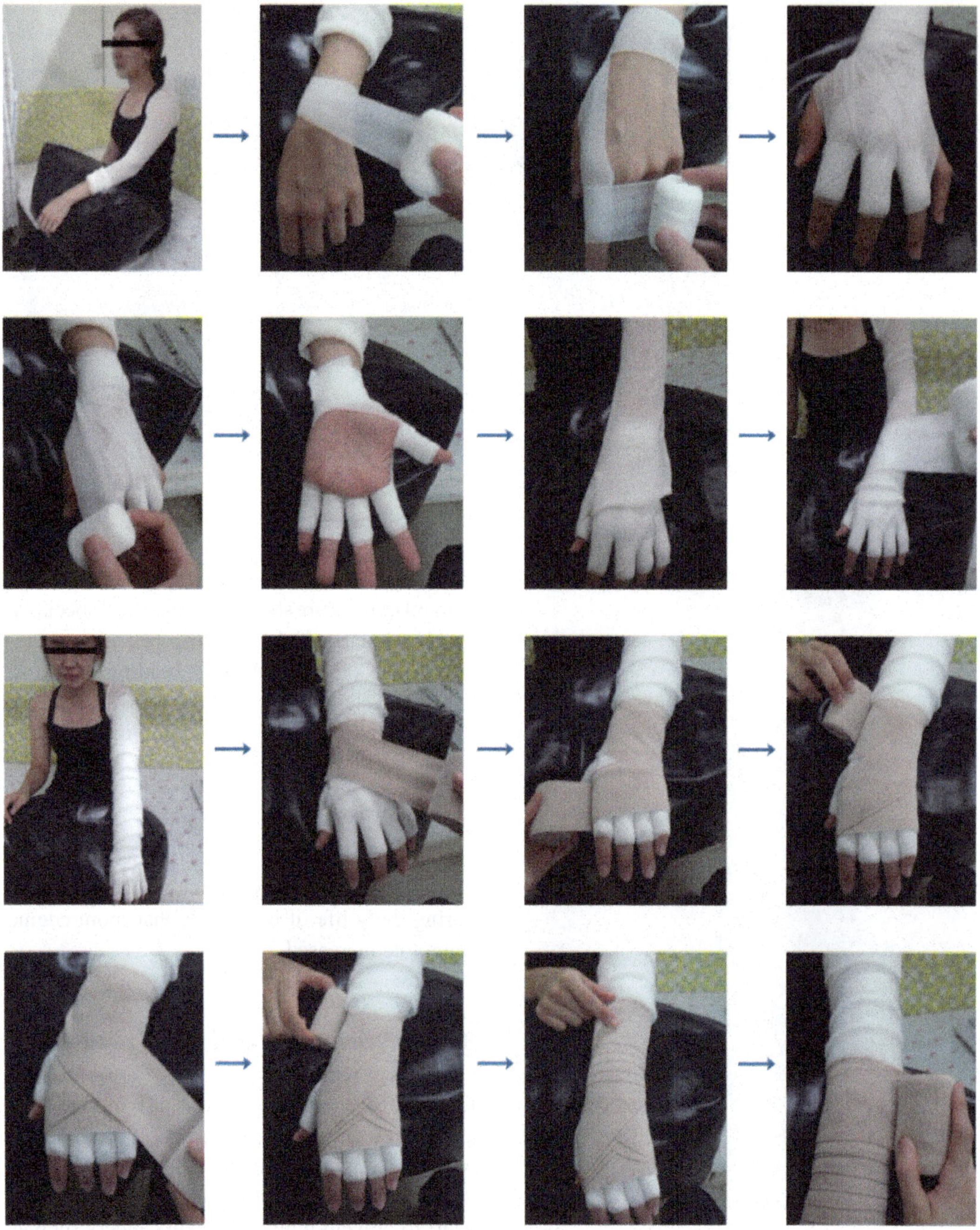

Fig. 8.26 Compress bandage winding order to prevent edema

stocking or elastic bandages worn in terms of simple prevention.

8.4.3.1 Prevention of Lymphedema

1. Maintain the arms and legs higher than heart (use a cushion or a pillow).
2. Avoid increasing blood circulation of the arms and legs (do not use hot pack and hot water).
3. Keep the skin of the arms and legs clean and maintain skin moisture (however, keep the feet dry).

4. Be careful of inflammation and injury of the arms and leg(do not inject to the region of edema).
5. Do not give excessive pressure on the arms and legs(do not sit with legs crossed).
6. Regularly measure the circumference of the arms and legs.
7. Maintain appropriate weight with moderate amount of exercise.
8. Meet medical staff regularly, and in case of severe edema, inform them of it immediately.

8.4.3.2 Management of Lymphedema

1. Lymphedema patients should care for lymphedema after learning treatment methods.
2. Using low-elastic bandages or pressure stocking helps body fluid reabsorbed (if there is erythema or itching on the skin, ask the medical staff).
3. Symptom of inflammation such as hot flush or pain exacerbates edema, so treat it right away.
4. The region where lymphedema is severe results in pain if there is a sense of skin being hard and wrinkles occur in the region of swelling.
5. If you do a strenuous exercise or adopt a bad posture with insufficient strength, swelling may become aggravated, so be careful. (Immoderate exercise, stair climb, sitting with legs crossed, squats should be avoided.)

8.4.3.3 Patient/Carer Education

Since lymphedema can be prevented for it not to turn into a grave disease depending on how well people exercise caution, roles of guardians as well as those of patients are very important.

Therefore, all patients and guardians should be educated about prevention and care.

Especially, always keep the region of edema in the arms and legs clean and apply lotion or ointment to the skin for it not to be dry. However, keeping the feet dry is a principle and it is necessary to give information to wear antisweat cotton clothing. Also, to prevent inflammation in the arms and legs, it is important to wear gloves during working hours, and when doing outdoor activities, wearing socks and shoes is required, and do not go around with bare feet (Lee et al. 2012).

Nail cleaning should be done by not cutting near the skin and toenail should be cut in line.

By having people informed of their own methods of measurement about the region of edema and having people taking their arms and legs measurement regularly (every day or every week), have them regularly (mostly in the morning) check if there is edema.

Advices for Physical Therapists

1. Physical therapists should pay special attention to the potential symptoms and signs of skin cancer and check dermal thickness and scar formation resulting from skin cancer in advance.
2. Eczema, psoriasis, and seborrheic dermatitis occur in over the half of skin cancer patients, more frequently than in the ordinary people. However, although a pale pink spot occurs in skin cancer, it is not important, and explaining it to patients well is important.
3. Physical therapists should minimize friction and contact caused by rough skin resulting from skin cancer, prevent the secondary hemorrhage, and pay special attention to spots of the skin that is locally subject to sunlight.
4. Changes such as color, size, shape, ulcer, hemorrhage, and uredo that appear at lump or moles occurring on the skin should be referred to and examined by doctors.
5. If people underwent lymphangiectomy, physical therapists should plan measures about remaining lymphedema or draw up measures to minimize it.
6. It is important for physical therapists to prevent skin cancer patients' pain and reduce level of pain, and scar care of the skin should be accompanied by thorough checking and care.
7. Because reduction in circulation of blood and the secondary problems of necrosis can occur when giving very strong pressure in care of lymphedema, care is required during the treatment.

8.5 Problem Solving

8.5.1 Skin Cancer and Lymphedema

Select one physical intervention method or potential test in each question.

Question 1
Mr. A, who is 36 years old and was diagnosed with skin cancer 2 years ago, has been regularly managed for his skin cancer. He, whose body has been recovered recently, works. However, he requires the help of physical therapists, visiting their place. That is because his working environment requires much sedentary work, and he feels heavy and suffers from pain with a little restrained movement. So, he wants to work continuously for the job, and what method is needed to lessen his problems?

1. Posture change
2. Pressure stocking
3. Use of ondol bed
4. Walking on treadmill
5. Wearing of a suture splinter

Question 2
Ms. A, who is 45 years old and was reported to suffer from squamous cell carcinoma, suffered from depression, anxiety about recurrence, and decreased body function 1 month before. What guidance do physical therapists need to take ahead of the physical therapy interference after the contact to doctor in charge?

1. Consult with a doctor
2. The optimal sunlight
3. Wearing of fabric clothes
4. The use of sunblock above SPF 15
5. The program to increase maximum amount of oxygen uptake

Question 3
Mr. A, who is 50 years old and was reported to suffer from squamous cell carcinoma, contacted physical therapy room by the prescription of his doctor after feeling pain. What physical factor interference is needed to facilitate lymph fluid and vein circulation?

1. Heliotherapy
2. Pressure therapy
3. Whirlpool bath
4. Aerobic exercise
5. Ultrasound therapy

Question 4
Ms. A, who is 50 years old and suffers from lymphedema after skin cancer diagnosis, requires physical therapy. What physical therapy interference method is needed for her?

1. Put the upper limbs and limbs lower than the position of the body.
2. Use copper medicine during iontophoresis.
3. Conduct pneumatic therapy twice a day for 2 h.
4. Teach abdominal breathing to facilitate lymph fluid.
5. Progress stroking lymph from the hands and feet to the body.

Question 5
Ms. A who is 50 years old and was operated 3 months before since her diagnosis of breast cancer is reported to suffer from poor blood circulation and decreased entire mobility. To intervene it, she requested physical therapy by surgery. What physical therapy interference method is needed for her?

1. Balance exercise
2. Manual therapy
3. Coordination movement
4. Acupressure massage
5. Circulatory promotion exercise

Answer
Question 1-②, Question 2-⑤, Question 3-②, Question 4-⑤, Question 5-⑤

References

An SG, et al. Korean common skin disease diagnose and therapy. Doctor's Book; 2009.
Catherine CG, Kenda SF. Pathology for therapists. 3rd ed. E-Public; 2010.
Choi YH. The aged and health. HyeonMunSa; 2010.

Fauci AS, Braunwald E, Kasper DL, Hauser SL, Longo DL, Jameson JL, Loscalzo J. Harrison internal medicine. The McGraw-Hill Professional; 2010.
Hildebrandt B, Wust P, Ahlers O. The cellular and molecular basis of hyperthermia. Crit Rev Oncol Hematol. 2002;43(1):33–56.
Jung JH. Easy human pathology. JungDam Media; 2010.
Jung Dam. CIBA a series of primary-color illustration medicine. CIBA a series of primary-color illustration medicine, vol 8, part III. CIBA a series of primary-color illustration medicine editing commission; 2010.
Jung SH, et al. One clinical study instance of second lymphedema examination for ovarian cancer and breast cancer using lymph-massage. Korea Orient Gynaecol Acad J. 2001;14(2):250–63.
Kim TH, Gwon OY, et al. Geriatric physiotherapy. Top Mediopia; 2008.
Lee GC, et al. Rehabilitation medicine. HyeonMunSa; 2012.
Lee JH, et al. Skin physical therapy. Jungdam Media; 2013. http://www.kostro.ok.kr.
Myers BA. Wound management: principles and practice (3rd Edition). Pearson; 2011.
Park JH, et al. Daily activities. HyeonMunSa; 2010.
Park JH, et al. Musculoskeletal diagnostics. HyeonMunSa; 2013a.
Park JH, et al. Musculoskeletal physical therapy intervention. HyeonMunSa; 2013b.
Park JH, et al. Musculoskeletal-disease physical therapy. HyeonMunSa; 2013c.
van der Zee J. Heating the patient: a promising approach? Ann Oncol. 2002;13(8):1173–84.
Wust P, Hildebrandt B, Sreenivasa G. Hyperthermia in combined treatment of cancer. Lancet Oncol. 2002;3(8):487–97.

Reference Sites

American National Cancer Institute. http://www.cancer.gov.
ICD10 data. http://www.icd10data.com.
ICD10 Version 2015. http://apps.who.int/classifications/icd10/browse/2015/en.
International Lymphology Academy. www.u.arizona.edu/~witte/ISL.htm.
Korea Centers for Disease Control and Prevention. www.cdc.go.kr.
Korean Lymphedema Academy. http://www.kslymph.or.kr/.
Korea National Cancerous Technology Information Center. http://www.cancer.go.kr/mbs/cancer/subview.jsp?id=cancer_030206030300.
Korean Radiation Oncology Academy. http://www.kostro.or.kr/.
Lymphnote Com. http://www.lymphnotes.com/article.php/id/474/.
Medcity. www.medcity.com.
Ministry of Health and Welfare. www.mw.go.kr.
University Medical Society. www.kams.or.kr.

Obesity

9

Eun Jeong Kim

ICD-10 Code
E65 Obesity
E66.0 Obesity due to excess calories
E66.1 Drug-induced obesity
E66.2 Extreme obesity with alveolar hypoventilation
Pickwickian syndrome
E66.8 Other obesities
Morbid obesity
E66.9 Obesity, unspecified
Simple obesity NOS

Learning Outcomes
After completing this chapter, you should be able to describe the following:

- Explain the concept of obesity.
- Explain the causes and symptoms of obesity.
- Conduct assessment and diagnosis.
- Conduct the physical therapy intervention of obesity.
- Solve the clinical trial problems of obesity.

E.J. Kim
Daejeon Health Institute of Technology,
Daejeon, South Korea
e-mail: muhasim@hanmail.net

Keywords
Hypothyroidism
Obesity
Triglyceride
Body mass index, BMI
Cushing's syndrome

9.1 Obesity

9.1.1 Overview

Obesity is defined as fat accumulated in the body more than a normal range which triggers a metabolic disorder caused by abnormal accumulation of body fat. WHO defined obesity as the abnormal excessive fat accumulation causing health problems. Body mass index (BMI) greater than 25 kg/m^2 is defined as overweight and greater than 30 kg/m^2 as obesity (http://www.who.int/en/).

Adipose tissues are widely distributed in the body storing excessive energy in a form of triglyceride, and it is released as a form of free fatty acid playing an important role in defense mechanisms. However, the energy imbalance caused by living conditions and exercise habits results in obesity by excessive energy accumulation. Obesity is one of the chronic diseases rapidly increasing worldwide resulting in increased risk of mortality and morbidity (Im 2013). The impacts of obesity are identified by 5Ds: disfigure, discomfort, disable, disease, and death.

J.-W. Park, D.-I. Jung (eds.), *Integumentary Physical Therapy*, DOI 10.1007/978-3-662-47380-1_9

9.1.2 Causes

9.1.2.1 Environmental Factors

Family eating habits or social and cultural factors are closely related to the occurrence of obesity. Typically, the dietary habits such as fast food, overeating, high-calorie diet, and social environment such as an education level, occupation, income, and residential environments affect in body weight changes. The incidence of obesity in low economic level population is 7~12 times higher than that of high-income population. In addition, obesity may result in any age, but it is different depending on the age groups and gender. Obesity is increased by smoking during pregnancy, gestational diabetes, low birth weight, and reduced frequency of breastfeeding. The body weight increases during pregnancy and menopause in women, while men's weight increases until their 50s, and due to the reduced physical activities, after 55, there are no body weight changes.

9.1.2.2 Genetic and Congenital Factors

Genes causing obesity are ob, pro-opiomelanocortin (POMC), and melanocortin-4 receptor (MC4R). Bardet-Biedl syndrome or Prader-Willi syndrome, congenital diseases caused by chromosomal abnormality, leads to obesity. If both parents are obese, 80 % of their children are possibly obese; if one parent is obese, the probability is 50 %; and if both parents are in normal weight, the probability is 10 %. Genetic factors are important in obesity but the mechanisms or specific obesity-related genes are not yet precisely identified (https://www.england.nhs.uk/).

Table 9.1 The secondary causes of obesity

Classification	Causes
Congenital diseases associated with obesity	Genes known to cause genetic and congenital obesity ob, POMC, MC4R, etc.
	Bardet-Biedl syndrome
	Prader-Willi syndrome
	Ahlstrom syndrome
	Cohen syndrome
Neurological and endocrine diseases	Hypothyroidism
	Cushing's syndrome
	Insulinoma
	Polycystic ovary syndrome
	Adult growth hormone deficiency
	Hypothalamic obesity: tumor, surgery, elevated intracranial pressure, infectious disease, trauma
Medications	Antipsychotic drugs: olanzapine, risperidone, quetiapine, thioridazine, clozapine
	Antiepileptic drugs: carbamazepine, valproate, gabapentin
	Antidiabetic drugs: insulin, glinide compounds, thiazolidinediones, sulfonylureas
	Tricyclic antidepressants: nortriptyline, amitriptyline
	Alpha-2 antagonists: mirtazapine, imipramine
	Selective serotonin reuptake inhibitors (SSRI): paroxetine
	Antihistamine: cyproheptadine
	Corticosteroids: glucocorticoid compounds, oral contraceptives
Mental disorders	Binge-eating disorder
	Seasonal affective disorder
	Bulimia nervosa

9.1.2.3 Neurological and Endocrine Disorders

If neurological and endocrine diseases such as hypothyroidism or Cushing's syndrome is suspected, physical examinations should be preceded (Table 9.1) (Kang et al. 2009).

Hypothyroidism

Hypothyroidism is a disorder with decreased thyroid hormones. Thyroid hormone is an iodine-containing hormone secreted by the thyroid glands. It regulates the basal metabolic rate of the body, the body temperature, and catabolism of carbohydrates, proteins, and lipids in cells. It also promotes the growth by releasing growth hormones. Therefore, if the hormone secretion is decreased, fatigue, lethargy, and sensitivity to cold increase due to the decreased body metabolism rate. The lower part of the neck is raised, and obesity might occur due to the body weight gain (Fig. 9.1).

Cushing's Syndrome

Cushing's syndrome is a disorder generated when the excessive glucocorticoid is secreted from the human body or the overdose of glucocorticoid is taken (Ahn et al. 2009). As a form of central obesity, the excessive subcutaneous fat is accumulated on the face, neck, shoulders, and trunk. Relatively, the arms and legs become thinner without fat accumulation. Unlike adults, childhood obesity is systemic instead of central obesity. In addition, protein degradation, facial blushing, hypertension, hyperglycemia, and musculoskeletal symptoms such as osteoporosis or myasthenia, striae rubra due to dermal collagen fibers weakened and ruptured, and the symptom easily forming bruise occur on the skin (Fig. 9.2).

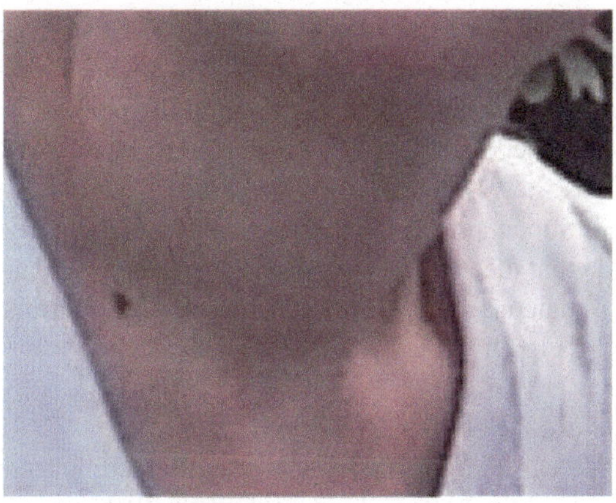

Fig. 9.1 Hypothyroidism

9.1.2.4 Medications

Steroid, some antidepressants, antipsychotic medications, and diabetic drugs cause weight gain. Antipsychotic drugs such as sertindole or risperidone cause more than 2 kg of weight gain and clozapine causes about 4.4 kg of weight gain. Antidepressants such as amitriptyline or cyproheptadine show similar pattern (Table 9.1).

9.1.2.5 Psychological Factors

Excessive stress, lack of love, anxiety, tension, and loneliness lead to obesity caused by overeating. Obesity causes mental problems such as social phobia and severe depression which further aggravate obesity.

Bulimia Nervosa

Bulimia nervosa is repeatedly eating large amounts of food quickly in a short period of time and emptying the stomach by inducing vomiting. Due to the repetitive vomiting, the salivary glands become enlarged, the teeth and esophagus are damaged by backflow of gastric fluid, and the stomach is damaged by excessive food intake.

Binge-Eating Disorder

Binge-eating disorder is binge eating in a long or short period of time. It mainly appears to people who experienced failed attempts to lose weight

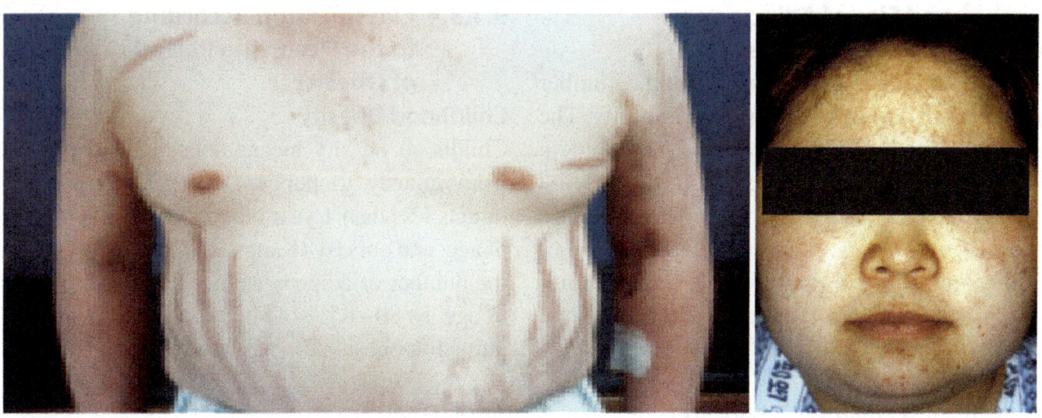

Fig. 9.2 Appearance of Cushing's syndrome

for several times. Binge-eating disorder does not empty the stomach after overeating which is different from bulimia nervosa.

9.1.3 Classification

9.1.3.1 Classification by Causes of Obesity

Simple Obesity

Simple obesity is also known as primary or exogenous obesity without specific causes. It is caused by overeating, lack of exercise, and bad lifestyle, and more than 90 % of obesity belongs to it. The calorie intake exceeds the calorie consumed. The excess nutrients are converted into glycogen and the remainings are stored in adipose tissues of the liver or subcutaneous in a form of triglycerides resulting in body fat increase. Among the daily total energy consumption, the calorie consumption is different depending on the amount of energy required by physical metabolic activities, the basal metabolic activity at the rest state, and digesting food.

Secondary Obesity

Obesity caused by specific diseases is called secondary obesity or endogenous obesity consisting less than 10 % of the total obesity. The diseases causing obesity are hypothyroidism, insulinoma, Cushing's syndrome, polycystic ovary syndrome (PCOS), etc.

9.1.3.2 Classification by the Number and Size of Adipocytes

Obesity with Adipogenesis

The size of adipocytes is normal but the number is increased during adipogenesis in obesity. The number of adipocytes is rapidly increased in between 30 weeks of the gestation to the first year of the birth, and it gradually increases until the age of 6 years. The increased number of adipocytes does not diminish and this phenomenon is closely associated with childhood obesity.

Obesity with Enlarged Adipocytes

The number of adipocytes is nearly normal, but obesity is caused by enlarged adipocytes.

Combined Obesity

Both number and size of adipocytes are increased.

9.1.3.3 Classification According to the Distribution of Adipose Tissues in the Body

Abdominal Obesity

Abdominal obesity is mainly in the form of fat accumulated in the abdomen and waist called central, android, or apple-shaped obesity (Fig. 9.3a). Fat accumulated in the abdomen is closely located to the hepatic portal vein, so it migrates to the liver and triggers low density lipoprotein (LDL) formation causing the coronary artery diseases, hyperlipidemia, hypertension, cardiac diseases, and diabetes (Kim 2003).

① Visceral fat obesity

Visceral fat obesity is fat accumulated in abdominal mesentery and greater omentum, and the morbidity of visceral fat obesity is higher than that of subcutaneous fat obesity (Fig. 9.4).

② Subcutaneous fat obesity is abdominal obesity that the adipose tissues accumulated in subcutaneous tissues between muscles and dermis (Fig. 9.4).

Gluteal-Femoral Obesity

Gluteal-femoral obesity is fat mainly accumulated around the bottom, hips, or thighs called bottom, gynoid, or pear-shaped obesity (Fig. 9.3b).

9.1.3.4 Classification According to the Occurring Period of Obesity

Childhood Obesity

Childhood obesity means obesity that occurred from infancy to puberty. It usually occurs in infants less than 1 year old, children in 5–6 years of age, and puberty (Kang et al. 2008). Especially, the number of adipocytes increases until 6 years of age, so 80 ~ 85 % of childhood obesity persists into adult obesity.

Adult Obesity

Body mass index (BMI) greater than 30 kg/m^2 after 20 years old is referred to as adult obesity.

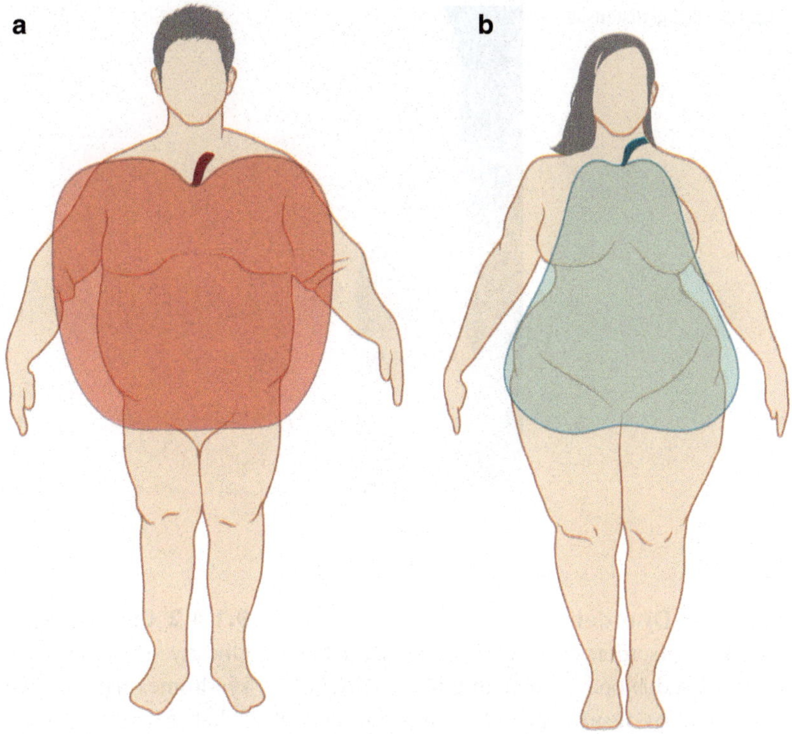

Fig. 9.3 (**a**) Abdominal obesity. (**b**) Buttocks obesity

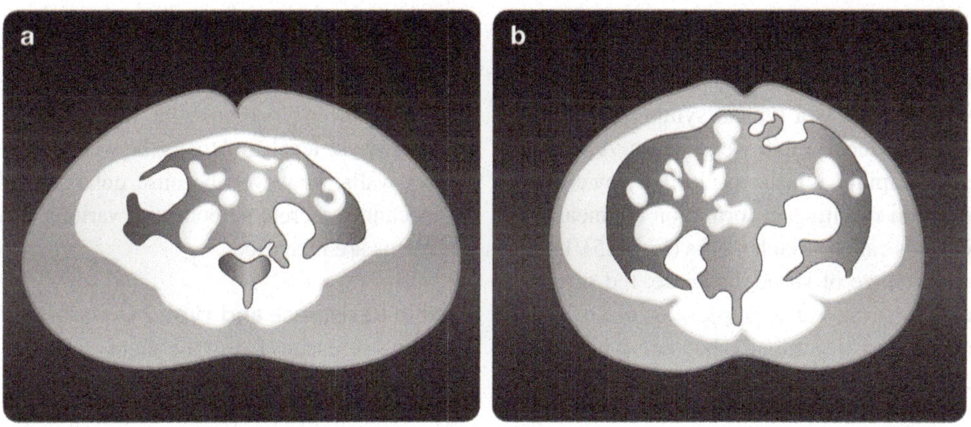

Fig. 9.4 (**a**) Subcutaneous fat obesity. (**b**) Visceral obesity

Women seem to gain weight due to physiological factors such as pregnancy and after menopause mostly occurring after the puberty. Particularly after menopause, obesity is caused by the change of body fat distribution due to reduced estrogen and progesterone secretion (Kopelman 2008). In general, men gain weight until their 50s, but the body weight does not change from their mid-50s and gradually it decreases after their mid-60s.

9.1.4 Symptoms and Complications

9.1.4.1 The Symptoms of Obesity

The common symptoms caused by obesity are gastroesophageal reflux disease, pectoralgia after eating a meal, gastralgia, edema, diaphoresis, dyspnea, fatigue, and arthralgia. Sleep apnea, menstrual irregularity, and contact dermatitis are shown in highly obese people due to excessive skin chafing of enlarged body.

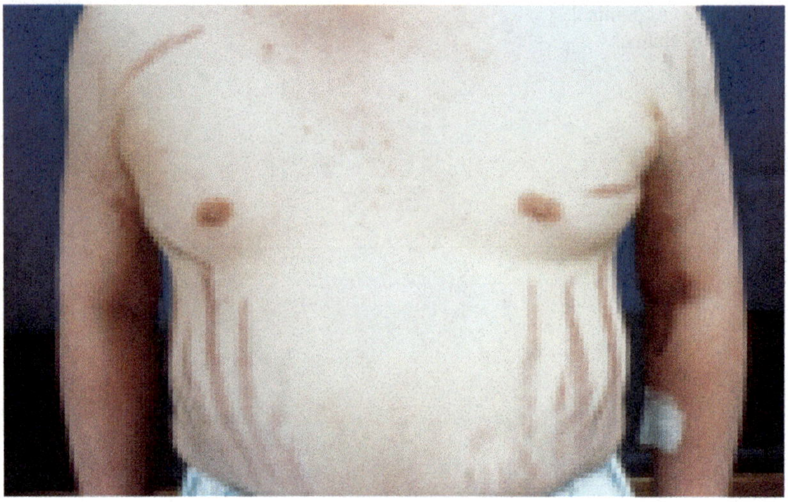

Fig. 9.5 Striae distensae

Breathing Disorders

Breathing disorders caused by obesity are defined as increased blood carbon dioxide and hypoxemia state by insufficient blood oxygen, called obesity hypoventilation syndrome or Pickwickian syndrome.

Striae Distensae

Striae distensae is a typical symptom appearing on the skin due to rapid weight gain. As the skin stretches rapidly, it loses its elasticity by collagen destruction resulting in formation of linear atrophic bands called stretch marks (Fig. 9.5). During the early stage of striae distensae, red or purple bands of striae rubra appear as elastic fibers decrease, and it gradually become white, wrinkled, and atrophic skin called striae alba.

Cellulite

Cellulite is excess fat accumulated in the subcutaneous tissues of the skin pushed along the dermis making the skin raised and bumpy. It causes impaired local blood flow followed by fluid retention and skin degeneration by coagulation of accumulated adipocytes and a globule of fat. It is caused by various factors, and especially it is formed in femoral region, gluteal region, abdomen, and brachial region due to the excessive fat accumulation (Fig. 9.6).

9.1.4.2 Complication of Obesity

Obesity increases the incidence of metabolic syndromes including insulin resistance (IR) type 2 diabetes, hypertension, coronary artery diseases, and hyperlipidemia. In general, normal adipocytes secrete various physiologically active substances including adipocytokines. Among the adipocytokines, adiponectin improves the resistance to insulin; reduces blood pressure, triglycerides, and blood glucose level; and treats the wounded blood vessel walls. However, because enlarged adipocytes cannot secrete adiponectin, various clinical problems are increased.

Insulin Resistance and Type 2 Diabetes

Insulin, released from the beta cells of the pancreas, reduces blood glucose level when it is increased. Glucagon, released from the alpha cells of the pancreas, stops the glucose production in the liver. Insulin resistance (IR) is defined as the state that the muscles and adipocytes cannot burn off the glucose caused by reduced function of insulin (Kim et al. 2009). If insulin resistance increases, the body secretes excess insulin triggering a high blood glucose level, hyperinsulinemia, and diabetes. If the body weight is increased by 30 ~ 40 %, the insulin sensitivity reduces by 30 ~ 40 %. The body weight gain over the

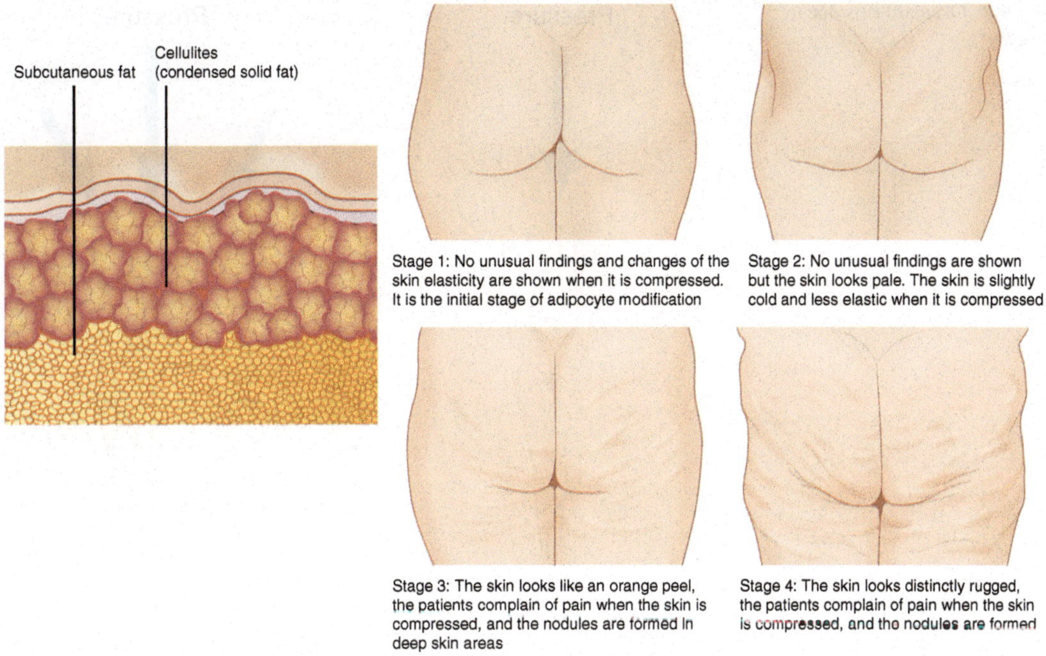

Fig. 9.6 Cellulites

years due to the increased insulin resistance and type 2 diabetes occurred by worsened insulin resistance.

High Blood Pressure and Coronary Heart Diseases

Obesity increases insulin resistance, hyperinsulinemia, and sodium reabsorption in the kidneys. The fluid absorption into blood vessels by increased blood sodium concentration triggers the sympathetic stimulation followed by increased heart rate. Angiotensinogen, the malicious cytokine, is released by enlarged adipocytes and causes hypertension due to vasoconstriction. The excessive secretion of other cytokines, plasminogen activator inhibitory-1 (PAI-1), causes thrombosis. If excessive heparin-binding epidermal growth factor (HB-EGF) is released, the incidence of hypertension and coronary heart diseases increases by narrowed blood vessels caused by growth of vascular endothelial cells. In addition, released tumor necrosis factor-a (TNF-a) causes diabetes by triggering insulin resistance.

Dyslipidemia

Dyslipidemia is defined as increased cholesterol or triglycerides compared with the normal range. The triglycerides and cholesterol in the blood are not soluble in water, but they are surrounded by apoprotein called lipoprotein. It is divided into very low density lipoprotein (VLDL), low density lipoprotein (LDL), and high density lipoproteins (HDL) according to the density. LDL plays a role in delivering cholesterol to various tissues, but its high deposition on the blood vessel wall causes arteriosclerosis. HDL, unlike LDL which carries cholesterol, usually delivers cholesterol from tissues to the liver for degradation preventing arteriosclerosis. Obesity is the cause of LDL increase, and if it persists for a long term, atherosclerosis may occur followed by narrowed blood vessels and reduced elasticity and blood flow. Reduced blood flow hinders oxygen and nutrient transport to various organs. It causes ischemic heart disease or stroke when lasting for a long time (http://www.mohw.go.kr/front_new/index.jsp).

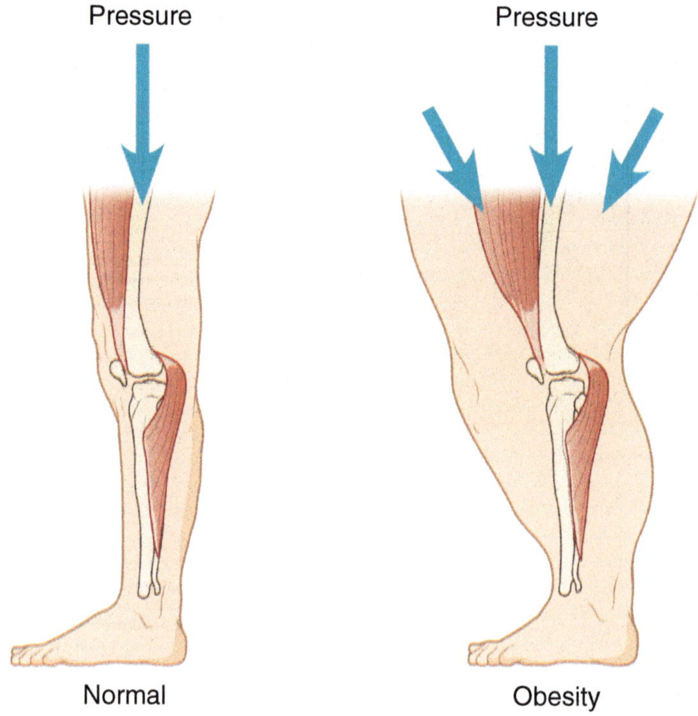

Fig. 9.7 Osteoarthritis due to obesity

Osteoarthritis

Weight gain gives burden to locomotive organs, especially bones and joints which support the body. Overload of weight-bearing joints causes cartilage damages and osteoarthritis by obesity-related hormone, leptin (Fig. 9.7). The incidence of osteoarthritis increases if BMI is greater than 25 kg/m^2. The pain becomes severe as becoming severely obese by increased load on the knees and causes obesity progressed by lack of exercise (Park et al. 2013).

Respiratory Disorders

Total lung and vital capacity is reduced in obesity. Also, expiratory reserve volume (ERV), resting end expiratory volume, and functional residual capacity (FRC) are reduced. The respiratory problems are caused by reduced maximum expiratory flow (MEF) in male. The fat accumulated in the abdomen and thoraces compresses the diaphragm and increases resistance of the respiratory system due to the reduced elasticity of the lower thoraces. In addition, the reduced area of the upper airway causes sleep apnea.

Others

Obesity raises the incidence of cancers such as pancreatic cancer, renal cancer, endometrial cancer, breast cancer, colon cancer, bladder cancer, and esophageal cancer. In addition, complications are caused including gout, fatty liver, polycystic ovary syndrome, female infertility, and intrahepatic stones.

9.1.5 Diagnosis and Assessment

9.1.5.1 Methods Using Weight and Height Indices

Body Mass Index

One of the methods widely used worldwide to evaluate overweight and obesity is body mass index (BMI) (http://www.nhlbi.nih.gov/). The score is calculated by the body weight over the square of the height. The body mass index is correlated with body fat, and as the score becomes higher, the relative morbidity and mortality of the cardiovascular diseases increase. The Centers for Disease Control and Prevention (CDC) defined BMI 25 ~ 29.9 as overweight and BMI greater than 30 as adult obesity, while South Korea assesses BMI greater than 23 kg/m^2 as overweight and greater than 25 kg/m^2 as obesity (Tables 9.2 and 9.3). BMI is correlated with body fat, but it does not directly measure the body fat and might be changed according to gender, race, and age. The considerations are as follows.

① Females might have more fat than males with the same BMI.
② Older people might have more fat than younger people with the same BMI.
③ BMI might be higher than the actual body fat in people with developed musculoskeletal system.

In general, obesity is defined as only BMI in adults older than age 20 years. However, since BMI increases depending on the body growth and age in people younger than age 20 years, BMI alone cannot be used to define obesity. The child growth percentile charts with the record of the intersection of age and height are used as a reference to determine the childhood obesity (Fig. 9.8).

The Relative Weight

The relative weight is the standard method for evaluating and classifying overweight and obesity which is calculated by the actual weight over the standard weight multiplied by 100 (Table 9.4). In Korea, the standard weight is calculated using modified Broca method and the formula changes depending on the height (Table 9.5).

9.1.5.2 Evaluation Method by Fat Distribution

Since the percentage of the medical risk is different in diseases including hypertension, diabetes, hyperlipidemia, coronary artery disease, and stroke depending on the areas where fat is accumulated in obesity, the evaluation by fat distribution is important.

In general, fat distribution patterns appear differently depending on gender, age, and hormonal status.

Waist Circumference

The waist circumference is measured as an indicator reflecting the risk of visceral fat, metabolic complications, and other cardiovascular diseases. The method used in WHO is breathing in a standing position with feet 25 ~ 30 cm apart and measuring the lowest ribs and the middle part of the iliac crest horizontal to the ground using a tapeline (Fig. 9.9). Male with waist circumference greater than 102 cm and women greater than 88 cm is at risk of metabolic complications. Even though BMI is lower than 25 kg/cm^2, the abdominal obesity with the high waist circumference causes cardiovascular diseases.

Waist-to-Hip Ratio Measurement Method

In waist-to-hip ratio measurement, the hip circumference is measured at the most protruding part of the hips, and the waist circumference is measured in the same manner as the waist circumference method. The calculated ratio is

Table 9.2 The adult BMI of centers for disease control and prevention

BMI	Weight status
<18.5	Underweight
18.5 ~ 24.9	Standard
25.0 ~ 29.9	Overweight
>30	Obesity

Table 9.3 Weight classification of Koreans according to BMI and the risk of associated diseases

		Waist circumference (cm)	The risk of associated diseases
Classification	BMI (kg/m^2)	<90 (male) <85 (female)	>90 (male) >85 (female)
Underweight	<18.5	Low	Moderate
Normal weight	18.5~22.9	Moderate	Increased
Overweight	23~24.9	Increased	Moderate
Obese class I	25~29.9	Increased	Severe
Obese class II	>30	Severe	Very severe

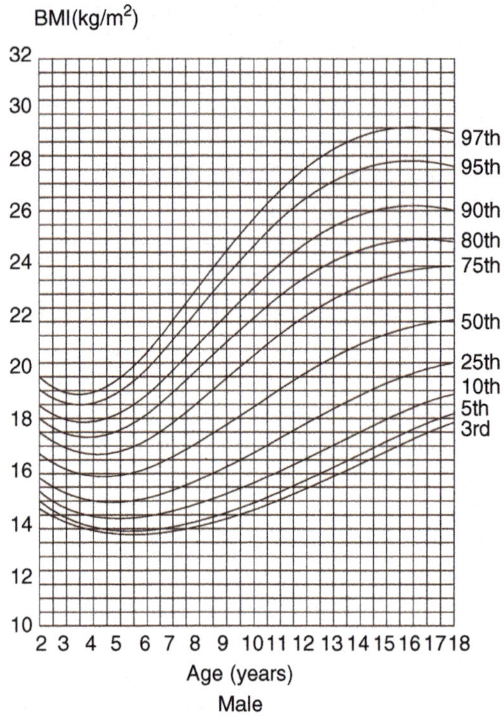

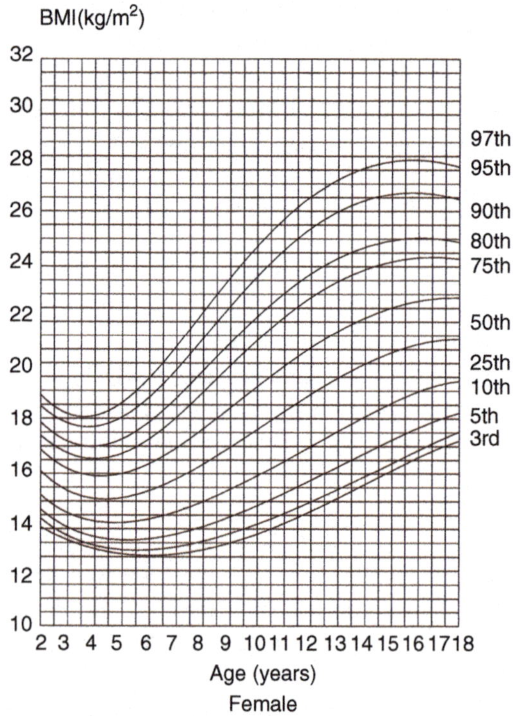

Fig. 9.8 BMI percentile. (**a**) Male. (**b**) Female

Table 9.4 Classification of obesity according to relative weight

Classification	Relative weight (%)
Underweight	<90
Normal	90–110
Overweight	110–120
Mild obesity	120–140
Moderate obesity	140–200
Severe obesity	>200

Table 9.5 Standard weight calculation by Broca formula according to height

Height (cm)	Formula
>160	(Height − 100) × 0.9
160~150	(Height − 150)/2 + 50
<150	(Height − 100) × 1.0

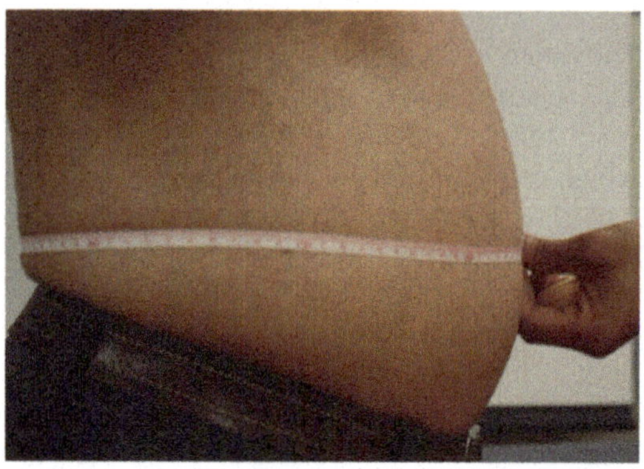

Fig. 9.9 Waist measurement

widely used in evaluating abdominal obesity. In general, the ratio of the hip circumference over the waist circumference exceeding 1.0 in male and 0.85 in female is define by abdominal obesity, and the ratio more than 1.0 in male and 0.85 in female is define by obesity in the buttocks.

Skinfold Thickness Measurement

Skinfold thickness measurement is a method measuring body fat by holding the specific parts of the skin with the thumb and index finger using a caliper. The total body fat is estimated by measuring the biceps brachii, lower triceps brachii,

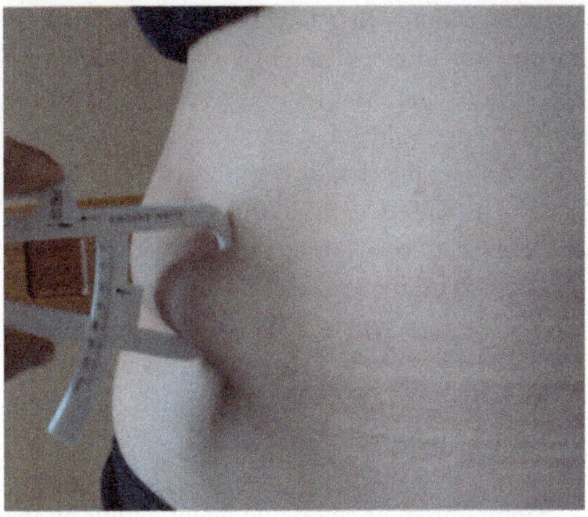

Fig. 9.10 Skinfold thickness measurement by caliper

Table 9.6 Classification of obesity according to skinfold thickness

Classification	Skinfold thickness (cm)	
	Male	Female
Moderate	>60	>37
Severe obesity	>74	>43

scapula, and upper iliac crest (Fig. 9.10, Table 9.6).

9.1.5.3 Other Methods Measuring Body Fat

Other methods are total body electrical conductivity (TOBEC), isotope dilution, whole-body moisture measurement, and whole-body potassium count, and the methods commonly used are described as follows.

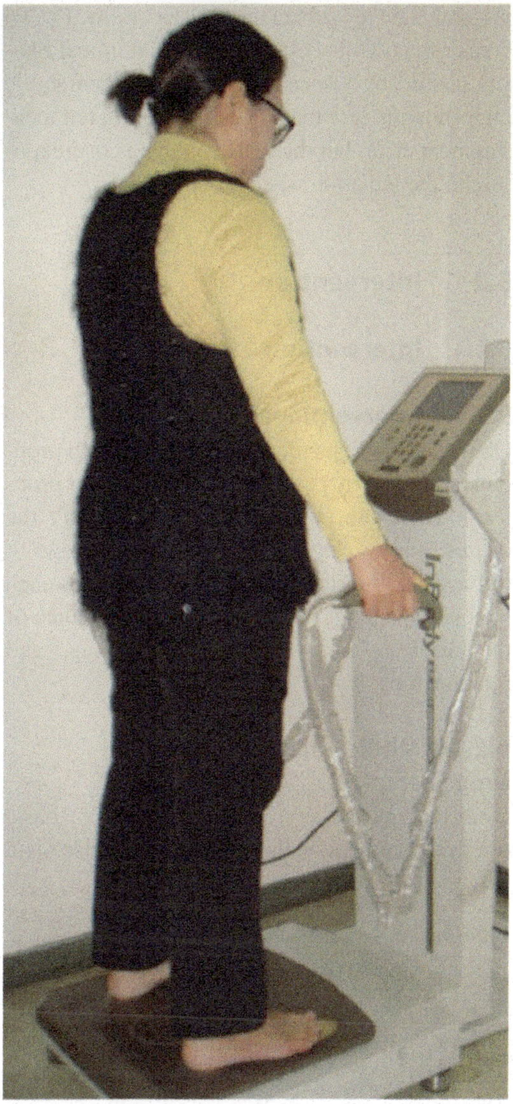

Fig. 9.11 Bioelectrical impedance analysis measurement

Bioelectrical Impedance Analysis

Bioelectrical impedance analysis (BIA) is defined by measuring the degree of obesity by analyzing the resistance of the current passing through the human body, which is composed of more than 70 % of water. It is widely used in clinic with the brand name inbady because it is easy and safe to measure body fat mass, lean mass, and moisture contents (Fig. 9.11). The measurement error occurs because of fluid intake and urination before the measurement, so measurement carried out under the same time and conditions is necessary at each measurement. The classification of obesity according to body fat measurement is shown in Table 9.7.

Computed Tomography

Computed tomography is a method calculating the area of the visceral fat and subcutaneous fat by taking images between the fourth and fifth lumbar vertebra. After calculating the total fat area, subcutaneous fat area is recalculated, and the subcutaneous fat area subtracted by the total fat area is the visceral fat area (VFA) (Fig. 9.12). The calculated visceral fat area greater than 100 cm^2 or the visceral fat to subcutaneous fat ratio (VSR) greater than 0.4 is determined as abdominal obesity caused by visceral obesity. The accuracy is high showing less than 1 % of visceral area measurement error, but the disadvantage is overexposure to the radiation when taking images.

9.2 Intervention

9.2.1 Intervention

9.2.1.1 Interventional Approaches

Obesity is a chronic disease causing health problems followed by psychological and social problems. Therefore, it is important to identify the causes and types of obesity and manage it through long-term treatment specific for each patient depending on the presence or absence of the disease, diet, occupation, hobbies, and relationships.

9.2.1.2 Medical Treatment

Drug Therapy

Drug therapy is the secondary method of basic obesity treatment including diet, exercise, and behavior therapy. It gives the satiety, suppresses appetite, or induces weight loss by reducing fat absorption. The drug therapy is conducted if the weight is not reduced even after 24 weeks of diet and exercise, the risk of complications continues in patients with BMI 25 ~ 29.9 kg/m^2, or the sleep apnea and complications such as hypertension, diabetes, and hyperlipidemia are accompanied with BMI 23 kg/m^2. If there is no 3 ~ 10 % of weight loss and no improvement of accompanied diseases within 3 months of drug use, changing of the drug is recommended.

① Sibutramine, an anorectic agent acting on the central nervous system, induces satiety and leads to weight loss by increasing heat production. In about 2 ~ 4 % of patients, hydrodipsomania, headache, constipation, and insomnia occurred. Its use is prohibited for hypertension patients who have difficulty in controlling blood pressure because the drug can increase blood pressure 1 ~ 3 mmHg and heart rate 4 ~ 5 per minute.

② Orlistat reversibly blocks pancreatic lipase required for the absorption and degradation of triglyceride to suppress the amount of calorie absorption by the small intestine and reduce the body weight. Absorption of fat-soluble vitamins can be suppressed as well, so fat-soluble vitamins A, D, E, and K supply are required for a long-term application of the drug. The gastrointestinal side effects such as steatorrhea, defecation, or fecal incontinence can occur.

Table 9.7 Body fat and obesity

	Body fat (%)	
Classification	Male	Female
Normal	15 ~ 18	20 ~ 25
Boundary	19 ~ 25	26 ~ 30
Obesity	>25	>30

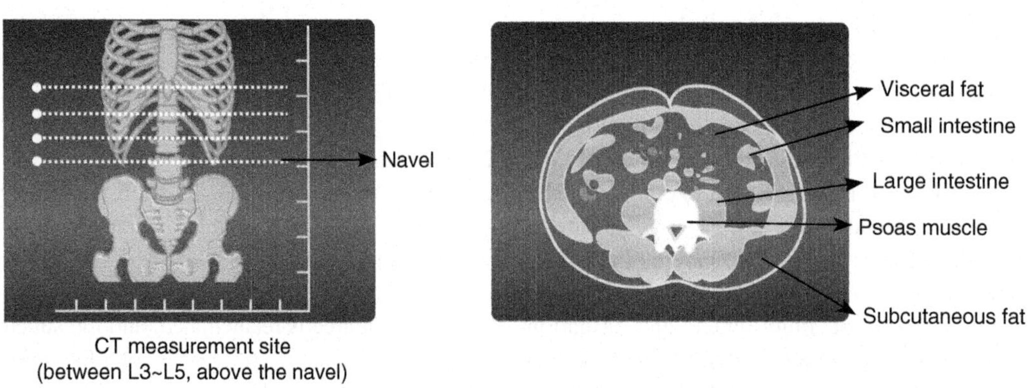

Fig. 9.12 Computed tomography

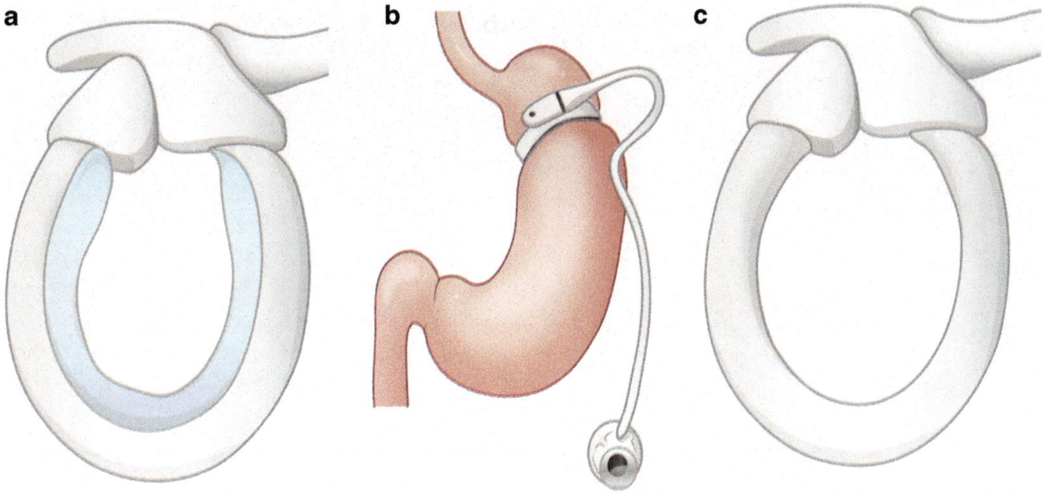

Fig. 9.13 Adjustable gastric banding. (**a**) Band with saline. (**b**) Surgery schematic diagram. (**c**) Band without saline

③ Phentermine is a short-term treatment of diet, exercise, and behavior therapy used in patients with BMI greater than 30 kg.m^2 or 27 kg.m^2 accompanied with risk factors. The side effects are headache, sleep disorder, anxiety, tachycardia, and palpitation.

Surgical Treatment

Surgical treatment is conducted to treat severe obesity. Severe obesity is defined as BMI greater than 40 kg/m^2 or BMI greater than 35 kg/m^2 with accompanied diseases caused by obesity. Surgical treatment largely consists of restrictive and malabsorptive surgery.

① Adjustable gastric banding

Adjustable gastric banding is winding an artificial band between the esophagus and stomach and implanting access port in the abdominal wall which can adjust the volume of the band where the brine can be added or emptied. It is a restrictive surgery leading to weight loss by controlling the amount of food inflow. The operation time is within 1 h and it can be adjusted depending on the nutritional status and weight loss. It is safer than other types of surgery, but weight loss after the surgery is relatively slow. Therefore, for the sustainable weight loss and maintenance, the band has to be adjusted (Fig. 9.13). The complications such as acute band congestion, band erosion, band slippage, esophageal expansion or reflux, and malfunction of the tube connected to the port or band and infection might occur.

② Sleeve gastrectomy

Sleeve gastrectomy is a restrictive surgery reducing the volume of the stomach and limiting food intake by stomach resection along the longitudinal axis of the stomach (Fig. 9.14a). The operation time is about 2 h. The prevalence of complications is low including burning sensation of the stomach, but the effects of weight loss is low, and regain of the body weight often occurs.

③ Roux-en-Y gastric bypass surgery

Roux-en-Y gastric bypass surgery is a surgery dissecting the stomach leaving 15~20 cc from the esophagus and connecting it to the small intestine. The clipped part is also connected to the small intestine where the food passes directly to the small intestine restricting the amount of food intake and nutrient absorption (Fig. 9.14b). Although the effect of weight loss is high, the surgery is complicated and takes about 2~4 h. The complications include malnutrition, metabolic disorders, diarrhea, anemia, and dumping syndrome.

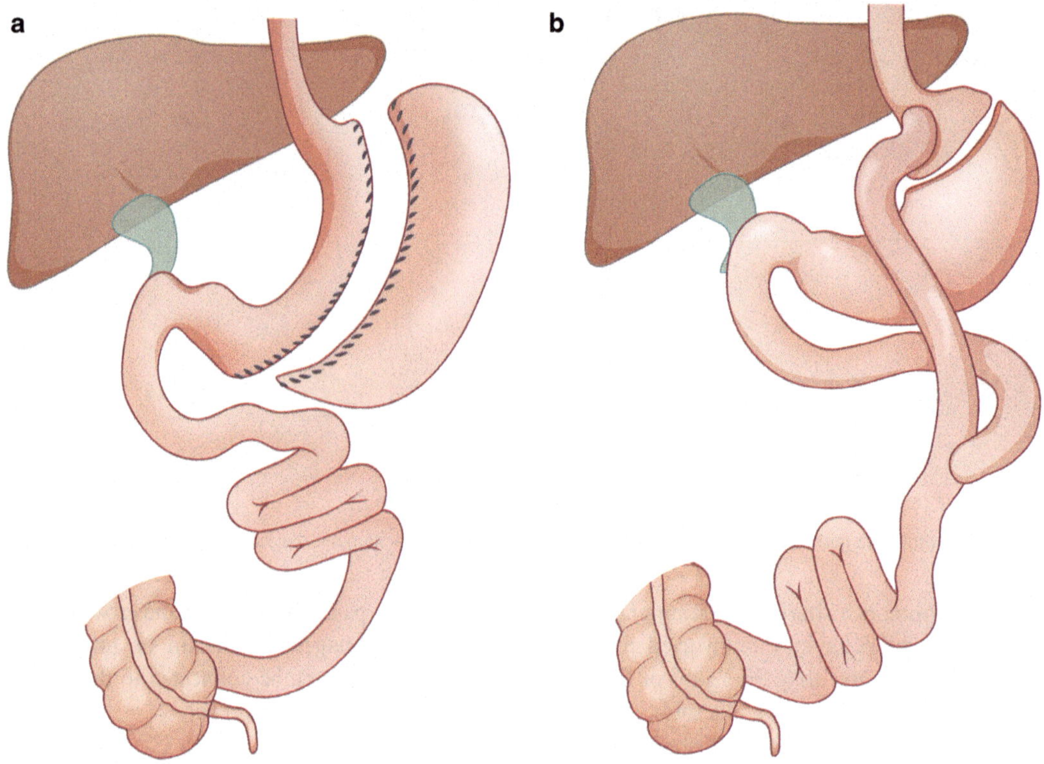

Fig. 9.14 (**a**) Sleeve gastrectomy. (**b**) Roux-en-Y gastric bypass surgery

Dietary Treatment

Dietary treatment limits the amount of the calorie intake by diet and induces body fat reduction by consuming energy from the body fat. However, the intake of essential nutrients such as vitamins and minerals might be reduced due to the limited calorie intake by diet, so dietary treatment should be prescribed according to the nutritional standards. Also, following the recommendations for the prevention and management of complications of obesity and various metabolic disorders is important. The method, intensity, and period of dietary treatment are determined considering the accurate nutritional assessment, physiologically functioning factors, and psychological factors (Song et al. 2010).

The prescription dietary treatment in obese patients is shown in Fig. 9.15.

① Dietary assessment

Understanding the usual amount of food and nutrition intake is important to carry out diet. Food record, 24 h retrospective method, and eating frequency method are used for nutritional assessment, and the patients should be careful to not miss out any food intake through repetitive questions or retrospection because 20 ~ 30 % less food intake has been reported in obesity.

② Calorie restriction

Generally, 1000 ~ 1200 kcal per day for women and 1200 ~ 1500 kcal per day for man is recommended. Lower than 1200 kcal is not recommended.

Low-calorie diet (LCD) is a method restricting 500 ~ 1000 kcal less than the calorie needed to maintain the body weight. The effects are about 0.5 ~ 1 kg weight loss and reduced abdominal and waist circumferences. It is a recommended method to lose weight because it almost does not accompany health problems. If this method is performed for 6 months, the weight loss effect is about 10 % of the body weight.

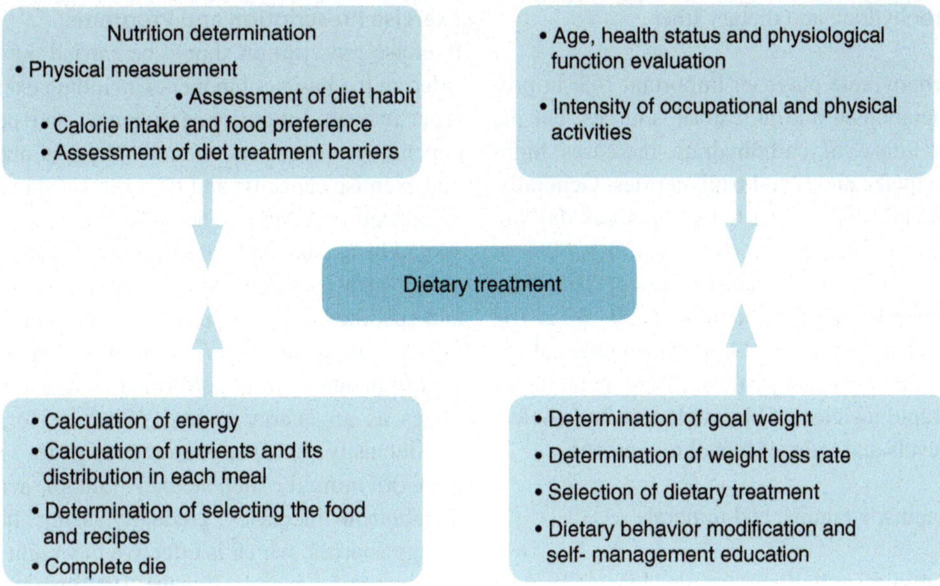

Fig. 9.15 Dietary treatment

Very low-calorie diet (VLCD) limiting the calorie intake at about 400 ~ 800 kcal per day performed for 12 weeks has an effect of reducing 20 kg of the body weight and mortality, but it may result in hair loss, headache, dizziness, fatigue, constipation, muscle cramps, dehydration, gallstones, and arrhythmia. Mifflin-St. Jeor equation is widely used to measure the energy needed per day because this equation is the most accurate.

Male: 103 weight (kg) 16.253 height (cm) 253 age (years) 15 kcal/day
Female: 103 weight (kg) 16.253 height (cm) 253 age (years) 2161 kcal/day

The daily energy requirements are calculated by the energy required at the rest state multiplied by the activity factor. Daily calorie intake is calculated by subtracting 500 kcal from the daily energy requirements (Table 9.8).

Table 9.8 Activity coefficient

Activity coefficient	Activity level	Activities
0.2	Very light activities	Mainly sedentary activities (sleeping, resting, etc.)
0.3	Light activities	Mainly sedentary activities, occasionally standing (office works, sedentary lifestyle, loading the car, slow walking, etc.)
0.5	Moderate activities	Mainly standing or walking (bicycling, cleaning, housework, cooking, etc.)
0.8	Vigorous activities	Regular activities can be exercised or exercise (aerobics, hiking, outdoor activities)

③ Fat

The risk of dyslipidemia has to be reduced by limiting the types and amounts of fat including saturated fat, cholesterol, and trans fat. The saturated fat intake should be limited to less than 6 % of the total calorie intake, and the trans fat intake should be minimized. The fat intake should not be exceeded by 25 % of the total calories. There are moderate-fat diets and low-fat diets. Since high-fat diets are high in calories and saturated fat, it leads to high blood lipid levels.

④ Carbohydrate and dietary fiber

Carbohydrate plays an important role in protein metabolism and as calorie sources, but the excess intake of carbohydrate increases high-calorie intake and blood triglycerides. Generally, more than 100 g of carbohydrates per day are required, but in the case of obesity, 50 ~ 60 % of the total calories are recommended. The daily recommendation of dietary fiber is 20 ~ 30 g. The calories can be regulated by lowering the calorie density and increasing satiety during meal. It prevents rapid increase of blood glucose and cholesterol levels and induces bowel movement.

⑤ Proteins, vitamins, and minerals

To minimize and prevent the loss of protein during the calorie-restricted dietary treatment, 1.0 ~ 1.5 g of protein intake per 1 kg of the body weight is recommended.

Insufficient intake of vitamins and minerals should be avoided during the dietary treatment because they are involved in antioxidant activity in the body; especially the intake should not be less than 1200 kcal per day.

Behavior Modification Therapy

Behavior modification therapy is an individual observing of their obesity-related habits and activities, identifying the stimulation and results affecting their behaviors, and then regulating their behaviors. Behavior modification therapy includes stimulus control technique, dietary behavior control, positive reinforces, self-observation, nutrition education, physical activity control, and cognitive restructuring techniques.

9.2.2 Physical Therapy Intervention

9.2.2.1 Exercise Therapy

Exercise therapy is performed to activate the lipolysis ability to increase the energy consumption of the body. Exercise programs should be properly applied depending on each type of patients after accurately evaluating their body composition and athletic ability

Exercise Prescription and Programs

Exercise prescription should be carried out considering the basic components including exercise type, intensity, duration, frequency, and period depending on each individual's physical activity and exercise capacity, and the exercise should be conducted regularly. The systematic planning should be established considering the basic principles such as safety, efficacy, progressiveness, and specificity. When performing high-intensity exercise in a short period of time, anaerobic energy metabolism is performed using carbohydrates as an energy source. When performing low-intensity exercise continuously for more than 30 min, the dependency rate of aerobic metabolism increases gradually using fat as energy sources, which is effective in weight loss. When starting exercise for the first time, regular light exercises, stretching, and aerobic exercise like walking for 20 ~ 30 min three times per week are recommended. After 2 ~ 3 weeks, gradual increase of exercise intensity to 30 ~ 45 min for 5 days per week is recommended. To prevent injuries due to exercise, warming up and cooling down should be performed thoroughly.

Types of Exercise

The types of exercise should be selected after consulting with patients considering the purpose of exercise therapy, exercise capacity, personal preference, and environmental factors. Aerobic exercises such as walking, jogging, cycling, climbing stairs, swimming, and aerobic dance can be performed to improve endurance, breathing, circulation, and muscle function. Weight training, 100 m running, and weightlifting are anaerobic exercise for the strength and endurance improvement. Depending on the load on the joints during the exercise, high-impact exercises such as jogging, running, and jumping rope and low-impact exercises such as swimming and bicycling are performed. Stretching, gymnastics, yoga, free gymnastics, and dance to improve flexibility are performed.

The Intensity of the Exercise

The intensity of the exercise is the amount of exercise performed in predetermined time, and it

Table 9.9 Intensity according to the type of exercise

Exercise intensity (MET)	Type of exercise
3 ~ 4	Walking (speed 4 km/h), gymnastics, stretching
4 ~ 5	Walking (speed 6 km/h), cycling (speed 16 km/h), swimming (slowly)
5 ~ 6	Walking (speed 6.5 km/h), badminton
6 ~ 7	Walking (speed 8 km/h), cycling (speed 17.5 km/h), hiking (lightly), basketball
7 ~ 8	Running (speed 8.5 km/h), cycling (speed 20 km/h), basketball tournament

is determined by the maximum heart rate within a range which does not bear on cardiorespiratory function and the maximum oxygen uptake (VO2max). And the heart rate and the metabolic equivalent (MET) are basic physiological index. The heart rate is commonly used as an index of the intensity of the exercise because it is easy to measure. The metabolic equivalent is oxygen consumption (VO2) of stably seated 70 kg 40-year-old man. 1METs is 3.5 mL/kg/min. Generally, for the target exercise intensity, the moderate strength exercise, maximum 50 ~ 80% of MET and 3.0 ~ 6.0 of MET range, is appropriate.

Select the type of exercise according to the exercise intensity (Table 9.9).

9.2.2.2 Manual Therapy

Obese people complain of pain by swelling and reduced circulation. Arthralgia and limited mobility are caused if obesity is severe. In this case, the physical therapists can perform myofascial therapy and massage to reduce pain and improve circulation.

Myofascial Therapy

The superficial fascia is a connective tissue including the musculature, blood vessels, nerves, and fat under the skin. Below, the deep fascia is continued with the superficial fascia (Park et al. 2014).

① Skin rolling

Skin rolling increases the mobility and circulation of superficial fascia by lifting the surface fat tissues with the therapist's thumbs and index fingers of both hands (Fig. 9.16).

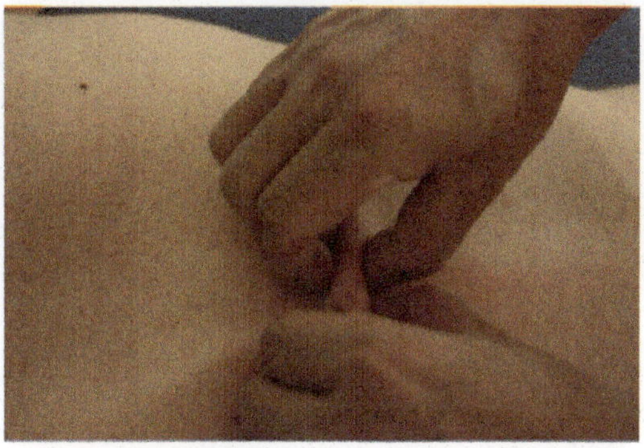

Fig. 9.16 Skin rolling

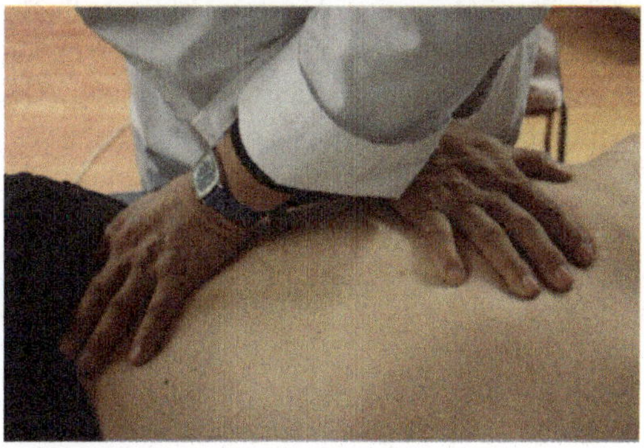

Fig. 9.17 Fascial relaxation

② Myofascial relaxation

Myofascial relaxation is a method slowly stretching the myofascia by crossing the therapist's hands to the direction where the therapists can easily move to hardened skin or tender points on the obese areas (Fig. 9.17). If the resistance of the stretch is felt by the therapist's hands, the pressure should be kept steady and wait for at least 90 ~ 120 s. If it is relaxed, the therapists feel heat, vibration, beating, and then smoothing under their hands. Until these feelings disappear, therapists should keep the pressure and stretching and then release.

Manual Lymph Drainage

Prior to the intervention of obesity, performing manual lymph drainage reduces elevated pressure

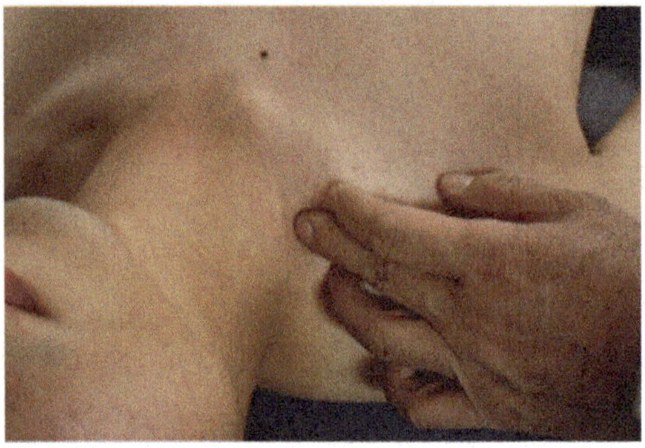

Fig. 9.18 Lymphatic drainage

of the dermis by active absorption of tissue fluids. It is also performed at the end of the intervention to induce the tissue elasticity and calming. The therapists release the lymph nodes and lymph vessels of the neck and trunk areas to facilitate the circulation of body fluids. It is conducted regularly at the pressure of about 20 ~ 40 mmHg five to seven times for 20 ~ 30 min (Fig. 9.18).

Meridian Massage

Meridian connects distal extremities of the human body and organs three dimensionally including the upper, lower, left, right, inside, and outside. It is a network distributing aeremia evenly throughout the body and includes the muscular system, nervous system, circulatory system, and all the physiological functions of the body. Obesity is a result of aeremia circulation disorders of systemic meridian. Therefore, the recovery of the systemic metabolism by meridian massage helps in degrading subcutaneous fat (Lee 2005). In addition, among the meridians, the massage of the stomach meridian and spleen meridian is directly related to digestion and obesity. Acupuncture points used for the restoration of metabolism are the bladder meridian distributed on the back of the body including Feishu (Lung Point, BL 13), Xinshu (Heart Point, BL 15), Ganshu (Liver Point, BL 18), Danshu (Gallbladder Point, BL 19), Pishu (Spleen Point, BL 20), Weishu (Stomach Point, BL 21), Yinmen (Gate of Abundance, BL 37), Heyang (Confluence of Yang, BL 55), and Chengshan (Support the Mountain, BL 57). Acupuncture points related to the digestive function are Zhongwan (Middle of the Stomach, CV 12), Zhangmen (Screen Door, LR 13), Zusanli (Leg Three Miles, ST 36), and Dabao (Great Wrapping, SP 21) (Fig. 9.19) (WHO 2008).

9.2.2.3 Physical Agent Modalities

Hydrotherapy

Depending on the presence of the comorbidities by obesity, the physical therapists should be able to determine the type of hydrotherapy. Russian bath, Nauheim bath, foam bath, hydrogen carbonate bath, Radon bath, brine or salt bath, and oscillation medical bath are effective hydrotherapy (Park et al. 2010).

① Russian bath

It is a bath mixed with air and moisture vapor, and usually it is performed at 46 °C (114.8 °F) for 5 ~ 10 min. It is performed for obese patients without hypertension, diabetes, and heart disorders caused by obesity. It is effective in improving metabolism and circulation and relieving pain by significant expansion of peripheral blood vessels (Fig. 9.20).

② Brine bath

It is salt water having osmotic effects, so it is effective in weight loss by reducing food intake in obese people. The artificial salt is made by 2.27 ~ 13.6 kg of sodium chloride dissolved into 151 L of water. If 2.27 ~ 2.72 kg of sodium chloride is dissolved, it become salt water like 1 ~ 7 % of the natural seawater. 4 ~ 20 min in above 20 °C (68 °F) is appropriate.

③ Low-frequency oscillation bath

Low-frequency oscillation bath makes oscillation in water by frequency of 40 ~ 57 Hz. The low-frequency operation reduces pain by increasing microcirculation. The oscillation is transmitted through the body inducing degradation and metabolism of lipid, therefore, burning off the fat accumulated in the body (Fig. 9.21).

Electrical Therapy

① Ultrasound therapy

Ultrasound effectively heats deep areas of the skin and subcutaneous fascia without energy loss. The temperature increases by 4 ~ 5 °C (39.2 ~ 41 °F) in 5 cm depth of subcutaneous tissues. The absorption of the wave becomes

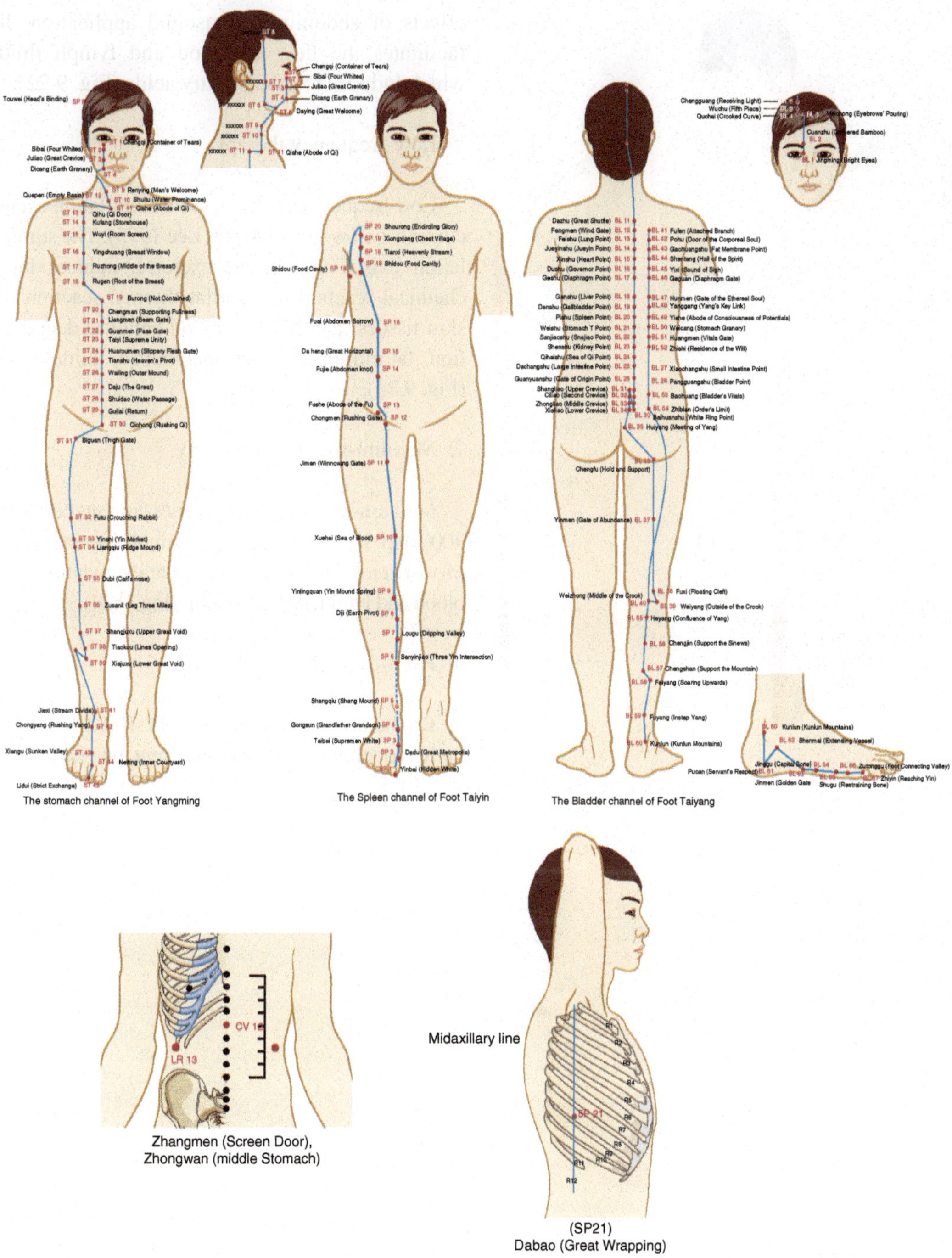

Fig. 9.19 Meridians and acupuncture points

higher in the boundary of the bones and muscles, so the tissue temperature increases by 46 °C. At this time, the absorbed ultrasound has micromassage effect due to the pressure change of the waves. The effect of micromassage includes increased diffusion through the cell membrane, massage effects between cells, reversible reduction of the viscosity in colloidal materials inside and outside of the cells, friction effects of producing heat, and effects on nerves and circulation mechanism. The lipids become in easily degradable condition by vibrational and thermal

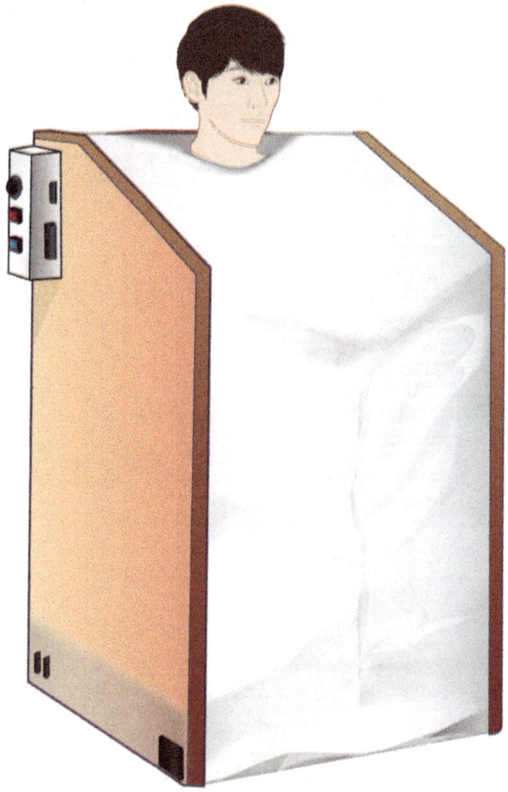

Fig. 9.20 Russian bath

effects of abdominal ultrasound application. It facilitates the flow of blood and lymph fluid which induces release of fatty acids (Fig. 9.22).

② Low-frequency therapy

Low frequency is an electrical stimulation using currents below 1 ~ 1,000 Hz (Lee 1995). The stimulation makes the muscle exercise, induces biochemical reaction and partial thermal reaction in skin tissues, and has effects on cellulite degradation, fat elimination, and metabolism stimulation (Fig. 9.23).

③ Medium-frequency therapy

Medium-frequency therapy uses currents between 4000 and 45,000 Hz smoothly stimulating the depth of wide areas and induces cellulite degradation and blood and lymphatic circulation (Fig. 9.24).

④ High-frequency diathermy

Diathermy converts more than 100,000 Hz of high frequency, an alternating current, into body heat

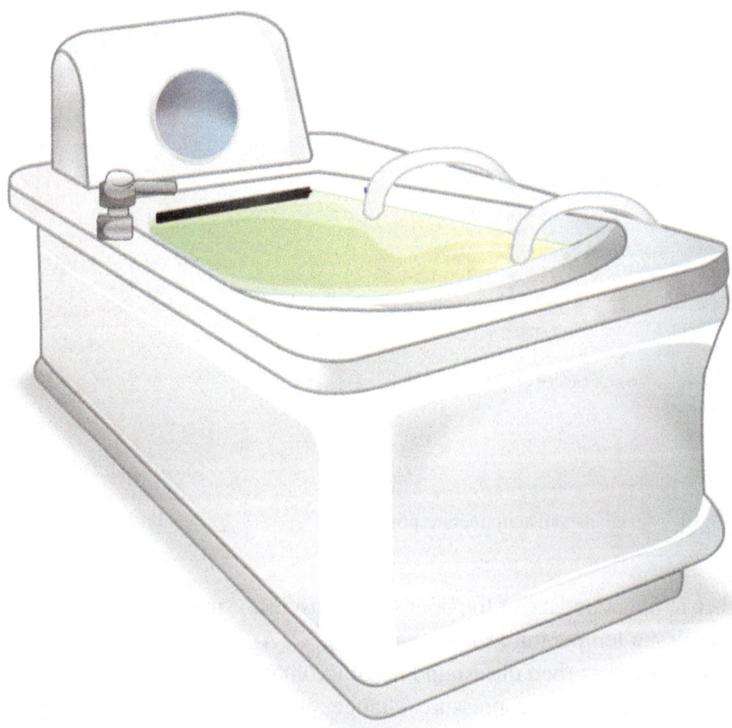

Fig. 9.21 Low-frequency vibration bath

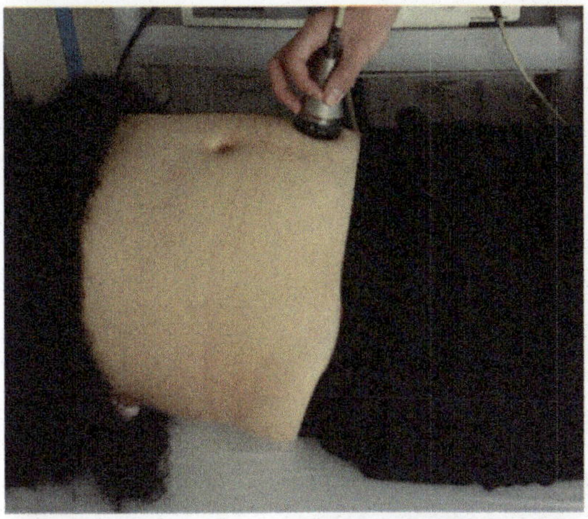

Fig. 9.22 Ultrasound

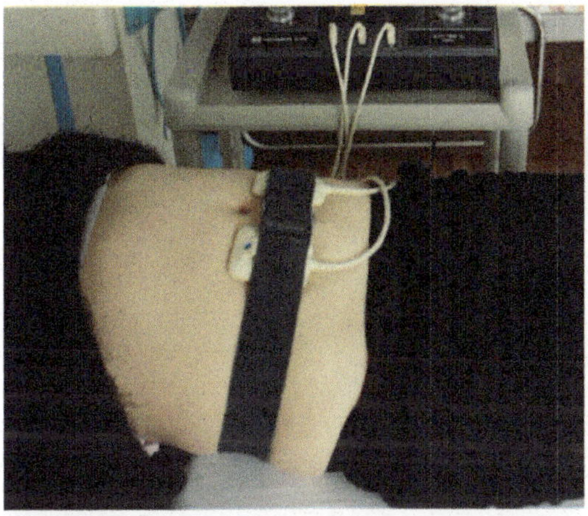

Fig. 9.23 Low frequency

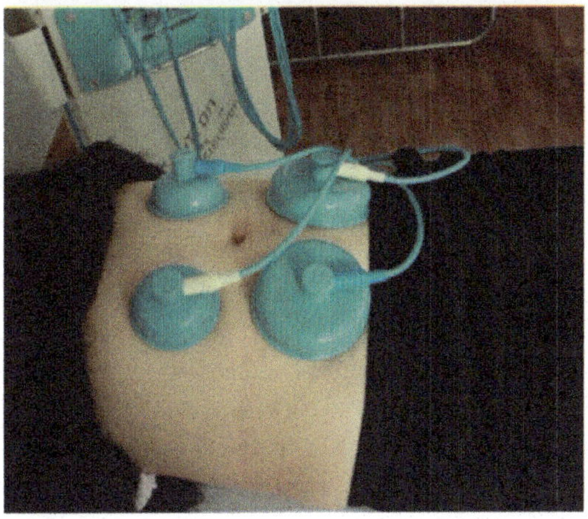

Fig. 9.24 Mid-frequency

in the skin or tissues (Shin et al. 2006). It is a therapeutic method using thermal effect of diathermy, and 0.5 MHz of frequency is commonly used in treating obesity. When the high-frequency current is applied to the body, it increases the local temperature of deep tissues by 40 °C (104 °F) causing blood flow to the capillaries, promoting metabolism and blood circulation, and facilitating fat degradation by oxygen supply. Lipids are degraded by high-frequency diathermy and discharged through sweat glands and urine (Figs. 9.22 and 9.25).

⑤ Extracorporeal shock wave therapy, ESWT

Extracorporeal shock wave therapy, ESWT, generates ultrasonic waves with 1 ~ 2 Hz of the frequency and relieves pain by transmitting a mechanical stimulation to the body. The ultrasound penetrates into 15 mm below the epidermis and destroys adipocyte masses, and the adipocytes are eliminated through the normal metabolism of the body (Fig. 9.26). It is applied to patients with localized obesity or dietary treatment that is no longer effective.

9.2.3 Prevention and Management

9.2.3.1 Prevention

1. Obesity caused by energy imbalance can be prevented by identifying the factors causing lack of exercise and usual physical activities and by accurate assessment of the energy consumption.
2. Since the food intake is a personal preference and habit, inducing balanced energy consumption by selecting healthy and nutritious diet is needed.
3. It is important having a habit of participating in a various physical activity from the early age, and preventing obesity by recognizing the importance of exercise and practice even after becoming an adult

9.2.3.2 Management

1. During weight loss, it is important to lose weight for a long period of time by consistent management rather than losing it in a short

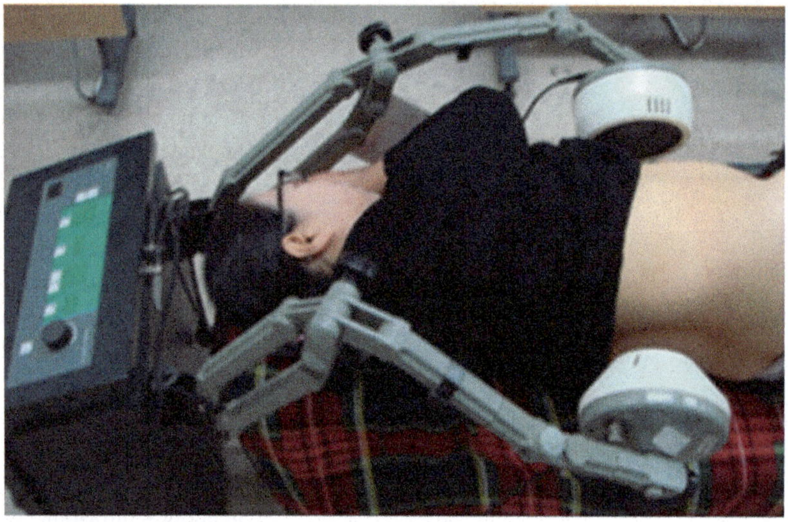

Fig. 9.25 High-frequency diathermy

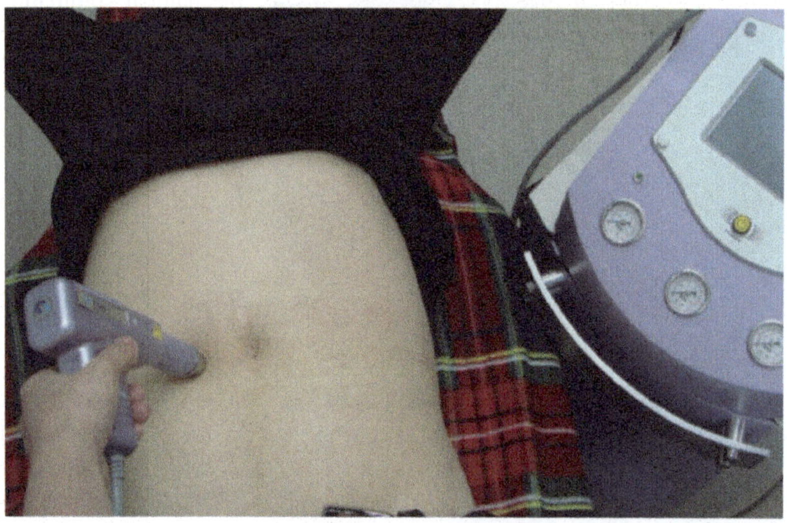

Fig. 9.26 Extracorporeal shock wave

period of time, so aiming for gradual weight loss is more appropriate.

2. When there are obesity-related complications, examining in every 3 months or every 6 months if there are no complications is recommended.
3. Weight loss and long-term management should be emphasized for obese patients.

9.2.3.3 Patients/Caregiver Education

1. Generally, it is important that obese patients with high dependence on others and low compliance know that active participation is an effective therapy.
2. Many factors are involved in preventing and managing obesity such as correct understanding of the body weight, motivation and the practice of weight control, and the presence or absence of the diseases. Therefore, educating patients according to the realistic goal and therapeutic methods of each patient is necessary.
3. It is necessary to lead patients to monitor their body weight and activities in a regular basis.

Advice for Physical Therapists

1. Physical therapists give professional advice to obese patients about therapeutic interventions and also play an important role in progressing treatment for obesity by managing obesity and providing appropriate exercises.
2. It is very important that obese patients understand the risks of obesity in treatment and exercise, so the physical therapists should conduct observation, advice, and revaluation consistently. The therapists should observe whether the patients have risk factors of obesity, perform exercise properly, and control their emotion.
3. It is important to treat striae distensae or contact dermatitis in their early stages, so therapists should advice obese patients about the sanitation and moisturizing of the skin.

9.3 Problem Solving

9.3.1 Obesity

Choose a possible examination or physical therapy intervention from each question.

Question 1

"A" is a 57-year-old woman and had symptoms of gaining fat on the face and shoulders, easily bruising, showing reddish complexion, and increased blood pressure. She thought that the symptoms were caused by aging and menopause. But she was diagnosed with osteoporosis and obesity when she was hospitalized due to the pain on the knees and back. What is the suspected disease for this patient before performing physical therapy intervention for the pain on the knees and back?

1. Diabetes
2. Insulinoma
3. Cushing's syndrome
4. Dyslipidemia
5. Hypothyroidism

Question 2

"A" with a BMI of 36 kg/m^2 is severely obese and was diagnosed with hypertension and dyslipidemia. Recently, he was also diagnosed with sleep disorder due to sleep apnea accompanied by fatigue and depression. What is the correct intervention for this patient?

1. Roux-en-Y gastric bypass surgery
2. Nutrition education and dietary therapy
3. Lifestyle modification and behavioral therapy
4. Drug therapy such as obesity treatment
5. Hydrotherapy to improve circulation

Question 3

"A" is 5 years old and his parents are obese. "A" was diagnosed with childhood obesity with a BMI of 30 kg/m^2. What type of obesity is "A" showing?

1. Obesity with enlarged adipocytes with the low risk to proceed into adult obesity
2. Obesity with adipogenesis with the high risk to proceed into adult obesity
3. Obesity with adipogenesis with the low risk of morbidity
4. Obesity with enlarged adipocytes showing increased cell size and number with the high risk to proceed into adult obesity
5. Combined obesity with increased cell size and number so the management is easy and has low risk to proceed into adult obesity

Question 4

"A" was diagnosed with metabolic syndrome by 102 cm of waist circumference in a hospital. What is the correct intervention to reduce waist circumference?

1. Adjustable gastric banding
2. Ultrasound therapy
3. Infrared therapy

4. Anaerobic exercise
5. High-intensity exercise therapy

Question 5

As shown in Fig. 9.5, "A" is a Cushing's syndrome patient with central obesity due to the steroid side effect. What is the correct intervention?

1. Muscle endurance
2. Muscle relaxation
3. Muscle strengthening
4. Anaerobic exercise
5. Range of motion exercise

Answer

Question 1-③, Question 2-①, Question 3-②, Question 4-②, Question 5-①

References

Ahn S, et al. Common skin disease of Koreans: diagnosis and treatment. Seoul: Doctor's Book; 2009.

Im H. Antiobesity effects of Jeju Citrus unshiu and Citrus sphaerocarpa peel extracts in 3T3-L1, Myongji University Graduate School, Department of food and nutrition Master's thesis; 2013.

Kang JH, et al. Clinical obesity. Seoul: Korean Medical Book Publishing Co; 2008.

Kang JH, et al. Guidelines for treating obesity. Seoul: Chungwoon Publishing Co; 2009.

Kim JY. Guidelines for the management of obesity. Seoul: Hanmi Medical Publishing Co; 2003.

Kim JH, et al. Measurement and clinical application of insulin resistance. Seoul. J Korean Endocr Soc. 2009;24(1):75–83.

Kopelman PG. Clinical obesity. Seoul: Gabon; 2008.

Lee DH. Yakson therapy. Seoul: Mindvision; 2005.

Lee JH. Electrotherapy. Seoul: Daehak Publishing Co; 1995.

Park JH, et al. The physical therapy of musculoskeletal disease. Seoul: Hyunmoon Publishing Co; 2013.

Park JH, et al. The physical therapy of musculoskeletal disease. Seoul: Hyunmoon Publishing Co; 2014.

Park JC, et al. The principles and practices of manual therapy. Seoul: Hyunmoon Publishing Co; 2010.

Shin S-U, et al. Effects of high frequency therapy on localized obesity. J Kor Orient Assoc Study Obes. 2006;6(2);75–83.

Shin SU, et al. Effects of high frequency therapy on localized obesity. J Kor Orient Assoc Study Obes. 2006;6(2);75–83.

Song NY, et al. Comparison of frequency and amount of dishes reported in semi-quantitative dish-based frequency questionnaire vs. 12-day dietary records. Korean J Nutr. 2010;43(6):638–52.

WHO Western Pacific Region. WHO standard acupuncture point locations. Seoul: Korean Edition. Medbook; 2008.

Reference Sites

Ministry of Health and Welfare. http://www.mohw.go.kr/front_new/index.jsp.

U.S National Heart, Lung, and Blood Institute. http://www.nhlbi.nih.gov/.

UK National Health Service. https://www.england.nhs.uk/.

World Health Organization. http://www.who.int/en/.

10 Other Skin Diseases (Psoriasis, Herpes Zoster, Dermatophytosis, Vitiligo)

Nam Jeong Cho

ICD-10 Code
B02 Zoster [herpes zoster]
B02.0† ~ B02.9
B35 Dermatophytosis
B35.0 ~ B35.9
L40 Psoriasis
L40.0 ~ L40.9
L80 Vitiligo

Learning Outcomes
After completing this chapter, you should be able to do the following:

- Explain the types of other skin diseases.
- Explain the causes, symptoms, and classification of each skin disease.
- Explain the diagnosis and assessment of each skin disease.
- Explain the physical therapy intervention of each skin disease.
- Explain the problem solving of each skin disease.

Key Terms
Psoriasis
Herpes zoster
Dermatophytosis
Vitiligo
Psoriasis

10.1 Psoriasis

10.1.1 Overview

Psoriasis is a noncontagious chronic skin disease. It is a papulosa lesion with red swellings and scaling of the skin. Psoriasis mainly occurs in the head, elbow, and knees, but it can occur in other areas. Sometimes, it can be confused with dermatomycosis, and there is an unusual form of psoriasis called pustular psoriasis. Usually, it occurs in about 1.5–3 % of the population in Europe and North America, but it rarely occurs in Africa and Japan. The incidence rate in South Korea is 1 % which is lower than that of Caucasians, and it is a

N.J. Cho
Professor, Department of Physical Therapy,
Hanlyo University, Gwangyang, South Korea
e-mail: mjnj12@hanmail.net

J.-W. Park, D.-I. Jung (eds.), *Integumentary Physical Therapy*, DOI 10.1007/978-3-662-47380-1_10

common disease because it occurs in 0.5–2 % of the total population. There are no differences in genders, and generally the symptoms occur in early 20s (Ahn et al. 2009a).

10.1.2 Causes

The exact cause of psoriasis is not yet defined, but the stratum corneum of the skin tends to proliferate faster than that of the normal people. Genetic predispositions and environmental factors act together to cause psoriasis. Psoriasis is not contagious, and the disease is caused and worsened by bacterial infection (particularly by tonsillitis), skin wound, mental stress, impact of the seasons, and some medications.

10.1.3 Classification

The following description is about various types of psoriasis showing the typical characteristics. Psoriasis changes the skin into red for a long period of time and shows repeated mitigation and aggravation. Also, it can appear in any parts of the skin and may change to a different type of psoriasis. In some cases, various types of psoriasis can occur at the same time.

10.1.3.1 Plaque Psoriasis

Plaque psoriasis is the most common type of psoriasis. It is red lesions covered with silvery white scaling of the skin. Scaling of the skin is a phenomenon caused by the dead cells. The medical name of plaque psoriasis is psoriasis vulgaris. Plaque psoriasis can appear in anywhere on the skin, and the knees, elbows, head, and trunk are the most common areas (Fig. 10.1).

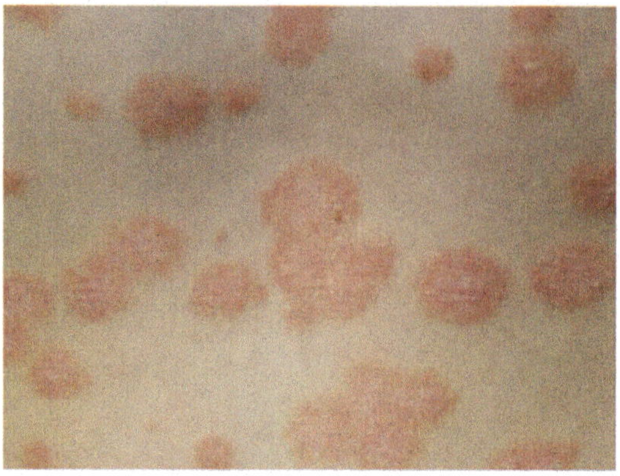

Fig. 10.1 Plaque psoriasis

10.1.3.2 Guttate Psoriasis

Guttate psoriasis is in small red dot (or drop) shape. The word guttate is derived from "gutta" meaning drop in Latin language. It mainly appears on the trunk and limbs. The scaling of the skin might form on the lesions.

10.1.3.3 Inverse Psoriasis

Inverse psoriasis appears mainly on the skinfolds such as armpits, inguinal area, and below the breast. It typically appears smooth without scaling of the skin, and it is itchy when rubbed the lesion and sweating.

10.1.3.4 Exfoliative Psoriasis

Erythrodermic psoriasis is characterized by fine red scaling of the skin broadly raised from the lesions, and severe itching, pain, and swelling may be accompanied.

10.1.3.5 Pustular Psoriasis

Pustular psoriasis is characterized by pustules (blister-like lesions of noninfectious pus) on the skin. It is not inflammatory and contagious. It appears on certain parts of the body such as hands and feet, and it also might be spread throughout the body. Pustular psoriasis tends to have a cycle of erythema, reddening of the skin; formation of pustules; and scaling of the skin (Fig. 10.2).

10.1.3.6 Psoriasis Arthritis

Psoriasis arthritis appears in a form of arthritis in approximately 10 % of the psoriasis patients. Psoriasis arthritis is accompanied by inflammation and swelling. Usually, it appears on hands and feet and can be spread to large joints such as the knees, buttocks, elbow, and spine. It is stiff and gives damage to the joints.

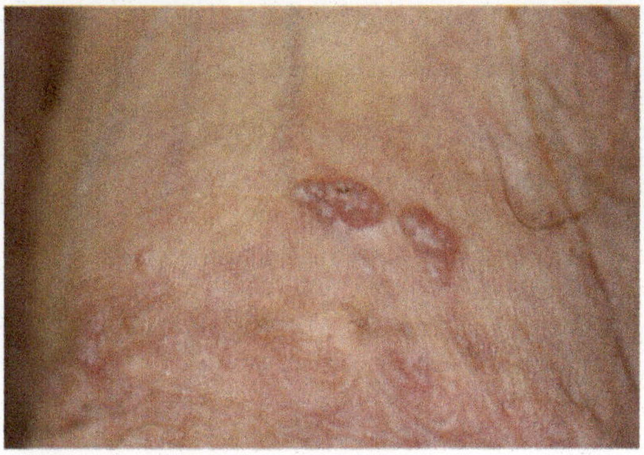

Fig. 10.2 Pustular psoriasis

Table 10.1 The symptoms of psoriasis

1. Complaint of itching of the skin
2. The redness of the skin disease becomes strong
3. The systemic fever is accompanied
4. Countless skin scales occur in the whole body
5. Pustules around the lesion occur (pockets of pus)
6. The whole body becomes flushed skin
7. Pustules increase in hands and soles
8. The existing lesion is spread rapidly to the surroundings
9. The lesion is extended rapidly to the face, genital organs, armpits, etc.

10.1.3.7 Scalp Psoriasis

Scalp psoriasis appears on the majority of the patients with psoriasis. Usually, it is covered with scaling of the skin and appears in a form of plaque psoriasis with red lesions.

10.1.3.8 Fingernail and Toenail Psoriasis

Hand and nail psoriasis mainly appears in a form of dent and occurs in various sizes, shapes, and depths. Occasionally, nails become yellow and thick. The nails are easily broken or become inflamed. It also causes the nails separated from the nail beds.

10.1.4 Symptoms and Complications

The early phase of psoriasis is characterized by slightly risen rash (papules) that appears as small millet less than 1 cm on the skin. The color is slightly red, and then the rash grows from the size of millet to a walnut and then to a chestnut and egg. And new millet like rash appears, grows, and fuses with others. Thus, the rash becomes a size of one large egg or palm. If the lesion is not treated properly, it spreads to the whole limbs and body. The white dead skin cells are piled up on top of the rash. The dead skin cells can be easily peeled off by fingernails, but sometimes it is hard to peel off due to its thickness. The color of the rash is generally red, but it differs in some degrees from strong to light red. In psoriasis, red rash gradually increases, fuses, and becomes a coin shape. Gradually, the distinctive white and thick skin peels appear on top of the rash. The skin peels gradually become thicker over time. The psoriasis occurs mainly on the knees, elbows, hips, and head (Table 10.1). Psoriasis induces arthritis and it is accompanied by 20–30 % of psoriasis patients. There are no differences between genders, and it appears in three types which are asymmetrical oligoarticular arthritis, symmetrical polyarthritis, and spondylitis. First, asymmetrical oligoarticular arthritis invades into a small number of joints, but the function is well maintained. Second, symmetrical polyarthritis is associated with transformation and functional degeneration. It is different from rheumatoid arthritis because it invades in the interphalangeal joint and shows negative in rheumatoid factors. Third, spondylitis is similar to ankylosing spondylitis, and it occurs either independently or in combination with arthritis of distal ends (Ahn et al. 2009b).

10.1.5 Test and Assessment

Unlike other diseases of internal organs, skin diseases and their shapes can be easily confirmed by naked eyes because they appear on the skin. Likewise, psoriasis that appeared on the skin can be diagnosed clinically. There are many types of psoriasis, and the treatment and prognosis are different depending on each type. The shape and area of the lesions, elapsed time, and medical history are the most essential factors in clinical diagnosis. The most important clinical manifestations of the underlying disease in diagnosis of psoriasis include few characteristics. They are millet-sized rash protruding from the skin, red pigment of rash, white skin scales on the rash, easily peeled off scales, thickening skin, and mild itching. This rash becomes large when the size of the lesion is increased and fused with other lesions. Likewise, the psoriasis with a typical shape is called plaque psoriasis, and the coin-shaped psoriasis is called psoriasis nummularis. Psoriasis is different depending on the individual and depending on the treatment and elapsed time in the same person. In some cases, strong red pigment and particularly many scales appear. Occasionally, the skin becomes unusually thick even with less scale and red pigments. Besides the typical plaque psoriasis, if the pustules appear on the whole body, it is called systemic pustular psoriasis, and if it appears specifically on hands and soles, it is called localized pustular psoriasis. Also, if the whole body skin is red and many scales are falling off, it is diagnosed with erythrodermic psoriasis.

10.2 Intervention

10.2.1 Intervention

10.2.1.1 Interventional Approach

Psoriasis is a chronic and recurrent disease causing not only physical problems but aesthetic and mental health problems even though psoriasis itself is not fatal. Psoriasis is a disease described as one of the oldest diseases in the history of the disease, of course; therefore, various treatments have been developed and advanced achieving innovative treatment therapies as a result recently. However, because of recurrence of psoriasis, the disease itself cannot be fully prevented but slows down the recurrence. Therefore, for the treatment of chronic recurrent psoriasis, effective treatments with fewer side effects are more desirable in long-term therapy.

10.2.1.2 Medical Treatment

Many methods are used in treating psoriasis. They are a topical treatment applying drugs, phototherapy, systemic treatment administering drugs, and combination therapy. Rarely, climate therapy, hyperthermia therapy, or dialysis is used as an alternative method. There are three types of major treatments. They are a treatment applying topical agents such as ointments, applying light, and administering drugs (Table 10.2).

Table 10.2 Treatment of psoriasis

1. Topical treatments: ointment application (steroids, emollients)
2. Phototherapy: UVB, UVA, PUVA
3. Systemic therapy: drug therapy (MTX (methotrexate), biological agents)
4. The combination therapy: combination of drug, ointment, UV light, etc.
5. Others: climate therapy, hyperthermia dialysis, traditional Chinese medicine, etc.

10.2.2 Physical Therapy Intervention

10.2.2.1 Postures

It is appropriate taking a correct posture from the beginning of the disease because the functional transformation might be accompanied by the lesion invading distal phalanx bone joints in psoriasis arthritis. In addition, since the postural abnormality similar to ankylosing spondylitis might occur, maintaining a functional posture is necessary.

10.2.2.2 Exercise Therapy

The complications by psoriasis are arthritis in the interphalangeal joint and in the spine. To minimize the functional disorder of the finger and the restricted range of motion, the active exercise for range of motion of fingers is performed. To prevent the rigidity of the joints and promote recovery, manual exercise at the beginning and gradually active assistive exercise are performed by therapists. Also, try to maintain normal muscle strength through muscle strengthening exercises of finger flexor and extensor muscles. For the catching function of the fingers, exercise using rubber ball more than three times per day, ten reps for one set for at least five sets, is appropriate. In the case of spondylitis, one of the complications of psoriasis, joint range of motion, can be maintained by bending and stretching the waist and lumbar movement. Lumbar alignment disorder can be prevented by strengthening exercise of erector spinae muscles (Fig. 10.3).

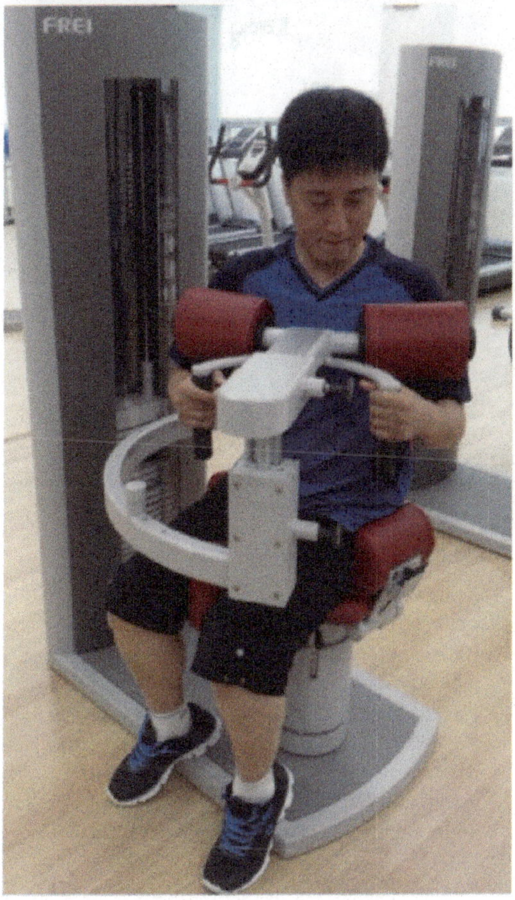

Fig. 10.3 Lumbar movement of spondylitis due to complications of psoriasis

10.2.2.3 Manual Therapy

If the transformation of the spinal column and interphalangeal joint by complications of psoriasis progresses, the normal articular rigidity must be restored through initial 1–2 grade of joint mobilization for pain relief and 2–3 grade of joint mobilization in progressive stage. To treat the soft tissue adhesion and muscle contracture around the transformed lumbar joint, muscle energy techniques are periodically performed 3–5 times per day (Fig. 10.4).

10.2.2.4 Physical Agent Modalities

Ultraviolet Treatment

It is a unique technique used only for the skin diseases in human diseases. It is applying beam on the psoriasis areas for 10–15 min using 3, 4° erythema doses. It is well known that psoriasis improves after the lesions are exposed to sunlight. Therefore, after analyzing sunlight, it is revealed that ultraviolet of the sunlight improves psoriasis. Phototherapy is a method applying this fact which emits ultraviolet light to the affected areas using artificial light similar to the fluorescent lamp (Fig. 10.5).

Photochemical Therapy

It is applying specific ultraviolet reacting with the drugs after administering a photosensitizer consisted with the components sensitive to light. It is called photochemical therapy because it is chemotherapy administering drugs combined with

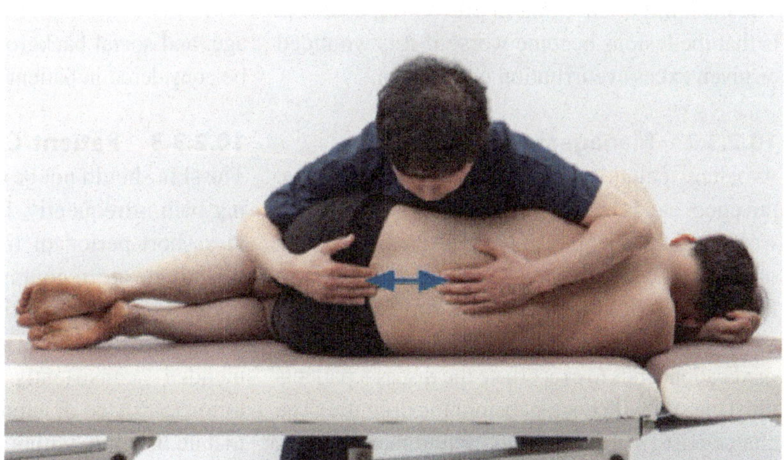

Fig. 10.4 Muscle energy techniques of erector spinae muscles. *Arrow* is treatment direction

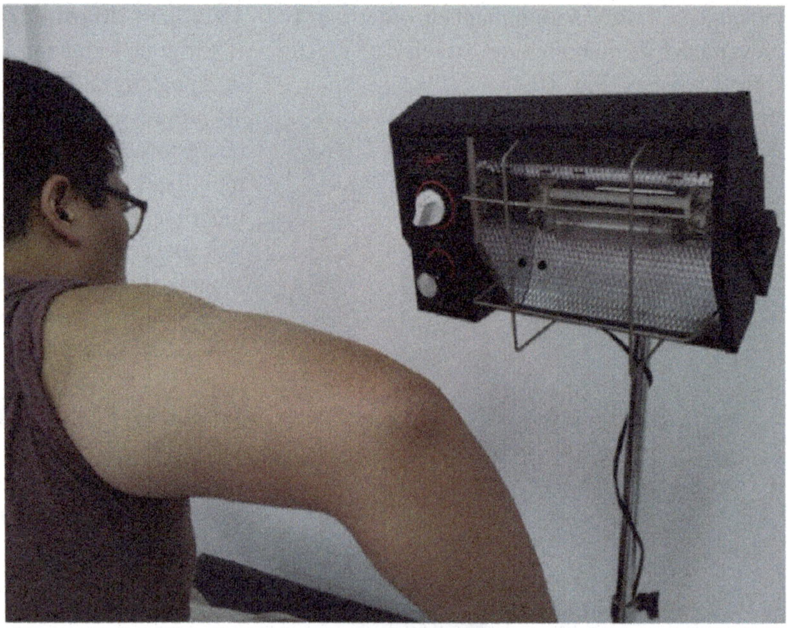

Fig. 10.5 UV therapy

light therapy. Photochemical therapies include a topical photochemical therapy using ultraviolet after applying photosensitizer, psoralen, on psoriasis areas, a systemic photochemical therapy using ultraviolet after administering photosensitizer (oral psoralen), and a bath photochemical therapy (bath-PUVA) using ultraviolet after performing the immersion bath where the photosensitizer is dissolved in water.

Table 10.3 Prevention of psoriasis

1. Avoid skin irritation or skin damage because they cause psoriasis or worsen the existing psoriasis
2. Beware of tonsillitis, pharyngitis, etc. because these inflammations can worsen psoriasis
3. Psoriasis worsens if the skin is dried so apply skin moisturizer often
4. Avoid mental stress and physical exhaustion because they worsen psoriasis
5. Various drugs can worsen psoriasis so avoid those drugs
6. Psoriasis patients are susceptible to the seasons; especially it worsens during the winter so beware of the season

10.2.3 Prevention and Management

10.2.3.1 Prevention

The most important point in preventing psoriasis is that the lesions become worse if it is wounded or given excessive irritation on the skin.

10.2.3.2 Management

Avoiding emotional stress, overwork, trauma, infection, etc. is needed because they may cause or worsen diseases (Table 10.3). Avoiding taking drugs that can exacerbate psoriasis is needed. Especially, steroid ointments and drugs temporarily improve the symptoms, but since stopping the medication tends to exacerbate the disease, patients must consult with doctors before the drug use. The characteristics of the diseases, requirements, range, age, and social background of the patients should be considered in patient's management.

10.2.3.3 Patient/Caregiver Education

The skin should not be dried. In other words, taking bath infrequently, finishing everyday shower in a short period of time, and not using rough washcloth are recommended. Applying enough body moisturizing lotion is appropriate before the body is dried after taking shower. It is recommended consistently applying moisturizing lotion consisted of natural products, which do not irritate the skin, without drug components.

10.3 Herpes Zoster

10.3.1 Overview

Herpes zoster (zoster, shingles) is a disease caused by virus and characterized by stripe-shaped blisters accompanied by painful rash (vesicles) appearing in one side of the body. It is caused by varicella-zoster virus (VZV) which also causes chicken pox. Varicella-zoster virus is hidden in nerve cells, brain or spinal ganglion, and autonomic and satellite cell ganglion without any symptoms. After years or decades of the varicella virus infection, the virus breaks out of the cell membrane, migrates along the nerve fibers, and infects the skin adjacent to the nerve. Virus is from more than one ganglion that belonged to the infected nerves, and it spreads within the same ganglion causing rash accompanied by pain. Usually, the rash is cured after 2–4 weeks, but some patients complain of neuralgia for months or years which is called postherpetic neuralgia. It is unknown how the virus becomes latent and how the virus occurred. The incidence rate of herpes zoster is 1.2–3.4 per 1000 healthy people per year, and it increases to 3.9–11.8 people after the age of 65 years worldwide (Cunningham et al. 2008).

10.3.2 Causes

Herpes zoster is a kind of viral skin disease causing inflammation in nerves by herpes zoster-varicella virus. Whoever had varicella in childhood can be susceptible to herpes zoster. After varicella, the virus becomes dormant in cells, and when the body resistance to the infection becomes weak, it suddenly proliferates and causes inflammation on the skin innervated by nerves. Children can get herpes zoster, but it commonly appears in adults after their 50s. Trauma or stress can be an inducer. Patients with decreased immunity (cancer patients, patients who have been on radiotherapy or immunosuppressive agents, etc.) are more susceptible to herpes zoster infection. However, even if the healthy people got herpes zoster, it is not necessary to worry about whether they have unknown serious diseases (Fig. 10.6) (Oxman et al. 2005a).

10.3.3 Symptoms and Complications

10.3.3.1 General Symptoms

If herpes zoster is infected, pain, irritation, and itching may occur in a certain area and one side of the body. Red spots appear after 1–3 days. In some cases, fever or headache might occur. The spots look like multiple blisters gathered together. It takes about 2–3 weeks that the blister gradually forms pus, becomes a scab, and is peeled away. The pain can last longer after the skin is recovered. Rarely, the pain only occurs without blisters or blisters without the pain (Fig. 10.7) (Oxman et al. 2005b).

10.3.3.2 Site of Origin

Blisters most often occur on the trunk and buttocks. However, blisters also can occur on the face, arms, and legs and at any sites of the body.

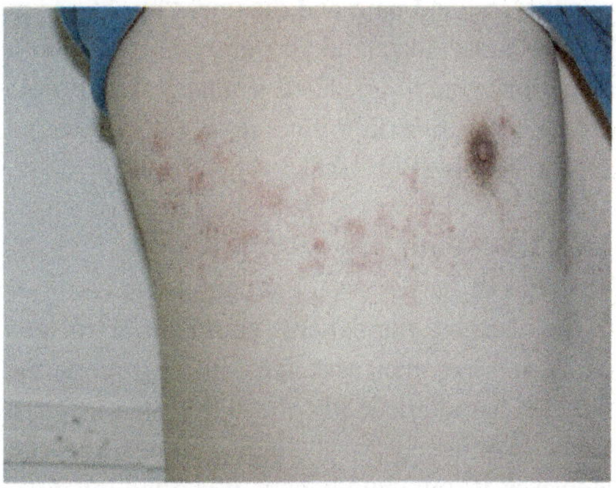

Fig. 10.6 Herpes zoster

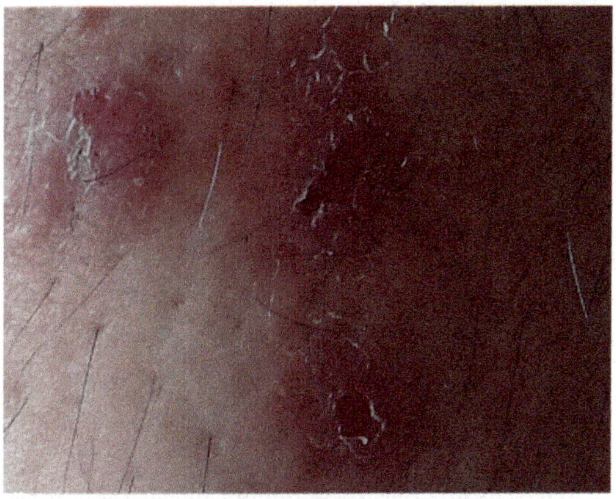

Fig. 10.7 Blister formation caused by herpes zoster

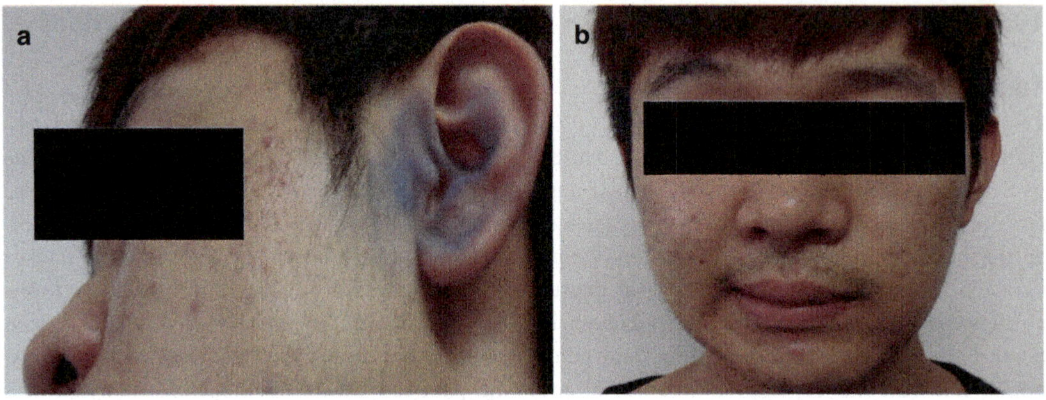

Fig. 10.8 Ramsay Hunt syndrome. (**a**) Herpes zoster in ears and (**b**) facial paralysis

Especially, if the blisters occur in eyes, the patients should seek medical treatment in ophthalmology because they might cause visual impairment.

If herpes zoster occurs in the ear, blisters might form, and pain and dizziness might occur. It may cause facial nerve paralysis and mouth alteration which is called Ramsay Hunt syndrome. After a certain time, it is often recovered spontaneously (Fig. 10.8).

10.3.3.3 Pain

The pain of herpes zoster occurs 4–5 days prior to the rash, but the patients complain of various pains, and in some cases, they suffer from paresthesia. Characteristically, the skin rash is enough to be diagnosed as a single clinical aspect. However, if only pain occurs, it is often misdiagnosed with other diseases, so the patients might receive unnecessary tests of treatments.

Therefore, if the pain or paresthesia is complained by patients, it helps to diagnose with herpes zoster before rash appears (Schmader et al. 2012).

10.3.3.4 Motor Disorder

Segmental zoster paresis is a motor disorder caused by herpes zoster. It is reported that it occurs in 0.5 % or 5 % of the patients. It is a rare complication typically occurring 2–3 weeks after the skin rash appeared, and it usually invades the muscle segments that match with the skin parts involved in herpes zoster.

Also, motor paralysis occurs in various areas. Generally, it most often occurs in dorsal part of the body and then numbness in the arms. Herpes zoster around the neck causes weakening of the arms. It most often occurs in cervical nerves 5–7, especially often limits extensor motions, and is rarely associated with the development of the diaphragm spasms.

Lumbosacral herpes zoster weakens legs, and it also accompanies bladder or intestinal dysfunction and abdominal muscle paralysis.

10.3.4 Test and Assessment

If the rash once appears, the disease can be diagnosed with naked eyes (differential diagnosis) because there are no diseases that have such distinctive shaped rash. It might be difficult to diagnose herpes zoster without rash (in the case of early and late herpes zoster, or zoster sine herpete). Other than rash, most symptoms can occur in other states.

Herpes zoster can be diagnosed by some pathological examinations. The most common examination is detecting immunoglobulin M (IgM) antibodies of varicella-zoster virus (VZV) from the blood. The antibodies cannot be detected when the herpes virus is in latency, and it can be detected when rash appeared by virus activities (Johnson and Dworkin 2003).

10.4 Intervention

10.4.1 Intervention

10.4.1.1 Interventional Approach

The purposes of the treatment are limiting pain and the duration of the pain and reducing the duration of herpes zoster and complications. The treatment according to the symptoms is necessary in the case of complications such as postherpetic neuralgia (Kennedy 2002).

10.4.1.2 Medical Treatment

According to the research on untreated herpes zoster, the pain that appeared after the rash disappeared is very rare in people under the age of 50, and it gradually disappears over time. The pain disappears slowly in older people, but even in 85 % of the patients older than 70, the pain disappears 1 year after herpes zoster.

Pain Reliever

The symptoms can be alleviated when lotion containing calamine is applied on rash or blisters. Sometimes, narcotic analgesics such as morphine might be needed for severe pain. Capsaicin cream can be applied after the scab has been formed. Lidocaine local anesthesia and blocking nerves also help to relieve the pain. Administration of gabapentin in combination with an antiviral agent is expected to alleviate the postherpetic neuralgia.

① Epidural Block

The lesions start from the nerve damage in dorsal root ganglions proceeding to peripheral and dorsal root spinal nerve. The use of the steroids with anti-inflammatory effects blocking epidural block, the use of topical anesthetics preventing depolarization of nerves by blocking the sodium channels, and the use of ketamine, an antagonist playing an important role in central sensitization, are the ideal methods preventing the mechanisms of chronic pain.

② Sympathetic nerve block

The damaged nerves activate the sympathetic nervous system, increase pain, and lead the disease into a chronic state, so sympathetic nerve block may have positive therapeutic effects.

③ Ganglion block and peripheral nerve block

Although no clinical studies have been reported, based on the results of pain mechanisms in animal models of neuropathic pain and based on the hypersensitivity and allodynia prevention after administering topical anesthetics to peripheral nerves, nerve ganglion block and peripheral nerve block are expected to prevent the peripheral and central sensitization (Dworkin et al. 2007).

Antiviral Agents

Antiviral agents can reduce pain and the duration of the disease when administered within 72 h after the rash caused by herpes zoster for 7–10 days. Antiviral drugs inhibit the varicella-zoster virus (VZV) replication and reduce the illness and the duration of herpes zoster with minimal side effects, but it does not prevent postherpetic neuralgia. Among the drugs, acyclovir is prescribed as a primary treatment, but the new drugs valacyclovir and famciclovir show similar or higher efficacy and safety. These drugs can be used for both prophylaxis and acute phases of the disease. The treatment using antiviral agents is recommended to all people over 50 years old with immunity who are suffering from herpes zoster. The drug efficacy is higher when administered within 72 h after the rash appeared.

The complications accompanied with herpes zoster in immunodeficient patients can be alleviated with intravenous acyclovir. Administration of oral acyclovir for 5 days is effective in the patients with high recurrence rates of herpes zoster.

10.4.2 Physical Therapy Intervention

10.4.2.1 Postures

The treatment of herpes zoster with mild symptoms is an allopathic treatment, and it is important to fully relax with a comfortable position. Particularly, if paralysis occurs, it is desirable to often change the positions with the neutral postures.

10.4.2.2 Exercise Therapy

It is necessary strengthening weakened muscles due to the segmental motor paralysis by herpes zoster. Herpes zoster in neck areas causes problems on the strength of the arms, so maintaining the muscle tension by isometric exercise of the muscles around the neck is necessary. Because the movement restriction occurs in the shoulder

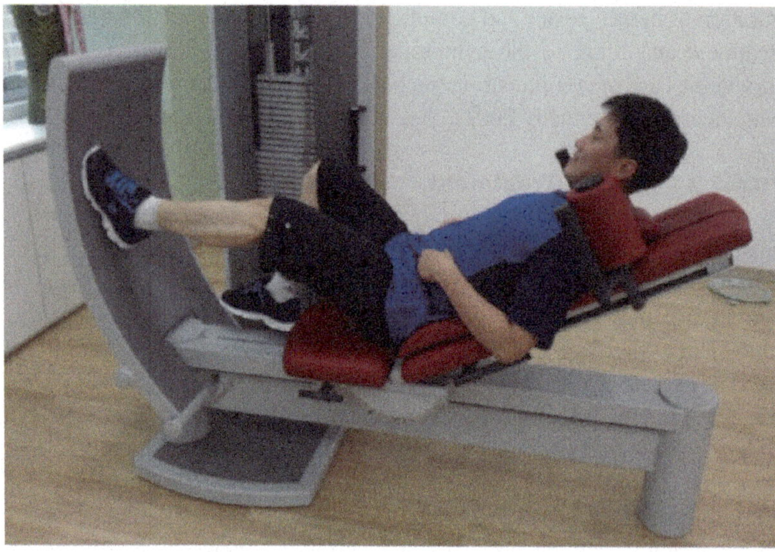

Fig. 10.9 Antigravity muscle movement

extensor muscles, extensor muscle strengthening around the shoulder rotator cuff such as the supraspinous muscle and deltoid muscle with light exercise of the neighboring muscles is necessary. For herpes zoster occurred in the dorsal part on the body, the rhomboid muscle strengthening exercise contributing in trapezius muscle and shoulder bone stabilization is performed. For the lumbosacral herpes zoster, isometric exercises, mainly for the weight-supporting joints, are performed to maintain antigravity muscles (Fig. 10.9).

10.4.2.3 Manual Therapy

The muscle weakness by herpes zoster can cause the joint contracture. Particularly, joint mobilization is applied due to the mobility restriction of the neck and dorsal part of the body.

To improve the mobility of lumbar joints, 1–2 grade of a gliding method with fast vibration is frequently applied 3–4 times for 1–2 min (Fig. 10.10).

10.4.2.4 Physical Agent Modalities

Infrared Therapy

Herpes zoster is a skin disease forming blisters, so to prevent the infection, using infrared light 3–4 times per week and 15–20 min at a time is more effective than using warm wet wrapping. The pain relief by infrared affects on terminal nerves of the skin. It relieves pain by soothing effect by mild heat and anti-stimulus effect by extreme heat. Particularly, since herpes zoster accompanies with the severe pain at the beginning of the disease, the early treatment is important (Fig. 10.11).

Transcutaneous Electrical Nerve Stimulation

High frequency-low intensity transcutaneous electrical nerve stimulation (TENS) based on a gait control theory is used to alleviate pain. The width of the pulse corresponds to the time of the low-frequency electric therapy stimulation. The range of 75–150 ms is known to be effective to stimulate the sensory nerves. The frequency approximately 3–100 pps is mainly used. Particularly, TENS is a useful and safe method to relieve postherpetic neuralgia (Fig. 10.12).

Laser Treatment

Recently, laser treatment is introduced to treat postherpetic neuralgia. The light energy is converted into the electrical and chemical energy when 600–1000 nm of the laser beam is applied on the body. The light reflected from between the cells exhibits biostimulating effects. Therefore, it

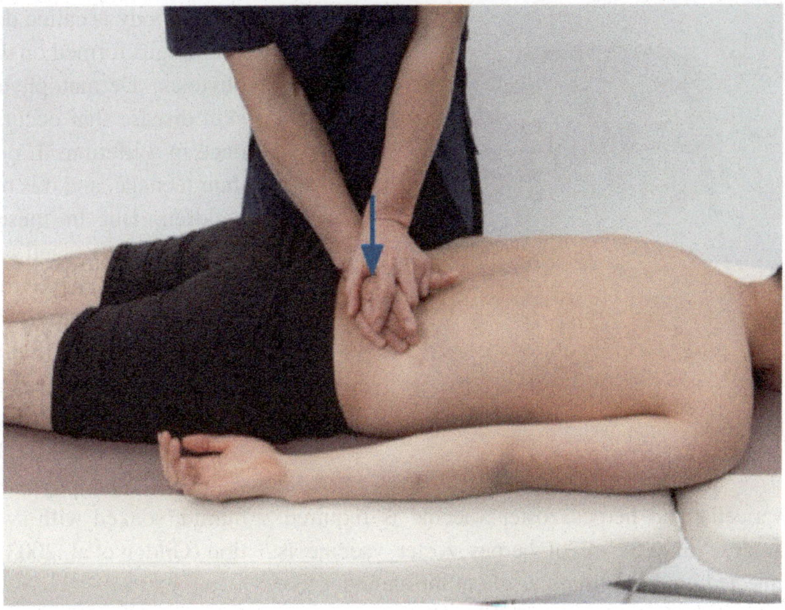

Fig. 10.10 Lumbar joint mobilization. *Arrow* is treatment direction

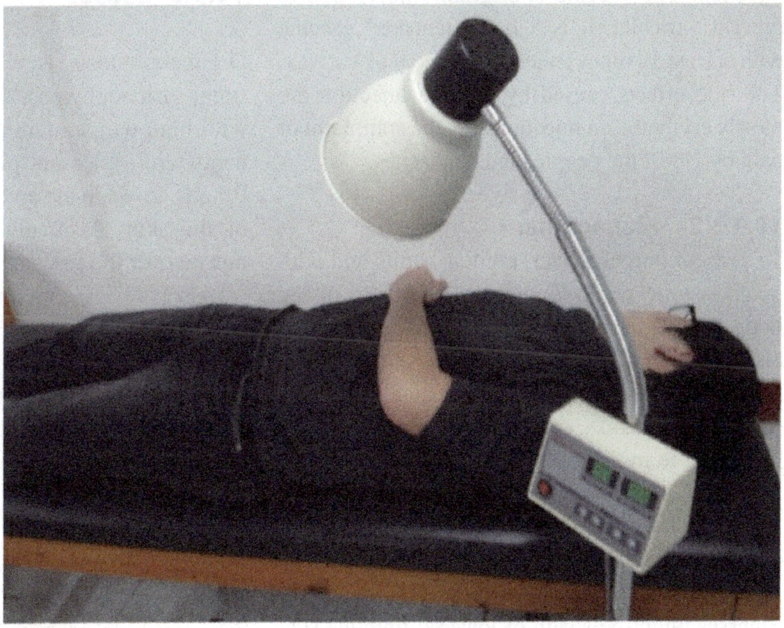

Fig. 10.11 Infrared therapy

increases the activity of the functionally depressed cells. There are a number of theories on the mechanisms of an analgesic effect of the laser. If the laser beam is applied on the pain region, it improves the blood vessel expansion and blood flow by stimulating autonomic nerves and relieves muscle tension.

10.4.3 Prevention and Management

10.4.3.1 Prevention

To prevent herpes zoster, regular habits and adequate rest are required, and the immunity of the body should be increased through regular exercise and a balanced diet. Also, the immunization by

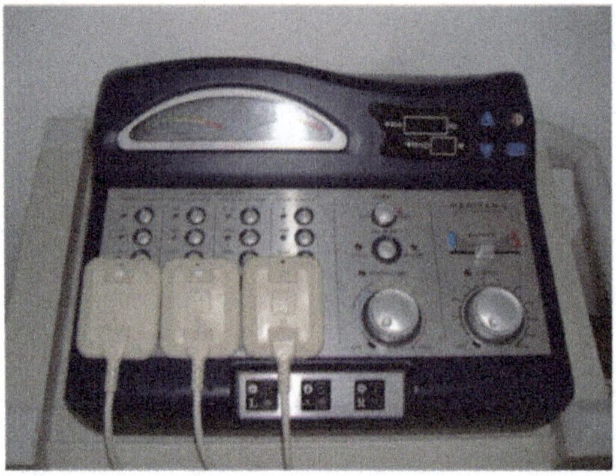

Fig. 10.12 Transcutaneous electrical nerve stimulation

varicella and herpes zoster vaccine is required. A dose of 0.65 ml of herpes zoster vaccine is injected on the deltoid muscle of the shoulder like a typical vaccine injected through subcutaneous injection. The vaccine is originally developed to prevent varicella. It is a live attenuated vaccine with at least 14 times enhanced potency of Varivax. The side effects caused by vaccine injection are mostly erythema on injection site, the complaint of pain by 1/3 of the people, and headaches.

10.4.3.2 Management

To prevent herpes zoster, regular habits and adequate rest are required, and the immunity of the body should be increased through regular exercise and a balanced diet. The meals should not be skipped. When busy, replacing a meal with porridge, health drinks, or nutritional supplements is necessary to maintain the immunity.

10.4.3.3 Patient/Caregiver Education

Patients and their careers should practice the minimum health rules. The occurrence of a few minor illnesses might be a sign of lowered immune system, so the individual should pay more attention.

10.5 Dermatophytosis

10.5.1 Overview

Dermatophytosis is a typical dermatomycosis. Dermatomycosis refers to the skin disease caused by eumycetes (fungus). Fungus formed on the human body is called dermatomycosis (or tinea), and fungus formed on the food is called dermatophytosis. Dermatophytosis is a very common skin disease that occurs in most people at least once in a lifetime. It occurs in male adults after their teenage, and it is not common in female and children. But in these days, dermatophytosis occurs in young aged people. The medical terminology of dermatophytosis is tinea pedis. Usually, the fungus causing dermatophytosis propagates on the human skin, but in some people, dermatophytosis does not occur although the fungus exists. Dermatophytosis does not occur in people walking with barefoot, but the fungus grows and causes dermatophytosis in the areas that are humid, soaked with sweat, and without ventilation (Gilden et al. 2003).

10.5.2 Causes

Dermatophytosis is a skin disease caused by fungi (trichophyton). The fungus likes places with high temperature and moisture, so feet and hands are a pleasant place for them. Therefore, fungus grows in the epidermis (stratum corneum) of the skin. Also, glucose-containing sweat is nutrient for the fungus.

Also, dermatophytosis is caused by several types of dermatomyces infections, and the most common causing agent is *Trichophyton rubrum*. It can be infected through direct skin contact with dermatophytosis patients, swimming pool, a foot towel in a public bath, and shoes (Fig. 10.13).

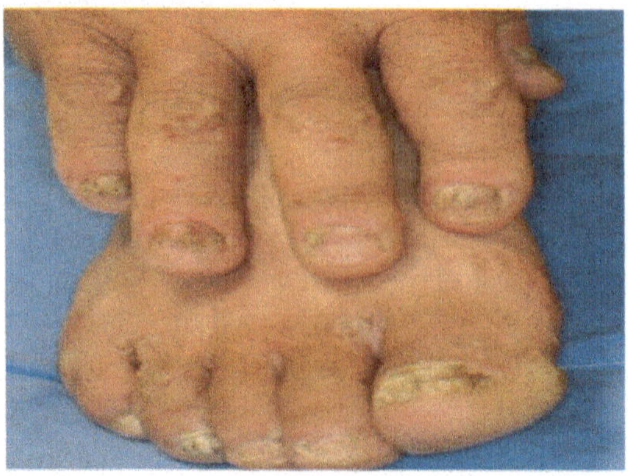

Fig. 10.13 Infected dermatophytosis

10.5.3 Symptoms and Complications

Dermatophytosis can be divided roughly into three types. They are vesiculobullous dermatophytosis forming blisters, interdigital dermatophytosis occurring between the toes, and moccasin dermatophytosis becoming a shape of scales. Vesiculobullous type is characterized by forming blisters or pus and causing pain and itching. In the severe case, the feet are swollen with severe pain. Interdigital dermatophytosis is usually formed between the fourth and fifth toes. The skin between toes is changed and the skin is peeled off and splitted. The symptoms include strong smell, swelling, and pain. Generally, dry dermatophytosis called moccasin type of dermatophytosis forms thick skin on soles and causes skin to be peeled off and splitted and pain. Dermatophytosis causes various symptoms depending on the people (Kim et al. 2006). The most common symptoms are the peeling of skin and cracked and formed dead skin between toes (usually the little toe) which is called interdigital type of dermatophytosis (Fig. 10.14). If dermatophytosis lasts for a long time without itching but forms white scales on soles (usually the heel) and the sole becomes thick, it is called moccasin type of dermatophytosis. Especially during the summer, blister formation, redness, and itching between toes or one side of the toe are called vesiculobullous type of dermatophytosis. When vesiculobullous type of dermatophytosis is not properly treated and the lesions are scratched, the secondary bacterial infection occurs followed by discharge secretion, swelling, and pain (Fig. 10.15).

10.5.4 Test and Assessment

10.5.4.1 Direct Smear Test

Scaling of the skin of the lesions is gathered and dissolved into 10 % of potassium hydroxide solution. It is observed under a microscope, and fungus is confirmed.

10.5.4.2 Fungal Culture Test

It is a method confirming dermatomyces by culturing the scales of the lesions for 3 weeks.

10.6 Intervention

10.6.1 Intervention

10.6.1.1 Interventional Approach

If dermatophytosis occurs, it is recommended to avoid drastic treatment but consistently apply and take drugs prescribed from the doctor. Although the lesion looks improved, the fungus can survive for a while and cause recurrence of dermatophytosis.

10.6.1.2 Medical Treatment

Once it is diagnosed, the immediate treatment is needed. In mild cases, applying dermatophytosis

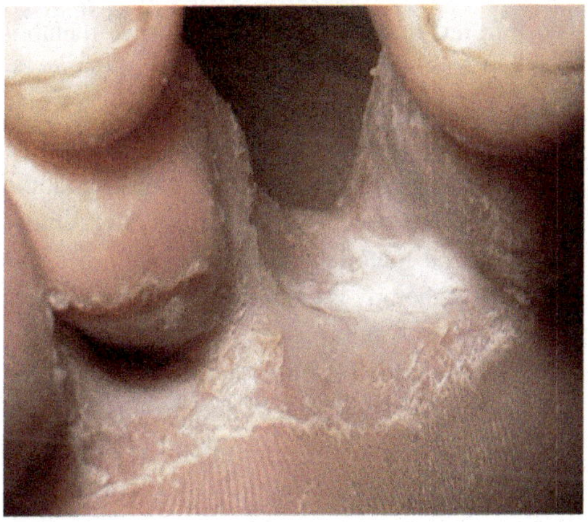

Fig. 10.14 Interdigital type of dermatophytosis

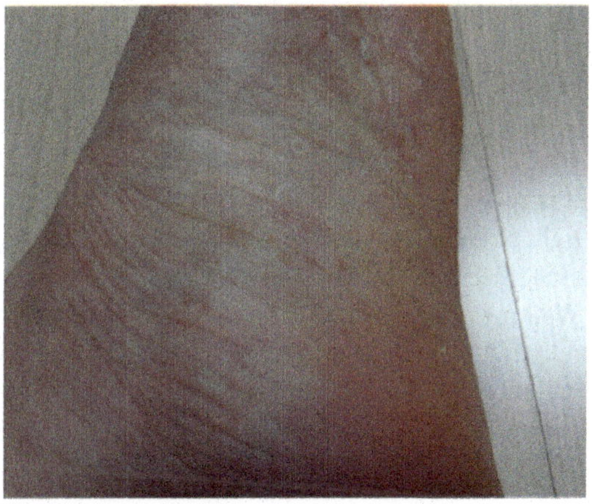

Fig. 10.15 Vesiculobullous type of dermatophytosis

drugs improves the symptoms. In severe cases, if blisters are formed, soaking feet in the drug-dissolved water to eliminate blisters is needed before applying ointments. In more severe cases, oral drugs of dermatophytosis are prescribed. However, before receiving a full-scale treatment, an accurate diagnosis has to be prioritized. Although it is dermatophytosis, the patients or pharmacists choose to use an eczema ointment which worsens the symptoms. It is also common that the patients apply ointments developed for all skin diseases which have compounds of dermatophytosis drugs and steroids. It delays or worsens the treatment. If the dermatophytosis is not properly treated, the secondary bacterial infection occurs. In this case, the drugs of dermatophytosis do not improve the symptoms. The secondary problems have to be treated for the fast recovery. Also, patients apply a strong keratolytic agent such as PM solution on dermatophytosis lesions for the fast recovery. If a strong keratolytic agent is applied, the skin of the lesions is peeled off, so itching symptoms can be alleviated. But it severely irritates the skin causing dermatitis and the secondary bacterial infection.

10.6.2 Physical Therapy Intervention

10.6.2.1 Postures

Patients should avoid wearing shoes smaller than their feet, and the environment with minimized humid and sweating conditions and posture are important. Overall, keeping the body dry is helpful.

10.6.2.2 Exercise Therapy

It is recommended walking on the treadmill and light stretching to prevent reduced immunity by skin diseases and improve blood circulation. Walking for 10–30 min with sufficient rehydration of the body according to the patients' condition, within the range that the patients do not become fatigue, is recommended (Fig. 10.16).

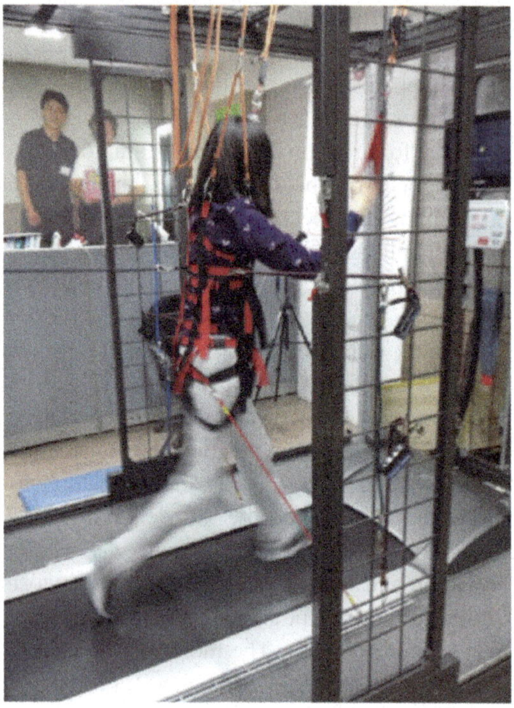

Fig. 10.16 Walking exercise to improve immunity

10.6.2.3 Manual Therapy

If there are problems in circulation and fatigue of the legs, the functional massage of the triceps muscle of the calf is performed. The therapists dorsiflex the ankle pushing the muscle belly of the triceps muscle of the calf toward the head. It is regularly performed 3–5 times per day and 3–5 days per week for 2–4 weeks (Fig. 10.17).

10.6.2.4 Physical Agent Modalities

The infrared light is applied to improve metabolism and sensory nerves and removal of the waste products. First, the clothing on the treatment site is removed and cold and warm reaction tests of the skin are performed. If there is no paresthesia, the infrared light is applied for 5–10 min after removing the metal materials from the body. The low-power laser therapy is performed for the treatment of infected sites and recovery of the wounded tissues. If it is applied for dermatophytosis, noncontact method is performed due to the risk of infection. The intensity of 1–6 J/cm^2 for 5–10 min is used to obtain anti-inflammatory effects.

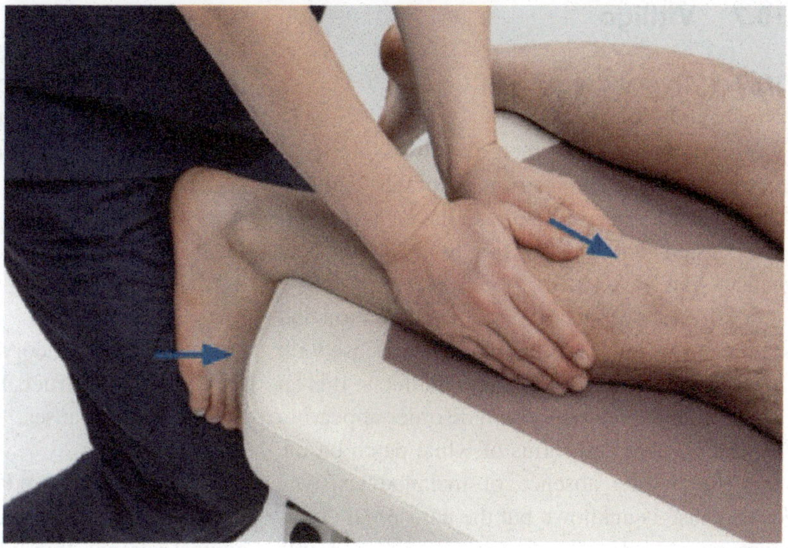

Fig. 10.17 Functional massage of the triceps muscle of the calf. *Arrow* is treatment direction

10.6.3 Prevention and Management

10.6.3.1 Prevention

Looking at the lifestyle habit preventing dermatophytosis, first, washing feet once a day or more often if sweating is recommended. In addition, the feet especially between the toes should be dried after washing and maintained in dry condition. Wiping sweat quickly and wearing socks to absorb the sweat are recommended. Well-ventilated toe-out shoes are more appropriate than tight shoes, and wearing comfortable and low-heeled shoes is recommended instead of wearing narrow and uncomfortable shoes. It is safe avoiding old and used shoes if possible (Table 10.4).

10.6.3.2 Management

The secondary infection including contact dermatitis and inflammation in tissues and lymphatic glands is caused if the lesions are unconditionally scratched due to itching. Also, fungus on feet can be spread to hands or nails. Blocking the environments for fungus proliferation should be prioritized if dermatophytosis is suspected. The best way is washing and drying feet thoroughly. When washing feet, avoiding the use of soap and washing in cold water for 10 min and removing the salt thoroughly are important. If the salt remains on the epidermis of the skin, it makes the skin absorb the moisture in the air by osmotic pressure and moistens the feet.

Table 10.4 Dermatophytosis prevention

1. Wash feet thoroughly, especially between the toes, and maintain feet dry all the time
2. Beware of the bathroom and swimming pool. Wash and dry feet thoroughly after visiting a public bath or swimming pool because the floor and foot towel of these places have fungus causing dermatophytosis
3. Avoid using slippers or a foot towel in public places where many people use together
4. If one of the family members has dermatophytosis, use a foot towel, slippers, or bath mat separately
5. Prepare more than two pairs of shoes and dry them in the sun
6. Coat the shoes with formalin if an individual wears the shoes for the whole day
7. Place the cotton in the shoes about a day or spray often antifungal agents used for car air conditioning
8. Avoid wearing tight clothes or shoes which cause sweating
9. Wear cotton socks which absorb sweat well

10.6.3.3 Patient/Caregiver Education

The infection pathway of dermatophytosis is a foot towel or carpet in a public bath, sand hared slippers. It can be infected by using the same foot towel with the dermatophytosis patients at home. Therefore, applying dermatophytosis drugs after taking shower is necessary to prevent further infection.

10.7 Vitiligo

10.7.1 Overview

Vitiligo is a disease characterized by white spots appearing on the skin. It is an incurable pigmentation disorder occurring due to the lack of melanocytes and abnormal function of melanocytes in human skin (Fig. 10.18).

Vitiligo appears in 10 % of the population and has been recognized as an incurable disease with low expectancy of the therapeutic effects. It is an acquired depigmentating skin disorder appearing in various sizes and forms of white patch on the skin due to the absence of melanocytes. The exact cause is unknown but the autosomal dominant genetic disorder is one of the possible causes. Mental disorders such as stress, physical disabilities, or sunburn can also act as secondary factors of vitiligo. The word vitiligo is a Western medical term. It is called bai dian feng (white patch wind) in traditional Chinese medicine, and the general public calls it as leucoma. Vitiligo occurs in 1–3 % of the population worldwide and there are no differences among the countries or ethnic groups. Unlike other diseases, vitiligo is not contagious and does not accompany with severe pain or reduced life expectancy.

However, because of whitening areas, many patients are under stress. Particularly in Korea, many patients are under serious stress due to the ignorance or prejudice about vitiligo and a closed social and cultural environment by the dense population. In recent years, the incidence rate of vitiligo increased due to the increased mental stress, pollution, and the destruction of the ozone layer. However, the exact causes and mechanisms of vitiligo are not identified, and also the treatment is not perfect (Korean Dermatological Association 2008).

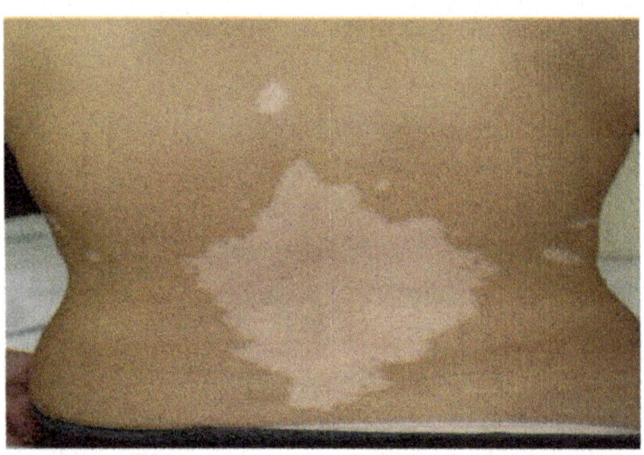

Fig. 10.18 Vitiligo

10.7.2 Causes

Immune system theory, nerve fluid theory, and melanin self-destruct theory are the convincing theories of the causes.

10.7.2.1 Immune Hypothesis

The incidence of producing self-antibodies against adrenal, thyroid, parietal, and pancreatic cells is high in vitiligo patients. Also, in some cases, it is often accompanied by autoimmune diseases. It has been reported that vitiligo occurs in 10–15 % of the autoimmune disease patients. The incidence rate is higher than 1 %, the incidence rate of the general population. Recently, it is described that it causes destruction or dysfunction of the melanocytes, and there are claims that the blood antibody level is proportional to the occurrence of vitiligo or the range of depigmentation. Also, specific antibodies show cytotoxicity to melanocytes, and melanocytes are destructed by secreted substances by cytotoxic lymphocytes and activated lymphocytes.

10.7.2.2 Neural Hypothesis

Melanocytes are originated from the neural crest. There is vitiligo distributed along the ganglions, and the case reports that vitiligo occurs after the nerve damage or mental stress which supports the nerve fluid theory. It explains that the cell death is derived from the inhibition of melanocyte reproduction by overexpressed neurochemical mediators closely located with melanocytes.

10.7.2.3 Self-Destruct Hypothesis

The intermediate molecules or metabolites produced in melanocyte formation are phenol complex, and they are accumulated in melanocytes and destruct them. However, instead of acting independently, these three theories act together to cause vitiligo. The symptoms are classified by local, systemic, and combined symptoms. It is a common disease occurring in 1 % of the population, and there are no differences between races or regions. The age varies from shortly after the birth to the old age, but it usually occurs between 10 and 30 years old. Also, about 40 % of the patients showed family history of vitiligo. The skin lesions start with various sized circles or irregularly shaped depigmentation and show clear boundaries and hyperpigmentation along the boundaries. Sometimes, erythematous boundaries are formed and the patients feel pruritus. There are no other epidemic symptoms or subjective symptoms except for the depigmentation, but the patients are hospitalized for the cosmetic defects. Sometimes, the hairs of the white patch areas look bleached, especially hairs and eyebrows, so the disease might be discovered as leukotrichia at first.

10.7.3 Symptoms and Complications

Vitiligo can occur at any site of the body, but it particularly occurs on the fingers or toes, protruding parts of the bones including knees and elbows, around the mouth and nose, back and front part of the legs, armpits, folded areas of the wrist, and tailbones. It also occurs on mucous membranes and frequently wounded sites. The distribution of vitiligo appears symmetrically or along with the ganglions. Besides depigmentation of the skin in vitiligo, depigmentation of the iris and the retina can be accompanied. Systemic diseases might be accompanied including diabetes, pernicious anemia, hypothyroidism or hyperthyroidism, and liver diseases. Particularly, autoimmune diseases can be accompanied.

10.7.4 Test and Assessment

Usually it can be easily diagnosed by observation with the naked eyes. If necessary, the disease can be differentiated from other diseases by skin biopsy, wood's lamp examination, and pigment examination.

Table 10.5 The causes of vitiligo

1. Vitiligo or a family history of autoimmune disease
2. Sun sensitivity or a personal medical history of other skin diseases
3. Rash appeared within 2–3 months of depigmentation, burns caused by the sun, other skin traumas
4. Records of atypical spots caused by melanoma
5. Symptoms of premature hair whitening (before 35 years old)
6. Stress or physical illness

The important factors in the medical history are shown in Table 10.5. The test methods are skin biopsy collecting a small portion of the lesion showing symptoms and blood test to check the blood cell number and thyroid function and the presence of the antinuclear antibodies (a kind of autoantibodies) showing the presence or absence of autoimmune diseases.

10.8 Intervention

10.8.1 Intervention

10.8.1.1 Interventional Approach

Long-wavelength ultraviolet light can be used for the treatment expecting high efficacy, but the treatment should be performed for a long time at least 100 times with the frequency of 2–3 times per week.

10.8.1.2 Medical Treatment

Long-term steroid therapy including topical and systemic administration is effective.

Sometimes, surgical transplantation of the skin and suction blister graft also show positive effects.

Treatment According to the Size and Condition of Vitiligo Areas

If the lesion is small or if it is an early phase of vitiligo, psychological stability, regulation of diet, and vitamin treatment are performed. If the lesion is medium size or it is a middle phase of vitiligo, photochemical treatment and herbal treatment can be performed. In addition, psychological stability, proper diet, and active lifestyle are important in all cases. Systemic vitiligo spread throughout the body is treated by photochemical therapy. "Bleaching" treatment eliminating the remaining pigments is used to make the whole body white. However, if the whole body pigments are bleached, it is impossible to regenerate pigments which cause increased sensitivity to sunlight or UV light, and the normal outdoor activities are difficult, so the decision should be made carefully. The current medical treatments for vitiligo are not sufficient to treat systemic vitiligo, but the treatment methods are improving, so enduring the current state for the future treatment can be one of the methods. Therefore, to overcome the severe skin conditions, maintaining and strengthening the active and positive psychological states are important. Also, to prevent worsening vitiligo and obtain better effects in the future, maintaining vitamin treatment, proper diet, and active lifestyle are necessary.

Steroid Therapy

Steroids may help returning the normal skin color (pigment regeneration). Particularly, the efficacy is higher when the treatment is started at the early phase of the disease. The mild steroid cream or ointment is prescribed to children or the people with wide spread of skin depigmentation. It takes about 3 months to see the changes of the skin color. The vitamin D derivative (calcipotriene, product name Dovonex) is used as a topical drug, and it is also used with steroids or UV light.

Immune Regulators

The topical ointments containing tacrolimus or pimecrolimus are effective when applied on smaller depigmentation areas, particularly the face and neck. It has fewer side effects than steroids and can be used with ultraviolet B (UVB) therapy. However, there is little research on this treatment which might increase the risk of skin cancer and lymphoma.

Depigmentation

If vitiligo appears on half of the skin of the patients, depigmentation can be one of the methods to treat vitiligo. Depigmentation treatment is whitening the skin color of the area in accordance with vitiligo appearing sites. The medication is applied to the skin where the pigment is still remained for twice a day. The treatment is continued until the dark skin matches with the already depigmented skin color.

Surgical Treatment

① Auto-skin Grafts

This method uses the patients' own tissue (autograft). The doctor removes a small part of the patient's body and attaches it to the other parts. This procedure is used occasionally when the spot is small. The doctor removes very small portion of the normal skin with pigments and fine hairs and attaches it on the site without the pigment. The complications include scars, gravel-shaped appearance, pigment spot, or depigmentation (Lee and Noh 2010).

② Suction blister graft

First, blisters are formed using suction on the skin with pigment. When the blister grows until the size of the grafting area, remove the part without pigment (make the same-sized blister there), and transplant the skin with pigment in this area. Suction blister graft may leave gravel-shaped scar and appearance, and the pigment might not regenerate on the transplanted area. However, the risk of forming scars is lower than other skin grafts (Park et al. 2014).

③ Tattoo Therapy

Tattoo is a method to plant pigment in the skin using a special tool. In vitiligo treatment, tattoo is the most effective treatment for around the lips and for the dark-skinned people. Sometimes, the tattoo color used might not be similar to the skin color. Also, the tattoo color gradually becomes lighter and the tattoo sites do not burn in the sun (http://www.apta.org).

10.8.2 Physical Therapy Intervention

10.8.2.1 Posture

The lesion appears and worsens when people are physically and mentally stressed, so maintaining the comfortable body and mind is important. Eye and inner ear disorder, thyroid diseases, and anemia might be accompanied, so receiving the tests and treatments in accordance with the instruction of the therapists is necessary.

10.8.2.2 Exercise Therapy

To improve the immune system, swimming and aerobic exercise such as walking are conducted at least 30–40 min per day, 3–5 times per week, and 85 % of the maximum heart rate for the age should be conducted.

10.8.2.3 Manual Therapy

After the skin graft, skin movements and pain relief can be improved by skin rolling and wound relaxation treatment (see Chap. 3, Manual Therapy for Decubitus Ulcer).

10.8.2.4 Physical Agent Modalities

Topical Psoralen and Ultraviolet A, PUVA

This therapy also known as photochemotherapy is effective in the patients with less than 20 % of skin depigmentation. The patients should visit the hospital 1–2 times per week for the treatment. A doctor or nurse applies a thin layer of psoralen and after 30 min, ultraviolet is applied. Psoralen makes the skin more sensitive to ultraviolet. Also, the skin becomes pink if it is exposed to ultraviolet, and then the skin is treated and becomes the normal skin color (Figs. 10.19). The use of psoralen and other therapies using psoralen is water bath PUVA (psoralen and ultraviolet A). Patients are soaked into the bath containing psoralen for 15 min before exposed to the light. After every treatment, the risk of the complications can be minimized by avoiding the direct sunlight, but the severe sunburn and blister formation might appear by the treatment as complications (www.cdc.go.kr).

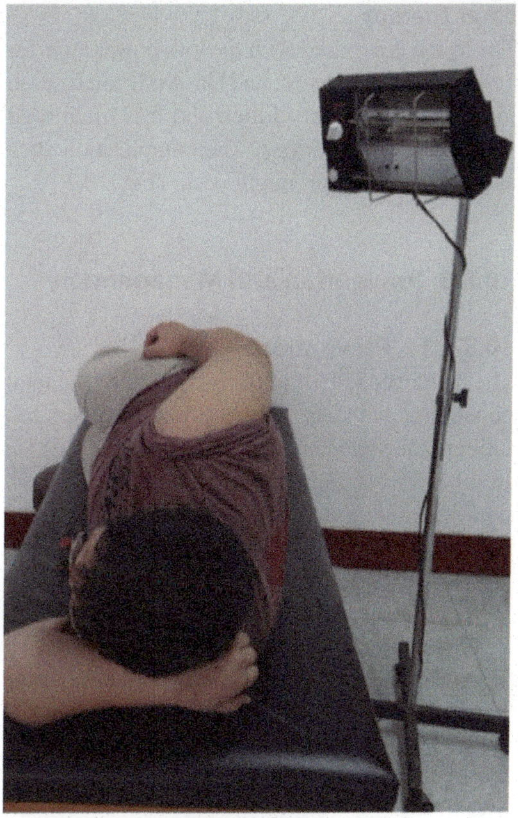

Fig. 10.19 UV therapy

Oral Psoralen (Oral PUVA) Therapy

If the depigmented skin of the patients is more than 20 % of the total body skin, oral psoralen is recommended. In this treatment, the patients take the oral psoralen 2 h before the ultraviolet. Receiving the treatment 2–3 times per week and leaving at least one day of interval are recommended. The treated skin turns pink after exposure to ultraviolet, and it gradually becomes lighter and then the normal skin color.

Narrowband Ultraviolet B Therapy

Narrowband UVB therapy is a special form of UVB using more specific UVB wavelengths as an alternative to PUVA. This treatment can be prescribed with PUVA and can be performed for 3 times per week. However, the procedure of the treatment is simple because there is no need to apply psoralen before the treatment. Phototherapy is widely used because the procedure is simple. The light used for the narrowband wavelength is also used with the strong light and laser, so it is applicable in treating smaller portions of vitiligo.

Laser Therapy

The lesion is exposed with the low-power laser for 15–30 min using He-Ne and Ga-As. It can be used in a small portion of vitiligo and it is often used with topical medications. The complication such as redness and blister might occur (Fig. 10.20).

10.8.3 Prevention and Management

10.8.3.1 Prevention

The incidence rate of vitiligo is 1.4 % of the total population, but if one of the family members has vitiligo, the incidence rate increases to 6.2–38 %. In other words, people with genetic predisposition are more susceptible to vitiligo compared with other people:

1. It might occur and worsen when people are physically and mentally tired and stressed, so the proper prevention is needed (www.kams.or.kr).
2. One should try to maintain and promote health.
3. Vitiligo needs regular monitoring and diagnosis.

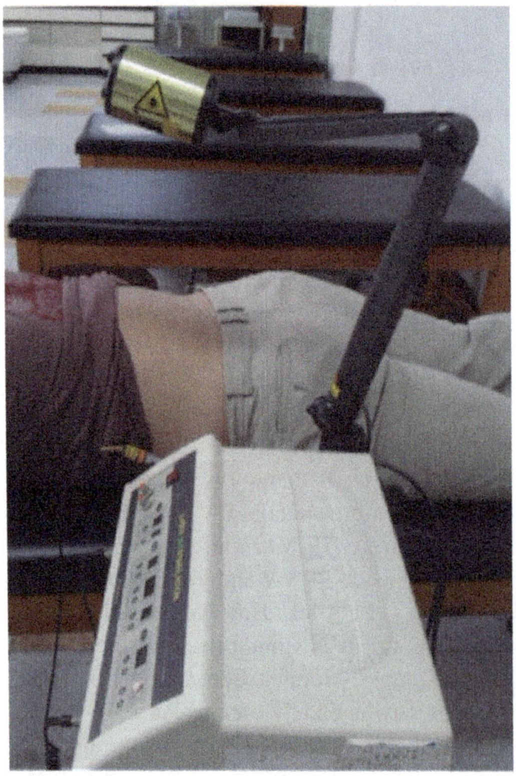

Fig. 10.20 Laser therapy

10.8.3.2 Management

If an individual spends most of the time outdoor, he or she should beware and pay more attention on excessive ultraviolet light caused by destroyed ozone layer of the Earth due to air pollution. UV light is a light used to treat vitiligo in Western medicine. But if it is misused or the skin is exposed to a large amount of the light, vitiligo might occur. In addition, if the chemicals such as hydroquinone paradioxybenzene used to develop photos, phenol, and catechol are used, one should avoid the direct contact with them.

10.8.3.3 Patient/Caregiver Education

Patients should eat a well-balanced diet, avoid wind, and maintain a stable life. In addition, the lesion tends to be worsened when it is severely irritated or the new lesion appears on wounded sites. Therefore, if vitiligo is in progress, rubbing and scratching by hands should be avoided.

Advices for Physical Therapists

The physical therapists should:

❶ Know about the causes and the classification of psoriasis, know the medical treatment, and promote the treatment through exercise therapy, manual therapy, and physical therapy modalities.

❷ Manage the pain and focus on physical therapy modalities for postherpetic neuralgia to alleviate the neuralgia. Beware and help the patients to return to society.

❸ Understand the psychological state of vitiligo patients who need psychological stabilities, and lead the patients to maintain their health by applying an appropriate photochemical therapy.

10.9 Problem Solving

10.9.1 Psoriasis, Herpes Zoster, Dermatophytosis, and Vitiligo

Choose the most appropriate symptoms and correct interventions from each question.

Question 1

A 55-year-old woman working in a restaurant near her home showed decreased immunity and often felt fatigue. A few days ago, she had blisters on her right ear accompanied with pain and dizziness. What is the correct diagnosis for this patient according to these symptoms?

Psoriasis

1. Dermatophytosis
2. Vitiligo
3. Herpes zoster
4. Contact dermatitis

Question 2

Office worker "A" had itching across the head. When she looked it on the mirror, stripe-shaped blisters were formed. It also caused pain, so she visited a pharmacy and bought painkillers. It alleviated the pain only for a moment and the symptoms did not disappear. One day, when she looked at the mirror, she found that her mouth is slightly skewed laterally with facial paralysis. Currently, she visited the hospital and waited for the blood test. What is the incorrect symptom of the disease in this case?

1. It is accompanied by inflammation and swelling of the joint.
2. It mainly appeared on the trunk and buttocks.
3. The pain appears 4–5 days before the rash appears.
4. If it occurs on the neck, it causes upper limb weakening.
5. Functional disorder of the bladder and intestine might occur depending on the occurring sites.

Question 3

Woman "A" working at a restaurant found fine red scaling of the skin raised widely on her calf. Also, itching and swelling symptoms were shown, so she visited the hospital and was prescribed with ointment and drugs. What is the correct physical therapy intervention for this disease?

1. Apply the functional massage to prevent adhesion.
2. Promote blood circulation by stimulating the disease sites.
3. Use UV light after soaking the body in photosensitizer-dissolved water.
4. Apply high frequency-high intensity low-frequency stimulation on lesions with swelling.
5. Conduct a strong resistance exercise therapy because arthritis might be accompanied as a complication.

Question 4

60-year-old woman "A" was hospitalized and diagnosed with dermatomycosis, a typical skin disease caused by fungus. Particularly, she complained of severe pain, swelling, and itching on her feet. What is the correct management and prevention for this disease?

1. Always maintain the feet moisturized.
2. Use a public bath more often than the private bath.
3. Take an immersion bath using hot water for a long period of time.
4. Choose slightly smaller-sized shoes.
5. Change the socks often, and keep the spaces between the toes.

Question 5

30-year-old man "A" had silvery white scaling of the skin that covered his elbow and then the red lesion was bulged. He was diagnosed with a noncontagious chronic skin disease which can appear anywhere of the skin; especially it occurs most commonly on the knees, elbow, scalp, trunk, etc. To treat this disease, chemotherapy administering drugs and special beam were applied. What is the correct intervention for this disease?

1. UV irradiation
2. Photochemical therapy
3. Iontophoresis
4. Infrared radiation
5. High-frequency therapy

Answer

Question 1-④, Question 2-①, Question 3-③, Question 4-⑤, Question 5-②

References

Ahn D, et al. Integumentary essentials applying the preferred physical therapist practice patterns. Philadelphia: Yeong Mun Publishing Inc.; 2009a.

Ahn S, et al. Common skin disease of Koreans: diagnosis and treatment. Seoul: Doctor's Book; 2009b.

Cunningham AL, Breuer J, Dwyer DE, Gronow DW, Helme RD, Litt JC, Levin MJ, Macintyre CR. The prevention and management of herpes zoster. Med J Aust. 2008;188(3):171–6.

Dworkin RH, Johnson RW, Breuer J, et al. Recommendations for the management of herpes zoster. Clin Infect Dis. 2007;44(Suppl 1):S1–26. doi:10.1086/510206.

Gilden DH, Cohrs RJ, Mahalingam R. Clinical and molecular pathogenesis of varicella virus infection. Viral Immunol. 2003;16(3):243–58. doi:10.1089/088282403322396073.

Johnson RW, Dworkin RH. Clinical review: treatment of herpes zoster and postherpetic neuralgia. BMJ. 2003;326(7392):748. doi:10.1136/bmj.326.7392.748.

Kennedy PG. Varicella-zoster virus latency in human ganglia. Rev Med Virol. 2002;12(5):327–34. doi:10.1002/rmv.362.

Kim H, Kim K, et al. Dermatology. 1st ed. Seoul: Koonja Publishing Inc.; 2006.

Korean Dermatological Association. Dermatology. Seoul: Ryo Moon Gak. P.Co; 2008.

Lee M, Noh H. Dermatology: an illustrated color text. Seoul: Koonja Publishing Inc.; 2010

Oxman MN, Levin MJ, Johnson GR, et al. A vaccine to prevent herpes zoster and postherpetic neuralgia in older adults. N Engl J Med. 2005a;352:2271–84.

Oxman MN, Levin MJ, Johnson GR, Schmader KE, Straus SE, Gelb LD, et al. A vaccine to prevent herpes zoster and postherpetic neuralgia in older adults. N Engl J Med. 2005b;253(22):2271–84. doi:10.1056/NEJMoa051016.

Park JH, et al. AAOS American academy of orthopaedic surgeon essentials of musculoskeletal care. 4th ed. Seoul: PanMun Education Publishing Inc; 2014.

Schmader KE, Levin MJ, Gnann Jr JW, et al. Efficacy, safety, and tolerability of herpes zoster vaccine in persons aged 50–59 years. Clin Infect Dis. 2012; 54:922–8.

Reference Sites

American Physical Therapy Association. http://www.apta.org.

Korea Centers for Disease Control and Prevention. www.cdc.go.kr.

Korean Academy of Medical Sciences. www.kams.or.kr.

Korean Dermatological Association. www.derma.or.kr.

Index

J.-W. Park, D.-I. Jung (eds.), *Integumentary Physical Therapy*, DOI 10.1007/978-3-662-47380-1

Printed by Printforce, the Netherlands